LIBREX-

DIAGNOSTIC IMAGING

PETER ARMSTRONG

MB, BS, FMed Sci, FRCP, FRCR

Professor of Radiology (retired)
Medical College of St Bartholomew's
and the Royal London Hospitals, London
Formerly Professor and Vice-Chairman
Department of Radiology, University of Virginia
Charlottesville, Virginia, USA

MARTIN L. WASTIE

MB, BChir, FRCP, FRCR

Late Professor of Radiology
University of Malaya Medical Centre
Kuala Lumpur, Malaysia
Formerly Consultant Radiologist
University Hospital, Nottingham

ANDREA G. ROCKALL

BSc, MB, BS, MRCP, FRCR

Consultant Radiologist
St Bartholomew's Hospital, London
Honorary Reader
Barts and the London School of Medicine and Dentistry, London

SIXTH EDITION

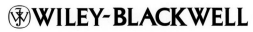

A John Wiley & Sons, Ltd., Publication

This edition first published 2009, © 2009 by P. Armstrong, M. Wastie, A. Rockall
Previous editions published 1981 (as *X-ray Diagnosis*), 1987, 1992, 1998, 2004

Blackwell Publishing was acquired by John Wiley & Sons in February 2007. Blackwell's publishing program has been merged with Wiley's global Scientific, Technical and Medical business to form Wiley-Blackwell.

Registered office: John Wiley & Sons Ltd, The Atrium, Southern Gate, Chichester, West Sussex, PO19 8SQ, UK

Editorial offices: 9600 Garsington Road, Oxford, OX4 2DQ, UK
The Atrium, Southern Gate, Chichester, West Sussex, PO19 8SQ, UK
111 River Street, Hoboken, NJ 07030-5774, USA

For details of our global editorial offices, for customer services and for information about how to apply for permission to reuse the copyright material in this book please see our website at www.wiley.com/wiley-blackwell

Library of Congress Cataloging-in-Publication Data

Armstrong, Peter, 1940–
    Diagnostic imaging / Peter Armstrong, Martin L. Wastie, Andrea G. Rockall. – 6th ed.
        p. ; cm.
    Includes index.
    ISBN 978-1-4051-7039-0
    1. Diagnostic imaging.   I. Wastie, Martin L.   II. Rockall, Andrea G.   III. Title.
    [DNLM: 1. Diagnostic Imaging. WN 180 A737d 2009]
    RC78.7.D53A76   2009
    616.07'54–dc22
                                        2008026357

ISBN: 978-1-4051-7039-0

A catalogue record for this book is available from the British Library.

Set in 9 on 12 pt Palatino by SNP Best-set Typesetter Ltd., Hong Kong
Printed in Singapore by Fabulous Printers Pte Ltd

2   2009

Contents

The colour plate sections can be found between pp. 8–9, pp. 104–105 and pp. 408–409.

Preface

Medical imaging has become central to many aspects of patient management and is increasing in importance. Medical students and junior doctors can be forgiven their bewilderment when faced with the daunting array of information which goes under the heading 'Diagnostic Imaging'. As plain film examinations remain the most frequently requested imaging investigations which non-radiologists may be called on to interpret at the time when medical decisions have to be made, we have once again given them due emphasis in this edition, along with relevant descriptions of ultrasound, computed tomography (CT), magnetic resonance imaging (MRI), radionuclide imaging, including positron emission tomography (PET), and interventional radiology.

With the widespread availability of the various imaging techniques, there are often several ways of investigating the same condition. We have avoided being too prescriptive as practice varies and so much depends on the personal preference of clinicians and radiologists as well as on the available equipment and expertise. It is important, however, to appreciate not only the advantages but also the limitations of modern medical imaging.

We have continued to try to meet the needs of the medical student and young doctor in training by explaining the techniques used in diagnostic imaging and the indications for their use. As in previous editions, much of the book is devoted to helping the reader understand the principles of interpretation of plain films and other imaging modalities. We have, however, responded to requests from readers of previous editions to include a heavily illustrated section on specific fractures in the chapter on skeletal trauma.

It is, unfortunately, beyond the scope of a small book such as this one to describe fully the pathology responsible for the various imaging appearances. Similarly, to cover adequately the role of imaging in clinical management would necessitate large sections on surgery, medicine and pathology. Consequently, this book cannot be read in isolation; it must be accompanied by the study of these other subjects.

Peter Armstrong
Martin L. Wastie
Andrea G. Rockall

Acknowledgements

It would not have been possible to prepare this edition without the help of the many radiologists who have given ideas, valuable comments and inspiration. We would like to thank particularly the staff of the Radiology Departments at the University Hospital, Nottingham, St Bartholomew's Hospital, London, University of Malaya Medical Centre, Kuala Lumpur and County Hospital, Lincoln for this and past edition illustrations. Our special thanks must go to Dr Tim Jaspan, who in this and previous editions has given unstinting help on the sections on neuroradiology. Dr Andrew Hatrick from Frimley Park Hospital made major contributions to the hepatobiliary and interventional radiology chapters.

The following kindly provided illustrations for this edition: Lorenzo Biassoni, John Bowe, Paul Clark, Siew Chen Chua, Andrew Hatrick, Peter Jackson, Jill Jacobs, Kasthoori Jayarani, Ranjit Kaur, Priya Narayanan, Steven Oscroft, Niall Power, Shaun Preston, Ian Rothwell, Peter Twining, Caroline Westerhout and Bob Wilcox.

We must also thank sincerely the photographers in the Department of Medical Illustration at St Bartholomew's Hospital, London.

This work would have been totally impossible without the superb secretarial help undertaken by Tiina Wastie and Julie Jessop.

Finally, we would like to express our gratitude to Karen Moore and the staff of Wiley-Blackwell.

1

Technical Considerations

The use of the imaging department

Good communication between clinicians and radiologists is vital because the radiology department needs to understand the clinical problem in order to carry out appropriate tests and to interpret the results in a meaningful way. Also, clinicians need to understand the strengths and limitations of the answers provided.

Sensible selection of imaging investigations is of great importance. There are two opposing philosophies. One approach is to request a battery of investigations, aimed in the direction of the patient's symptoms, in the hope that something will turn up. The other approach is 'trial and error': decide one or two likely diagnoses and carry out the appropriate test to support or refute these possibilities. Each course has its proponents; we favour the selective approach as there is little doubt that the answers are usually obtained less expensively and with less distress to the patient. This approach depends on critical clinical evaluation; the more experienced the doctor, the more accurate he or she becomes in choosing appropriate tests.

Laying down precise guidelines for requesting imaging examinations is difficult because patients are managed differently in different centres and the information required varies significantly.

• An examination should only be requested when there is a reasonable chance that it will affect the management of the patient. There should be a question attached to every request, e.g. for a chest examination – what is the cause of this patient's haemoptysis?

• The time interval between follow-up examinations should be sensible and related to the natural history of the disease in question, e.g. once pneumonia has been diagnosed, chest

examinations to assess progress can safely be left 7–14 days, unless clinical features suggest a complication.

• The localization of problems should be as specific as possible. Poor localization may lead to over-investigation or excessive radiation exposure.

• Careful consideration should be given to which diagnostic imaging procedure will give the relevant information most easily. It may be reasonable to construct a programme of investigations but the radiologist should always be asked to cancel any remaining tests once the desired positive result is obtained.

• Examinations which minimize or avoid ionizing radiation should be chosen whenever possible.

Conventional radiography

X-rays are absorbed to a variable extent as they pass through the body. The visibility of both normal structures and disease depends on this differential absorption. With conventional radiography there are four basic densities – gas, fat, all other soft tissues and calcified structures. X-rays that pass through air are least absorbed and, therefore, cause the most blackening of the radiograph, whereas calcium absorbs the most and so the bones and other calcified structures appear virtually white. The soft tissues, with the exception of fat, e.g. the solid viscera, muscle, blood, a variety of fluids, bowel wall, etc., all have similar absorptive capacity and appear the same shade of grey on conventional radiographs. Fat absorbs slightly fewer x-rays and, therefore, appears a little blacker than the other soft tissues. Images can be produced using a silver-based photographic emulsion or they can be recorded digitally and viewed on computer screens.

Projections are usually described by the path of the x-ray beam. Thus, the term PA (posteroanterior) view designates that the beam passes from the back to the front, the standard projection for a routine chest film. An AP

Diagnostic Imaging, 6th Edition. By Peter Armstrong, Martin Wastie and Andrea Rockall. Published 2009 by Blackwell Publishing. ISBN: 978-1-4051-7039.

(anteroposterior) view is one taken from the front. The term 'frontal' refers to either PA or AP projection. The image on an x-ray film is two-dimensional. All the structures along the path of the beam are projected on to the same portion of the film. Therefore, it is often necessary to take at least two views to gain information about the third dimension. These two views are usually at right angles to one another, e.g. the PA and lateral chest film. Sometimes two views at right angles are not appropriate and oblique views are substituted.

Portable x-ray machines can be used to take films of patients in bed or in the operating theatre. Such machines have limitations on the exposures they can achieve. This usually means longer exposure times and poorer quality films. The positioning and radiation protection of patients in bed is often inferior to that which can be achieved within the x-ray department. Consequently, portable films should only be requested when the patient cannot be moved safely or comfortably to the x-ray department.

Computed tomography

Computed tomography (CT) also relies on x-rays transmitted through the body. It differs from conventional radiography in that a more sensitive x-ray detection system is used, the images consist of sections (slices) through the body, and the data are manipulated by a computer. The x-ray tube and detectors rotate around the patient (Fig. 1.1). The outstanding feature of CT is that very small differences in x-ray absorption values can be visualized. Compared with conventional radiography, the range of densities recorded is increased approximately 10-fold. Not only can fat be distinguished from other soft tissues, but also gradations of density within soft tissues can be recognized, e.g. brain substance from cerebrospinal fluid, or tumour from surrounding normal tissues.

The patient lies with the body part to be examined within the gantry housing the x-ray tube and detectors. Although other planes are sometimes practicable, axial sections are

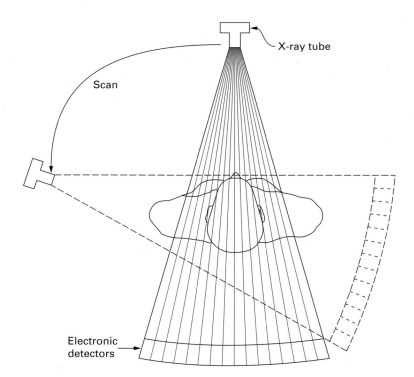

Fig. 1.1 Principle of CT. The x-ray tube and detectors move around the patient enabling a picture of x-ray absorption in different parts of the body to be built up. The time taken for the exposure is in the order of a second or so.

by far the most frequent. The operator selects the level and thickness to be imaged: the usual thickness is less than 1.25 mm (often viewed by aggregating adjacent sections so they become 5 mm thick). The patient is moved past an array of detectors within the machine. In effect, the data at multiple adjacent levels are collected continuously, during which time the x-ray beam traces a spiral path to create a 'volume of data' within the computer memory. Multidetector (multislice) CT is a relatively recent innovation whereby up to 64 or more sections (slices) can be acquired during one rotation of the x-ray tube. Multidetector CT enables the examination to be performed in a few seconds, thereby enabling hundreds of thin sections to be obtained in one breath-hold.

The data obtained from each set of exposures are reconstructed into an image by computer manipulation. The computer calculates the attenuation (absorption) value of each picture element (known in computer jargon as a pixel). Each pixel is 0.25–0.6 mm in diameter, depending on the resolution of the machine, with a height corresponding to the chosen section thickness. The resulting images are displayed on a monitor and can be photographed and/or stored electronically. The attenuation values are expressed on an arbitrary scale (Hounsfield units) with water density being zero, air density being minus 1000 units and bone density being plus 1000 units (Fig. 1.2). The range and level of densities to be displayed can be selected by controls on the computer. The range of densities visualized on a particular image is known as the *window width* and the mean level as the *window level* or *window centre*. Computed tomography is usually performed in the axial plane, but because attenuation values for every pixel are present in the computer memory it is possible to reconstruct excellent images in other planes, e.g. coronal (Fig. 1.3), sagittal or oblique, and even three-dimensional (3D) images (Fig. 1.4).

The human eye can only appreciate a limited number of shades of grey. With a wide window all the structures are visible, but fine details of density difference cannot be appreciated. With a narrow window width, variations of just a few Hounsfield units can be seen, but much of the image is either totally black or totally white and in these areas no useful information is provided. The effects of varying window width and level are illustrated in Figs 1.5 and 2.5, p. 21.

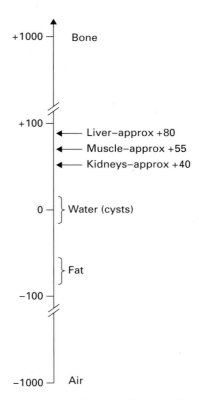

Fig. 1.2 Scale depicting the CT density (Hounsfield units) of various normal tissues in the body.

CT angiography

Rapid intravenous injections of contrast media result in significant opacification of blood vessels, which, with multiplanar or 3D reconstructions, can be exploited to produce angiograms. CT angiography, along with magnetic resonance angiography, is gradually replacing conventional angiography.

Artefacts

There are numerous CT artefacts. The most frequent are those produced by movement and those from objects of very high density, such as barium in the bowel, metal implants, dental fillings or surgical clips. Both types give rise to radiating linear streaks. The major problem is the resulting degradation of the image.

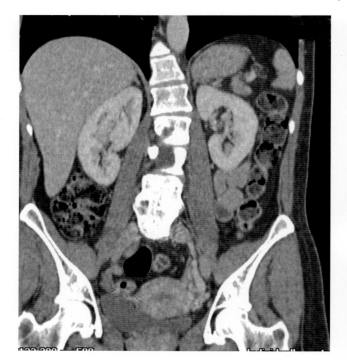

Fig. 1.3 Coronal reconstruction of CT of abdomen and pelvis. The images were obtained in the axial plane using very thin sections and then reconstructed into the desired plane – a coronal plane in this example. The illustrated section is through the posterior abdomen and shows the kidneys very well.

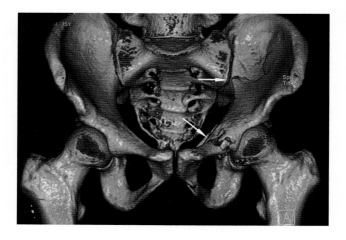

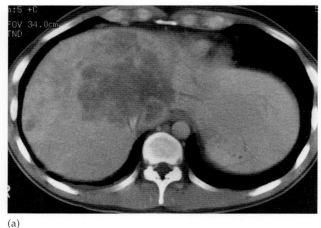

(a)

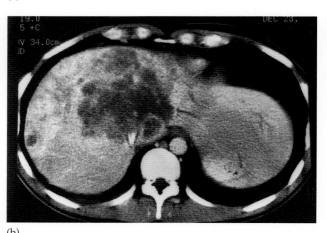

(b)

Fig. 1.5 Effect of varying window width on CT. In (a) and (b) the level has been kept constant at 65 Hounsfield units (HU). The window width in (a) is 500 whereas in (b) it is only 150 HU. Note that in the narrow window image (b), the metastases are better seen, but that structures other than the liver are better seen in (a).

Fig. 1.4 (*Left*) Shaded surface 3D CT reconstruction. The images can be viewed in any desired projection and give a better appreciation of the pelvis. Two fractures are demonstrated in the left innominate bone (arrows), which were hard to diagnose on the plain film. Further views of this fracture can be seen in Fig. 12.13, p. 379.

Contrast agents in conventional radiography and CT

Radiographic contrast agents are used to visualize structures or disease processes that would otherwise be invisible or difficult to see. Barium is widely used to outline the gastrointestinal tract; all the other radio-opaque media rely on iodine in solution to absorb x-rays. Iodine-containing solutions are used for urography, angiography and intravenous contrast enhancement at CT. Usually they are given in large doses, often with rapid rates of injection. As their only purpose is to produce opacification, ideally they should be pharmacologically inert. This has not yet been totally achieved, though the current low-osmolality agents, such as the non-ionic media, have exceedingly low complication rates.

Some patients experience a feeling of warmth spreading over the body as the iodinated contrast medium is injected. Contrast inadvertently injected outside the vein is painful and should be carefully guarded against. A few patients develop an urticarial rash, which usually subsides spontaneously.

Bronchospasm, laryngeal oedema or hypotension occasionally develop and may be so severe as to be life-threatening. It is therefore essential to be prepared for these dangerous reactions and to have available appropriate resuscitation equipment and drugs. Patients with known allergic manifestations, particularly asthma, are more likely to have an adverse reaction. Similarly, patients who have had a previous reaction to contrast agents have a higher than average risk of problems during the examination. Such patients are given non-ionic agents and premedicated with steroids. Intravenous contrast agents may have a deleterious effect on renal function in patients with impaired kidneys. Therefore, their use should be considered carefully on an individual basis and the patient should be well hydrated prior to injection.

Ultrasound

In diagnostic ultrasound examinations, very high frequency sound is directed into the body from a transducer placed in contact with the skin. In order to make good acoustic contact, the skin is smeared with a jelly-like substance. As the sound travels through the body, it is reflected by the tissue interfaces to produce echoes which are picked up by the same transducer and converted into an electrical signal.

As air, bone and other heavily calcified materials absorb nearly all the ultrasound beam, ultrasound plays little part in the diagnosis of lung or bone disease. The information from abdominal examinations may be significantly impaired by gas in the bowel that interferes with the transmission of sound.

Fluid is a good conductor of sound, and ultrasound is, therefore, a particularly good imaging modality for diagnosing cysts, examining fluid-filled structures such as the bladder and biliary system, and demonstrating the fetus in its amniotic sac. Ultrasound can also be used to demonstrate solid structures that have a different acoustic impedance from adjacent normal tissues, e.g. metastases.

Ultrasound is often used to determine whether a structure is solid or cystic (Fig. 1.6). Cysts or other fluid-filled structures produce large echoes from their walls but no echoes from the fluid contained within them. Also, more echoes than usual are received from the tissues behind the cyst, an effect known as *acoustic enhancement*. Conversely, with a calcified structure, e.g. a gall stone (Fig. 1.7), there is a great reduction in the sound that will pass through, so a band of reduced echoes, referred to as an *acoustic shadow*, is seen behind the stone.

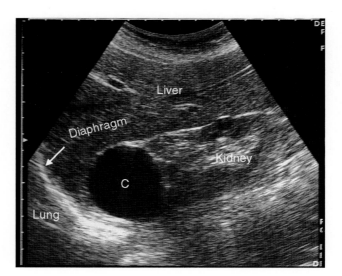

Fig. 1.6 Ultrasound scan of longitudinal section through the liver and right kidney. A cyst (C) is present in the upper pole of the kidney.

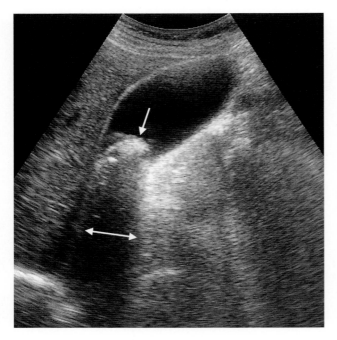

Fig. 1.7 Ultrasound scan of gall bladder showing a large stone in the neck of the gall bladder (downward pointing arrow). Note the acoustic shadow behind the stone (horizontal arrows).

Ultrasound is produced by causing a special crystal to oscillate at a predetermined frequency. Very short pulses of sound lasting about a millionth of a second are transmitted approximately 500 times each second. The crystal not only transmits the pulses of sound but also 'listens' to the returning echoes, which are electronically amplified to be recorded as signals on a television monitor. Photographic reproductions of the image can provide a permanent record.

The time taken for each echo to return to the transducer is proportional to the distance travelled. Knowledge of the depth of the interface responsible for the echoes allows an image to be produced. Also, by knowing the velocity of sound in tissues, it is possible to measure the distance between interfaces. This is of great practical importance in obstetrics, for example, where the measurement of the fetal head has become the standard method of estimating fetal age.

During the scan, the ultrasound beam is electronically swept through the patient's body and a section of the internal anatomy is instantaneously displayed. The resulting image is a slice, so in order to obtain a 3D assessment a number of slices must be created by moving or angling the transducer.

Unlike other imaging modalities, there are no fixed projections and the production of the images and their subsequent interpretation depend very much on the observations of the operator during the examination. Ultrasound images are capable of providing highly detailed information, e.g. very small lesions can be demonstrated (Fig. 1.8).

A recent advance is the development of small ultrasound probes which may be placed very close to the region of interest, thus producing highly detailed images but with a limited range of a few centimetres. Examples are rectal probes for examining the prostate and transvaginal probes for the examination of the pelvic structures. Tiny ultrasound probes may be incorporated in the end of an endoscope. Lesions of the oesophagus, heart and aorta may be demonstrated with an endoscope placed in the oesophagus, and lesions of the pancreas may be detected with an endoscope passed into the stomach and duodenum. Special ultrasound probes have also been developed that can be inserted into arteries to detect atheromatous disease.

Three-dimensional ultrasound has been recently developed and is used primarily in obstetrics to obtain 3D images of the fetus. A conventional ultrasound transducer is used, which is moved slowly across the body recording simultaneously the location and ultrasound image. A 3D image can be constructed from the data received.

At the energies and doses currently used in diagnostic ultrasound, no harmful effects on any tissues have been demonstrated.

Ultrasound contrast agents are currently being developed. These agents contain microscopic air bubbles that enhance the echoes received by the probe. The air bubbles are held in a stabilized form, so they persist for the duration of the examination and blood flow and perfusion to organs can be demonstrated. The technique is used to help characterize liver and renal abnormalities and in the investigation of cardiac disease.

Doppler effect

Sound reflected from a mobile structure shows a variation in frequency which corresponds to the speed of move-

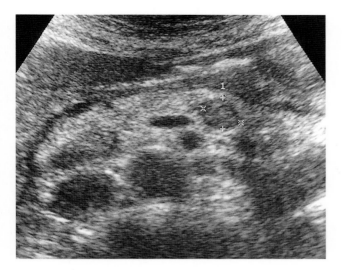

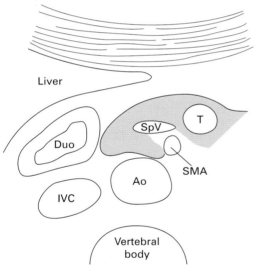

Fig. 1.8 Ultrasound scan of pancreas showing 1 cm tumour (T) (an insulinoma) at the junction of the head and body of the pancreas. The pancreas is shaded in the diagram. Ao, aorta; Duo, duodenum; IVC, inferior vena cava; SMA, superior mesenteric artery; SpV, splenic vein.

ment of the structure. This shift in frequency, which can be converted to an audible signal, is the principle underlying the Doppler probe used in obstetrics to listen to the fetal heart.

The Doppler effect can also be exploited to image blood flowing through the heart or blood vessels. Here the sound is reflected from the blood cells flowing in the vessels (Plate 1). If blood is flowing towards the transducer the received signal is of higher frequency than the transmitted frequency, whilst the opposite pertains if blood is flowing away from the transducer. The difference in frequency between the sound transmitted and received is known as the Doppler frequency shift.* The direction of blood flow can readily be determined and flow towards the transducer is, by convention, coloured red, whereas blue indicates flow away from the transducer.

When a patient is being scanned, the Doppler information in colour is superimposed onto a standard ultrasound image (Plate 3).

During the examination the flow velocity waveform can be displayed and recorded. As the waveforms from specific arteries and veins have characteristic shapes, flow abnormalities can be detected. If the Doppler angle (Plate 1a) is known then the velocity of the flowing blood can be calculated and blood flow can be calculated provided the diameter of the vessel is also known.

Doppler studies are used to detect venous thrombosis, arterial stenosis and occlusion, particularly in the carotid arteries. In the abdomen, Doppler techniques can determine whether a structure is a blood vessel and can help in assessing tumour blood flow. In obstetrics, Doppler ultrasound is used particularly to determine fetal blood flow through the umbilical artery. With Doppler echocardiography it is possible to demonstrate regurgitation through incompetent valves and pressure gradients across valves can be calculated.

Radionuclide imaging

The radioactive isotopes used in diagnostic imaging emit gamma-rays as they decay. Gamma rays are electromagnetic radiation, similar to x-rays, produced by radioactive

*The formula is:

$$\text{frequency shift} = \frac{2Fi \times V \times \cos\theta}{c}$$

(As c, the speed of sound in tissues, and Fi, the incident frequency of sound, are constant and if θ, the Doppler angle, is kept constant, the frequency shift depends directly on the blood flow velocity V.)

decay of the nucleus. Many naturally occurring radioactive isotopes, e.g. potassium-40, uranium-235, have half lives of hundreds of years and are, therefore, unsuitable for diagnostic imaging. The radioisotopes used in medical diagnosis are artificially produced and most have short half lives, usually a few hours or days. To keep the radiation dose to the patient at a minimum, the smallest possible dose of an isotope with a short half life should be used. Clearly, the radiopharmaceuticals should have no undesirable biological effects and should be rapidly excreted from the body following completion of the investigation.

Radionuclide imaging depends on the fact that certain substances concentrate selectively in different parts of the body. Radionuclides can be chemically tagged to these substances. Occasionally, the radionuclide in its ionic form will selectively concentrate in an organ, so there is no need to attach it to another compound. The radionuclide most commonly used is technetium-99m (^{99m}Tc). It is readily prepared, has a convenient half life of 6 hours and emits gamma-radiation of a suitable energy for easy detection. Other radionuclides that are used include indium-111, gallium-67, iodine-123 and thallium-201.

Technetium-99m can be used in ionic form (as the pertechnetate) to detect ectopic gastric mucosa in Meckel's diverticulum, but it is usually tagged to other substances. For example, a complex organic phosphate labelled with ^{99m}Tc will be taken up by the bones and can be used to visualize the skeleton (Fig. 1.9). Particles are used in lung perfusion images; macroaggregates of albumin with a particle size of 10–75 μm when injected intravenously are trapped in the pulmonary capillaries. If the macroaggregates are labelled with ^{99m}Tc, then the blood flow to the lungs can be visualized. It is also possible to label the patient's own red blood cells with ^{99m}Tc to assess cardiac function, or the white cells with indium-111 or ^{99m}Tc for abscess detection. Small quantities of radioactive gases, such as xenon-133, xenon-127 or krypton-81 m, can be inhaled to assess ventilation of the lungs. All these radiopharmaceuticals are free of side-effects.

The gamma rays emitted by the isotope are detected by a gamma camera, enabling an image to be produced. A gamma camera consists of a large sodium iodide crystal, usually 40 cm in diameter, coupled to a number of photomultiplier tubes. Light is produced when the gamma rays strike and activate the sodium iodide crystal, and the light is then electronically amplified and converted to an electrical pulse. The electrical pulse is further amplified and analyzed by a processing unit so that a recording can be made. Invariably, some form of computer is linked to the gamma camera to enable rapid serial images to be taken and to perform computer enhancement of the images when relevant.

In selected cases emission tomography is performed. In this technique, the gamma camera moves around the patient. A computer can analyze the information and produce sectional images similar to CT. Emission tomography can detect lesions not visible on the standard views. Because only one usable photon for each disintegration is emitted, this technique is also known as single photon emission computed tomography (SPECT).

Nuclear medicine techniques are used to measure function and to produce anatomical images. Even the anatomical images are dependent on function; for example, a bone scan depends on bone turnover. The anatomical information they provide, however, is limited by the relatively poor spatial resolution of the gamma camera compared with other imaging modalities.

Positron emission tomography

Positron emission tomography (PET) uses short-lived positron emitting isotopes, which are produced by a cyclotron immediately before use. Two gamma rays are produced from the annihilation of each positron and can be detected by a specialized gamma camera. The resulting images reflect the distribution of the isotope (Fig. 1.10a). By using isotopes of biologically important elements such as carbon or oxygen, PET can be used to study physiological processes such as blood perfusion of tissues, and metabolism of substances such as glucose, as well as complex biochemical pathways such as neurotransmitter storage and binding. The most commonly used agent is F-18 fluorodeoxyglucose (FDG). This is an analogue of glucose and is taken up by cells in proportion to glucose metabolism, which is increased in tumour cells. Because muscle activity results in the uptake of FDG, the patient rests quietly in the interval between injection of the FDG and scanning.

The images must be interpreted carefully as non-cancerous conditions may show uptake resembling cancer. Positron emission tomography using FDG is the most sensitive technique for staging solid tumours such as bronchial carcinoma (Plate 2) and in follow-up of malignancies,

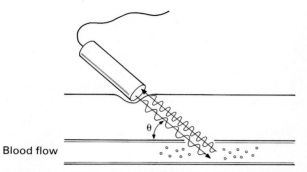

Blood flow

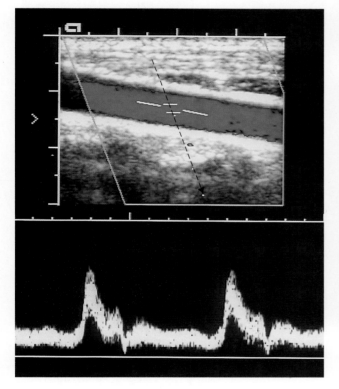

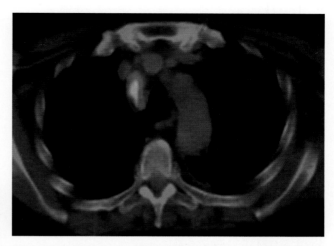

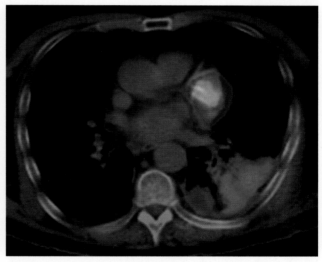

Plate 1   Principle of Doppler ultrasound. In this example, flowing blood is detected in a normal carotid artery in the neck. With blood flowing away from the transducer, the frequency of the received sound is reduced whereas with blood flowing towards the transducer, the frequency of the received sound is increased. For anatomical images, the flowing blood is colour coded according to the direction of flow. (θ is the angle between the vessel and the transmitted sound wave: an angle known as the Doppler angle; the angle of the beam is indicated by the fine zig-zag line across the image.) The flow-velocity waveform has been taken from the gate within the artery.The peaks represent systolic blood flow.

Plate 2   PET/CT of the chest in a patient with lung cancer (same patient as Fig 2.108, p. 92). These fused PET and CT images show how the increased PET activity, colour coded according to the magnitude of PET activity, can be precisely anatomically localized. The large lung cancer is shown lying posteriorly on the lower section (the high activity anteriorly over the heart is normal) and the metastases in the right paratracheal mediastinal lymph nodes are seen on the upper section.

(Facing p. 8)

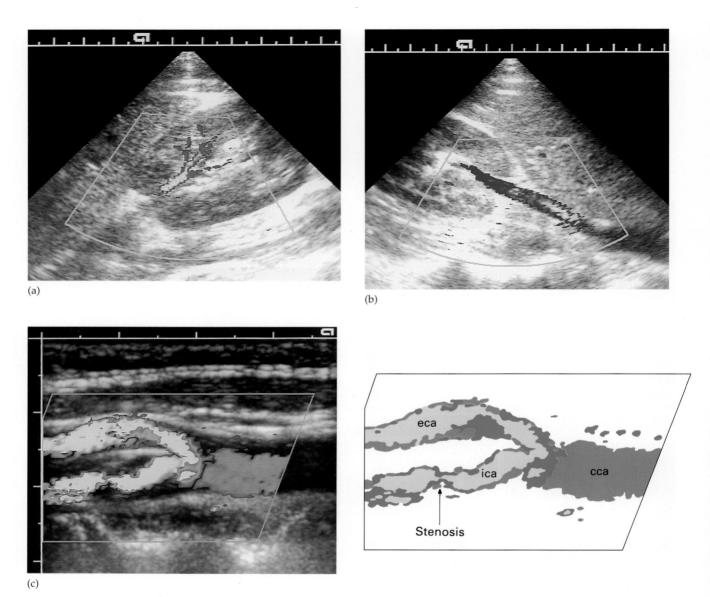

Plate 3 Colour Doppler. (a) Normal renal artery. (b) Normal renal vein. (c) Bifurcation of common carotid artery showing stenosis of internal carotid artery. The flowing blood is revealed by colour. The precise colour depends on the speed and direction of the blood flow. cca, common carotid artery; eca, external carotid artery; ica, internal carotid artery.

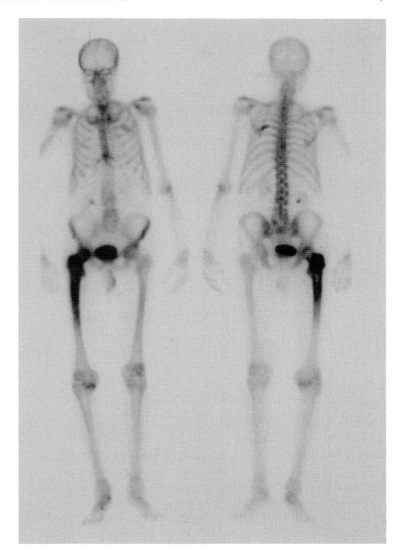

Fig. 1.9 Radionuclide bone scan. The patient has received an intravenous injection of a ^{99m}Tc-labelled bone scanning agent (a complex organic phosphate). This agent is taken up by bone in proportion to bone turnover and blood flow. The increased uptake in the femur in this patient was due to Paget's disease.

particularly lymphoma (Fig. 1.10b), where other imaging techniques may be unable to distinguish active disease from residual fibrosis.

Positron emission tomography is also used in the evaluation of ischaemic heart disease and in brain disorders such as dementia, epilepsy and Parkinson's disease.

PET demonstrates biological function while CT gives anatomical information. If PET and CT are fused, the lesions detected by PET can be precisely localized by CT (Plate 2). Modern equipment allows both PET and CT to be performed sequentially on the same machine.

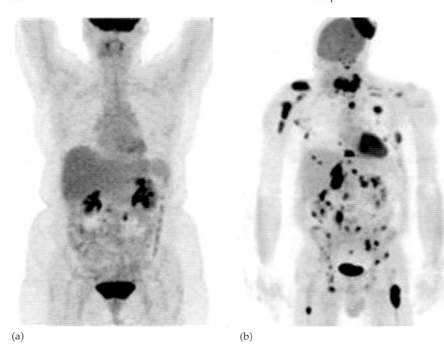

(a)   (b)

Fig. 1.10 FDG PET scans.
(a) Normal. There is intense uptake
in the brain. The neck uptake is in
the tonsils. The FDG is excreted
by the kidneys. (b) Lymphoma,
showing multiple visceral, nodal,
bone and scalp deposits.

Magnetic resonance imaging

The basic principles of magnetic resonance imaging (MRI) depend on the fact that the nuclei of certain elements align with the magnetic force when placed in a strong magnetic field. At the field strengths currently used in medical imaging, hydrogen nuclei (protons) in water molecules and lipids are responsible for producing anatomical images. If a radiofrequency pulse at the resonant frequency of hydrogen is applied, a proportion of the protons change alignment, flipping through a preset angle, and rotate in phase with one another. Following this radiofrequency pulse, the protons return (realign) to their original positions. As the protons realign (relax), they induce a radio signal which, although very weak, can be detected and localized by antenna coils placed around the patient. An image representing the distribution of the hydrogen protons can be built up (Fig. 1.11). The strength of the signal depends not only on proton density but also on two relaxation times, T1 and T2; T1 depends on the time the protons take to return to the axis of the magnetic field, and T2 depends on the

time the protons take to dephase. A T1-weighted image is one in which the contrast between tissues is due mainly to their T1 relaxation properties, while in a T2-weighted image the contrast is due to the T2 relaxation properties (see Box 1.1). Some sequences produce images which approximate mainly to proton density. Most pathological processes show increased T1 and T2 relaxation times and, therefore, these processes appear lower in signal (blacker) on a T1-weighted scan and higher in signal intensity (whiter) on a T2-weighted scan than the normal surrounding tissues. The

Box 1.1 Appearance of water and fat on different magnetic resonance (MR) sequences

Sequence	Water signal intensity	Fat signal intensity
T1-weighted	Low	High
T2-weighted	High	High
T1 with fat saturation	Low	Low
T2 with fat saturation	High	Low

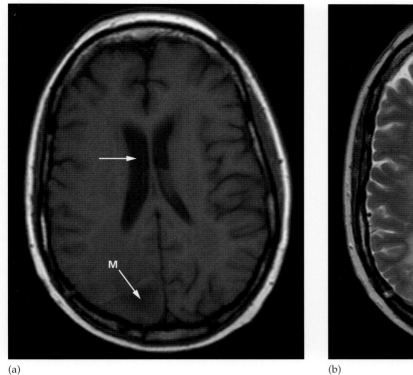

(a)

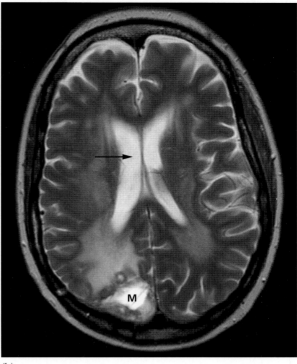

(b)

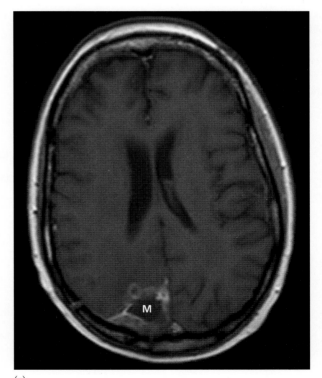

(c)

Fig. 1.11 MRI of the brain. (a) Axial T1-weighted image.
(b) Axial T2-weighted image. (c) Axial T1-weighted image
following gadolinium. Note that the cerebrospinal fluid within
the lateral ventricles is of low signal intensity on T1 and high
signal intensity on T2-weighted images (arrows). Note also that
the intensity of the white and grey matter of the brain differs on
the two images. There is a metastasis from a breast carcinoma
(M) in the right occipital pole, showing oedema around the
mass on the T2-weighted image and enhancement on the post
contrast image.

T1- and T2-weighting of an image can be selected by appropriately altering the timing and sequence of radiofrequency pulses.

There are many other sequences with a bewildering variety of names and acronyms. They are designed to highlight different tissue characteristics, e.g. to demonstrate water content (HASTE sequence), diminish the signal from fat and so highlight pathology or contrast enhancement (fat suppression or STIR sequence, see Fig. 4.43, p. 156), or demonstrate the combination of water and lipid content in the same voxel (chemical shift imaging, see Fig. 8.17, p. 283). Dynamic contrast-enhanced scans using gadolinium contrast medium (see below) may be used to demonstrate the anatomy of the large vessels as well as the enhancement characteristics of tumour angiogenesis (Fig. 1.11c). More recent developments include diffusion-weighted imaging and MR spectroscopy, which can further characterize tissues and are often used in tumour assessment.

A typical MRI scanner (Fig. 1.12) consists of a large circular magnet. Inside the magnet are the radiofrequency transmitter and receiver coils, as well as gradient coils to allow spatial localization of the MRI signal. Ancillary equipment converts the radio signal into a digital form, which the computer can manipulate to create an image. One advantage of MRI over CT is that the information can be directly imaged in any plane. In most instances, MRI requires a longer scan time (often several minutes) compared with CT, with the disadvantage that the patient has to keep still during the scanning procedure. Unavoidable movements from breathing, cardiac pulsation and peristalsis often degrade the image. Techniques to speed up scan times and limit the effect of motion by the use of various electronic methods have been introduced. Cardiac gating and breath-hold sequences are now readily available.

Magnetic resonance imaging gives very different information to CT. The earliest successful application was for scanning the brain and spinal cord, where MRI has significant advantages over CT and few disadvantages. Magnetic resonance imaging is now also an established technique for imaging the spine, bones, joints, pelvic organs, liver, biliary system, urinary tract and heart. At first sight it may seem rather surprising that MRI provides valuable information in skeletal disease as calcified tissues do not generate any signal at MRI. This seeming paradox is explained by the fact that MRI provides images of the bone marrow and the soft tissues inside and surrounding joints (Fig. 1.13).

The physical basis of imaging blood vessels with MRI is complicated and beyond the scope of this book. Suffice it to say that, with some sequences, fast-flowing blood produces no signal (Fig. 1.14), whereas with others it produces a bright signal. This 'motion effect' can be exploited to image blood vessels. Such flow-sensitive sequences are mostly used for head and neck imaging, for example, intracranial arteriovenous malformations and stenoses of the carotid arteries can be readily demonstrated without contrast media. The resulting images resemble a conventional angiogram (Fig 1.15).

Magnetic resonance imaging of the heart uses electronic gating to obtain images during a specific portion of the

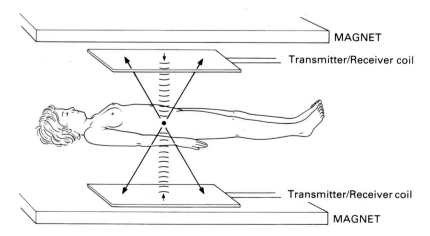

Fig. 1.12 Diagram of an MRI machine. The patient lies within a strong magnet (usually a cylindrical magnet). The radiofrequency transmitter coils send radiowaves into the patient and the same coils receive signals from within the patient. The intensity and source of these signals can be calculated and displayed as an image.

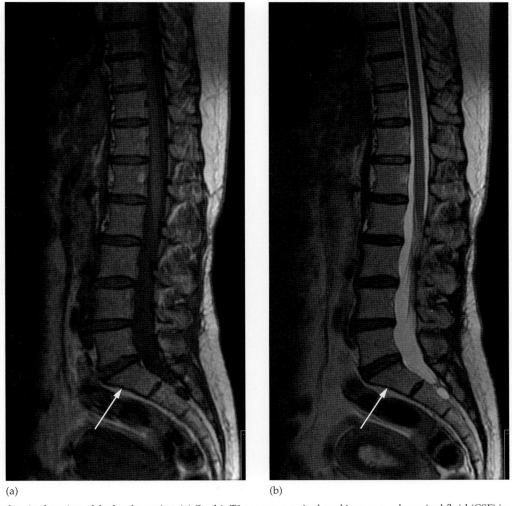

(a)   (b)

Fig. 1.13 MRI of sagittal section of the lumbar spine. (a) On this T1 sequence, spinal cord is grey, cerebrospinal fluid (CSF) is nearly black and subcutaneous fat is white. (b) T2-weighted sequence. Here the CSF is white. Cortical bone (arrow) returns no signal and appears as a black line on both sequences. The fat in the bone marrow produces a signal that enables the vertebrae to be visualized.

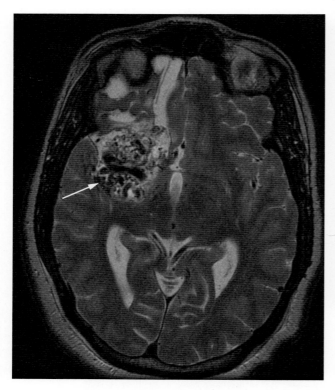

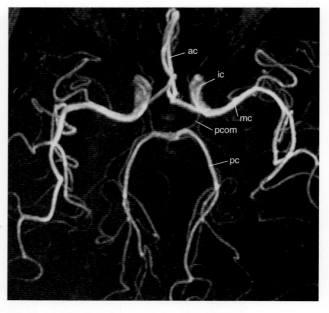

Fig. 1.15 MR angiogram of the intracranial arteries. No contrast medium was used to obtain this image. ac, anterior cerebral; ic, internal cerebral; mc, middle cerebral; pc, posterior cerebral; pcom, posterior communicating artery.

Fig. 1.14 MRI of brain showing an arteriovenous malformation (arrow) in the right cerebral hemisphere. The fast-flowing blood in the malformation is responsible for absence of signal (signal void). The image is a T2-weighted image, and is normal apart from the arteriovenous malformation and its consequences.

cardiac cycle. With this technique it is possible to limit the degradation of the image by cardiac motion and demonstrate the cardiac chambers, valves and myocardium. Alternatively, the beating heart can be directly visualized as a cine image.

One of the advantages of MRI is that it involves no ionizing radiation, and no adverse biological effects from diagnostic MRI have been demonstrated. The strong magnetic fields, however, mean that it is at present contraindicated in patients with certain implantable devices, including cardiac pacemakers, certain types of aneurysm clip and intraocular metallic foreign bodies.

Contrast agents for MRI

Just as contrast media have been of great value in CT, magnetic contrast materials are providing useful diagnostic information with MRI. The most widely used agents are gadolinium compounds which only cross the blood–brain barrier when it is damaged by disease (Fig. 1.11c), and which concentrate in tissues and disease processes with a high blood supply. Tissues which concentrate the agent show very high signal intensity (i.e. they appear white) on T1-weighted images. Tissue-specific media, such as iron-oxide agents for reticuloendothelial cell imaging, are also used. A particular application of contrast-enhanced MRI is magnetic resonance angiography (MRA), which along with CT angiography, is gradually replacing conventional angiography.

Gadolinium-based contrast agents are generally very safe and anaphylactic reactions are rare. They are contraindicated in pregnancy. Also, it has recently been recognized that patients in renal failure, on dialysis, or awaiting liver transplantation are at risk of developing nephrogenic systemic fibrosis (NSF), which can be fatal. In these patients, the MR scan is done without the use of gadolinium-based contrast agents.

Picture archiving and communication systems (PACS)

Digital recording has developed dramatically over the past two decades. CT, ultrasound, MRI, nuclear medicine and angiography are nowadays all digital techniques. Even conventional radiographs can be based on digital information.

Digital data can be processed by a computer which allows electronic transmission of images between buildings, towns and even countries, and most importantly allows computer storage. A fully digital department obviates the need for x-ray films; it enables images as well as their reports to be viewed on video screens.

Radiation hazards

X-rays used in conventional radiography and CT, as well as gamma-rays and other radionuclide emissions, are harmful. Natural radiation from the sun, radioactivity in the environment, together with atmospheric radioactivity from nuclear bombs and other man-made ionizing radiations contribute a genetic risk over which an individual doctor has no control. However, ionizing radiation for medical purposes is of several times greater magnitude than all other sources of man-made radiation and is under the control of doctors. It is their responsibility to limit the use of x-rays and other ionizing radiations to those situations where the benefit clearly outbalances the risks. Unnecessary radiation is to be deplored. The principle to be used is the so-called ALARA principle: 'as low as reasonably achievable'. This is achieved by the use of appropriate equipment and good technique – limiting the size of the x-ray beam to the required areas, limiting the number of films to those that are necessary, keeping repeat examinations to a minimum and ensuring that the examination has not already been performed. Just as important as these factors, all of which are really the province of those who work in the x-ray department, is the avoidance of unnecessary requests for x-ray examinations, particularly those that involve high radiation exposure such as barium enema, lumbar spine x-rays and CT examinations. If possible, alternative techniques such as ultrasound or MRI should be considered. In other words, the imaging examination being requested must be justified.

Radiation is particularly harmful to dividing cells. Genetically adverse mutations may occur following radiation of the gonads, resulting in congenital malformations and a genetic risk to the population. There is no threshold for the mutation rate, hence there is no such thing as a safe radiation dose.

Radiation to the developing fetus can have catastrophic effects. As well as the increased incidence of malformations induced in the developing fetus, it has been shown that the frequency with which leukaemia and other malignant neoplasms develop within the first 10 years of life is increased in children exposed to diagnostic x-rays while *in utero*, probably by about 40% compared with the normal population. X-raying a fetus should, therefore, be kept to the absolute minimum and preferably avoided.

Radiation-induced cancer is of general concern. It is not known whether exposures of the magnitude used for individual diagnostic examinations induces cancers, but recent estimates suggest that a standard CT examination might be associated with a risk of cancer induction of 1 in 2000. If all radiation-reducing methods were followed, including the elimination of unnecessary examinations, then in the UK it might be possible to reduce the number of cancer fatalities by over 100 cases per year.

2

Chest

THORACIC DISEASE

Imaging techniques

The plain chest radiograph

Routine chest radiography consists of a posteroanterior (PA) view, also known as a frontal view, with the optional addition of a lateral view (Fig. 2.1). Both should be exposed on full inspiration with the patient in the upright position. Films taken on expiration are difficult to interpret, because in expiration the lung bases appear hazy and the heart shadow increases in size (Fig. 2.2).

Even though chest films are the commonest x-ray examinations performed, they are amongst the most difficult to interpret. Trained radiologists often scan films in an apparently random fashion, but when an abnormality is found their thoughts are then structured, thinking of the possibilities for that particular shadow. For example, if a nodule representing a possible lung carcinoma is discovered, the shape of the nodule is analyzed and evidence of spread of disease to the hilum, pleura or rib cage, etc., is sought. This problem-orientated approach – the observer constantly asking questions, not only about the shadows but also about the patient's clinical findings – is the quickest and most accurate way of achieving a diagnosis. However, this approach takes time to

learn and, in the early stages, a routine is necessary in order to avoid overlooking valuable radiological signs. The order in which one looks at the structures is unimportant; what matters is to follow a routine, otherwise significant abnormalities will be missed. One approach to examining the frontal and lateral chest films is presented below.

Trace the diaphragm

The upper surfaces of the diaphragm should be clearly visible from one costophrenic angle to the other, except where the heart and mediastinum are in contact with the diaphragm. On a good inspiratory film, the dome of the right hemidiaphragm is at the level of the anterior end of the sixth rib, the right hemidiaphragm being up to 2.5 cm higher than the left.

Check the size and shape of the heart

See p. 97 for details.

Check the position of the heart and mediastinum

Normally, the trachea lies midway, or slightly to the right of the midpoint, between the medial ends of the clavicles. The position of the heart is very variable; on average one-third lies to the right of the midline.

Look at the mediastinum

The outline of the mediastinum and heart should be clearly seen, except where the heart lies in contact with the

Diagnostic Imaging, 6th Edition. By Peter Armstrong, Martin Wastie and Andrea Rockall. Published 2009 by Blackwell Publishing. ISBN: 978-1-4051-7039.

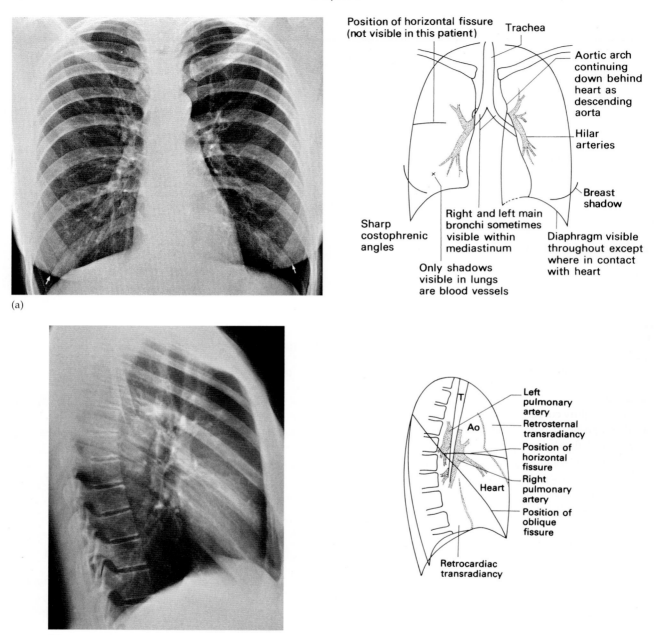

(a)

(b)

Fig. 2.1 Normal chest. (a) Posteroanterior (PA) view. The arrows point to the breast shadows of this female patient. (b) Lateral view. The vertebrae are more transradiant (i.e. blacker) as the eye travels down the spine, until the diaphragm is reached. Ao, aorta; T, trachea.

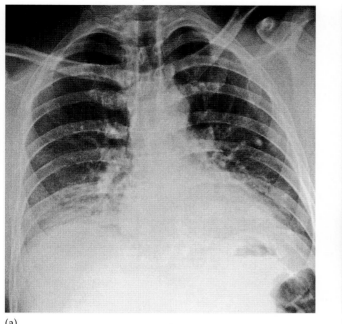

(a)

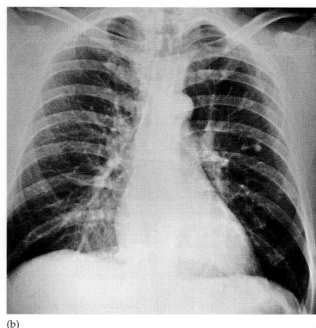

(b)

Fig. 2.2 Effect of expiration on chest film. Two films of the same patient taken one after the other. (a) Expiration. (b) Inspiration. On expiration the heart appears larger and the lung bases are hazy.

diaphragm. The right superior mediastinal border is usually straight or slightly curved as it passes downwards to merge with the right heart border. The left superior mediastinal border is ill-defined above the aortic arch. With increasing age, the aorta elongates. Elongation necessarily involves unfolding, because the aorta is fixed at the aortic valve and at the diaphragm. This unfolding results in the ascending aorta deviating to the right and the descending aorta to the left. In young children, the normal thymus is often clearly visualized. It may be very large and should not be mistaken for disease (Fig. 2.3).

Examine the hilar shadows

The hilar shadows represent the pulmonary arteries and veins. Air within the major bronchi can be recognized, but the walls of the bronchi are not usually visible. The hilar lymph nodes in the normal patient are too small to recognize as discrete shadows. The left hilum is usually slightly higher in position than the right.

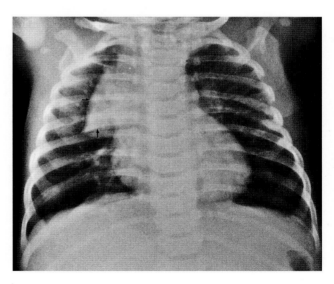

Fig. 2.3 Normal but prominent thymus in a child aged 3 months. The thymus shows the characteristic 'sail shape' projecting to the right of the mediastinum (arrows). This appearance should not be confused with right upper lobe consolidation or collapse.

Examine the lungs

The only structures that can be identified within normal lungs are the blood vessels, the interlobar fissures, and the walls of certain larger bronchi seen end-on. The fissures can only be seen if they lie along the line of the x-ray beam; they are, after all, composed of just two layers of pleura. Usually, only the horizontal fissure (minor fissure) is visible in the frontal projection, running from the right hilum to the sixth rib in the axilla. There is no equivalent to the horizontal fissure on the left. The oblique fissures (major fissures) are only visible on the lateral view. The fissures form the boundaries of the lobes, so knowing their position is essential for an appreciation of lobar anatomy (see Fig. 2.15, p. 30). In about 1% of people there is an extra fissure visible in the frontal view – the so-called azygos lobe fissure (Fig. 2.4).

Look for abnormal pulmonary opacities or translucencies. Do not mistake the pectoral muscles, breasts (Fig. 2.1) or plaits of hair for pulmonary shadows. Skin lumps or the nipples may mimic pulmonary nodules. The nipples are usually in the fifth anterior rib space, but they are, in practice, rarely misdiagnosed because, in general, if one nipple is visible the other should also be seen.

A good method of finding subtle shadows on the frontal film is to compare one lung with the other, zone by zone. Detecting ill-defined shadows on the lateral view can be difficult. A helpful and reliable feature is that as the eye travels down the thoracic vertebral bodies, each vertebral body should appear more lucent than the one above until the diaphragm is reached.

Check the integrity of the ribs, clavicles and spine and examine the soft tissues

The bones of the chest should be checked for fractures and metastases. Any rib notching should be noted as it may indicate coarctation of the aorta. In females, check that both breasts are present. Following mastectomy the breast shadow cannot be defined. The reduction in the soft tissue bulk leads to an increased transradiancy of that side of the chest, which should not be confused with pulmonary disease.

Assess the technical quality of the film

Technical factors are important as incorrect exposure may hide disease, and faulty centring or projection may mimic

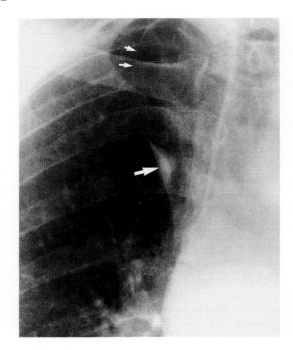

Fig. 2.4 The azygos lobe fissure. During normal intrauterine development the azygos vein migrates through the lung from the chest wall to lie within the mediastinum. In patients with an azygos 'lobe', the vein (large arrow) fails to reach the tracheobronchial angle and, therefore, lies in the lower end of the azygos fissure (small arrows). This variant is of no clinical significance.

pathology. The correctly exposed routine PA chest film is one in which the ribs and spine behind the heart can be identified but the lungs are not overexposed. Unless one can see through the heart, lower lobe lesions may be completely missed. A straight film is one where the medial ends of the clavicles are equidistant from the thoracic vertebrae.

Computed tomography

Technique

A routine chest computed tomography (CT) examination consists of contiguous sections. Intravenous contrast medium is given in many cases, particularly when the purpose of the examination is to visualize the mediastinum, the hila or the pulmonary blood vessels. The images

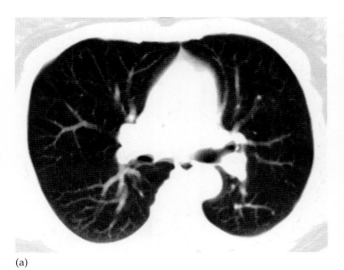 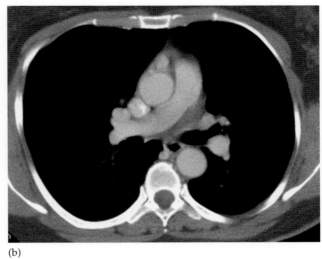

(a)   (b)

Fig. 2.5 Chest CT illustrating the different window centres (levels) used for the lungs and mediastinum. (a) Lung settings. A negative centre (minus 700 Hounsfield units [HU]) and a wide window width (1000 HU) shows the lungs to advantage, but there is no detail of mediastinal structures, the mediastinum being uniformly white. In this example, the lung vessels are the only identifiable shadows originating from within the lung. (b) Mediastinal settings. A centre close to average soft-tissue density (40 HU) and a narrow window width (400 HU) shows the structures within the mediastinum clearly, but the lungs are blacked out.

are usually viewed at both lung and mediastinal window settings (Fig. 2.5) (see p. 3 for explanation of CT windows and levels). If the CT scan has been performed to see bone lesions then bone settings are used.

Thin sections can be used to produce images with higher spatial resolution – so-called high resolution CT (HRCT). High resolution CT allows details of pulmonary parenchymal disease and bronchiectasis to be shown.

Indications

There are many indications for CT in chest disease, notably:
• Showing the presence and extent of mediastinal masses and other mediastinal abnormalities. Computed tomography is widely used to demonstrate enlarged lymph nodes when staging patients with neoplastic disease, particularly lung cancer and lymphoma. Sometimes CT can determine the likely nature of a mediastinal abnormality. Knowing the shape and the precise location of a mediastinal mass may make a particular diagnosis highly probable. One of the advantages of CT is that it can distinguish vascular from non-vascular structures (Fig. 2.6), e.g. an aneurysm from a solid mass. Also, CT allows fat to be recognized, which is useful for diagnosing fatty tumours or excluding significant abnormality when mediastinal widening is due merely to excess fat deposition.
• Showing the shape of an intrapulmonary or pleural opacity, or detecting calcification or cavitation, when the interpretation of plain chest radiographs is not straightforward.
• Localizing an opacity prior to biopsy.
• Demonstrating the presence of disease when an abnormality is uncertain or when the plain chest radiograph is normal but an intrathoracic abnormality is suspected on other grounds, e.g. detecting pulmonary metastases or demonstrating thymic tumours in patients with myasthenia gravis.
• Documenting the presence, extent and severity of bronchiectasis and other airway diseases.
• Diagnosing and assessing diffuse pulmonary disease.
• Diagnosing pulmonary emboli using CT pulmonary angiography (Fig. 2.7).

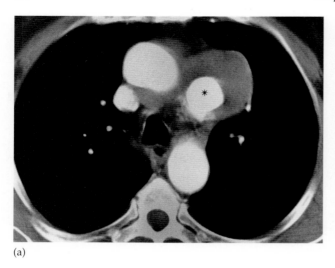

(a)

Fig. 2.6 Aortic aneurysm: example of the use of (a) contrast-enhanced CT to diagnose an aortic aneurysm. The lumen of the aneurysm (*) enhances brightly. Much of the aneurysm is lined by clot. (b) The plain chest radiograph shows a mass (arrows), but the precise diagnosis of aortic aneurysm cannot be made.

(b)

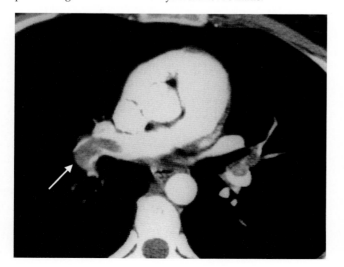

Fig. 2.7 CT pulmonary angiogram showing, in this example, bilateral filling defects owing to emboli in the central pulmonary arteries. The arrow points to the largest of these emboli.

Normal images

Just as on plain chest radiographs, the only structures seen on CT within the normal lungs are blood vessels, pleural fissures and the walls of bronchi. Vessels within the lung are recognized by their shape rather than by contrast opacification (see Fig. 2.5a). When seen in cross-section they appear round and may be indistinguishable from small lung nodules. Fortunately, most metastases and granulomas are located peripherally where the vessels are smallest.

The fissures may be seen as a line, or their position may be recognizable only as a relatively avascular zone within the lung. The CT appearances of the normal mediastinum and hila are discussed on p. 57.

Magnetic resonance imaging

Magnetic resonance imaging (MRI) has only a very small role in the management of pulmonary, pleural or mediastinal disease, although it is playing an increasingly large part in the diagnosis of cardiac and aortic diseases. Magnetic resonance imaging can be useful in selected patients with lung cancers, when the relevant questions cannot be answered by CT and can show the intraspinal extent of mediastinal neural tumours.

Radionuclide lung scanning

There are two major types of radionuclide lung scan: perfusion and ventilation scans.

Perfusion scans use small particles, approximately 30 μm in diameter, labelled with ^{99m}Tc, injected intravenously. These particles become trapped in the pulmonary capillaries; the distribution of radioactivity, when imaged by a gamma camera, accurately reflects blood flow (Fig. 2.8).

For ventilation scans, the patient inhales a radioactive gas such as xenon-133, xenon-127 or krypton-81 m and the distribution of radioactive gas is imaged using a gamma camera (Fig. 2.9).

The major indication for radionuclide lung scanning is to diagnose or exclude pulmonary embolism (see p. 86), but this indication has been superceded by CT pulmonary angiography.

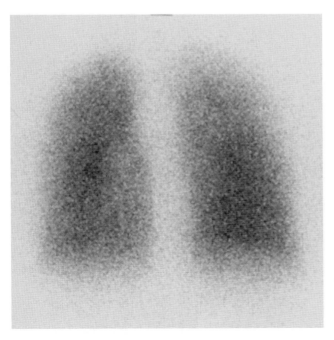

Fig. 2.8 Normal radionuclide perfusion scan using ^{99m}Tc-labelled macroaggregates of albumin. Posterior view.

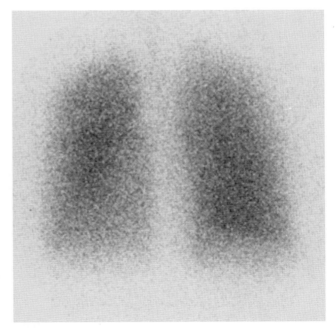

Fig. 2.9 Normal radionuclide ^{81m}Kr ventilation scan. Posterior view.

Positron emission tomography (PET scanning)

Fluorodeoxyglucose (FDG) (see p. 8 for a description of FDG) is taken up by a number of tumours, notably primary lung cancers, metastases and active lymphomatous tissue. Positron emission tomography (PET) of the thorax (Fig. 2.10) is, therefore, used to stage lung cancer or lymphoma and to diagnose recurrent lung cancer. It is also increasingly used to diagnose the malignant nature of a solitary pulmonary nodule. Unfortunately, inflammatory conditions also concentrate the agent, so the appearances are not entirely specific for neoplastic tissue.

Ultrasound of the thorax

The use of thoracic ultrasound, as opposed to cardiac ultrasound (see Chapter 3), is confined to the demonstration of processes in contact with the chest wall, notably pleural effusion, pleural masses and selected mediastinal masses. It can be very useful for guiding a needle to sample or drain loculated pleural fluid collections and for needle biopsy/ aspiration cytology of masses in contact with the chest wall. As ultrasound is absorbed by air in the lung, conventional ultrasound cannot be used to evaluate processes that lie deep to aerated lung tissue.

It is possible to pass a small ultrasound probe through an endoscope to visualize structures immediately adjacent to the oesophagus, e.g. para-oesophageal nodes and the descending aorta (see Fig. 2.70 and 2.71, pp. 65 and 66).

Diseases of the chest with a normal chest radiograph

Serious respiratory disease may exist in patients who have a normal chest radiograph. Sometimes it is only possible to detect abnormality by comparison with previous or later examinations, e.g. subtle pulmonary shadows from infection or pulmonary fibrosis. Chest disease with a normal chest radiograph occurs in:

Obstructive airways disease

Asthma and acute bronchiolitis may produce overinflation of the lungs, but in many cases the chest film is normal.

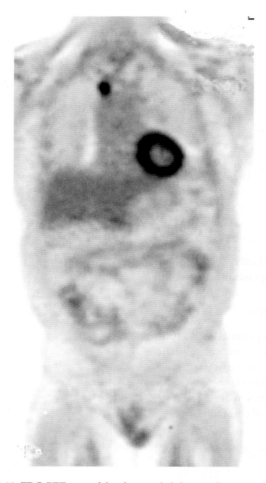

Fig. 2.10 FDG-PET scan of the chest and abdomen showing a focus of high activity in a mediastinal lymph node (metastasis from lung carcinoma). The remainder of the image is normal. The primary tumour is not shown on this section. The high activity in the myocardium is normal. Fused PET-CT images of this patient are shown in Plate 2.

Emphysema, when severe, gives rise to the signs described on p. 81, but, when the disease is moderate, the chest radiograph may be normal or very nearly so. Uncomplicated acute or chronic bronchitis does not usually produce any radiological signs, so if a patient with chronic bronchitis has an abnormal film, some other disease or a complication has developed, e.g. pneumonia or cor pulmonale. Many patients with productive cough due to bronchiectasis show no plain film abnormality.

Small lesions

It is usually impossible to see solitary lung masses or consolidations of less than 1 cm in diameter. Even 2–3 cm lung cancers may be very difficult to identify on routine films if they are hidden by ribs or clavicles or if they lie behind the heart or diaphragm.

Endobronchial lesions, such as carcinoma, cannot be diagnosed on routine films unless they cause collapse/consolidation.

Pulmonary emboli without infarction

The chest radiograph is often normal even when life-threatening emboli are present.

Infections

Most patients with acute bacterial pneumonia present with recognizable consolidation, but in other infections, notably *Pneumocystis carinii* pneumonia, obvious pulmonary consolidation may only develop after the onset of symptoms. Patients with miliary tuberculosis may initially have a normal chest film.

Diffuse pulmonary fibrosis

Widespread pulmonary fibrosis may be responsible for breathlessness with substantial alteration in lung function tests before any clear-cut abnormalities are evident on chest radiographs.

Pleural abnormality

Dry pleurisy does not produce any radiological findings and small amounts of pleural fluid may be impossible to recognize on standard PA and lateral chest films.

Mediastinal masses

Plain chest radiography is very insensitive for the diagnosis of mediastinal masses, lymph node enlargement and mediastinal fluid collections.

Abnormal chest

When viewing an abnormal examination of the chest, be it a plain film, CT or MRI, the first questions to ask are 'Where is the abnormality?' and 'How extensive is it?'. Only then can the question 'What is it?' be answered, because the differential diagnosis for pulmonary lesions is clearly quite different from that for mediastinal, pleural or chest wall disease.

The first step is to examine all available films. Usually, the location of a lesion will be obvious. If the abnormality is surrounded on all sides by aerated lung it must arise within the lung. Similarly, many masses are clearly within the mediastinum. However, when a lesion is in contact with the pleura or mediastinum it may be difficult to decide its origin.

If the shadow has a broad base with smooth convex borders projecting into the lung and a well-defined outline it is likely to be pleural, extrapleural or mediastinal in origin (Fig. 2.11).

The silhouette sign

The silhouette sign (Fig. 2.12) is an invaluable sign for localizing disease from plain chest radiographs. The information on a plain chest film is largely dependent on the contrast between air in the lungs compared with the opacity of the heart, blood vessels, mediastinum and diaphragm. An intrathoracic lesion touching the heart, aorta or diaphragm obliterates the border of the structure in question. This sign is known as the *silhouette sign* and has two important applications:
- It is often possible to localize a shadow by observing which borders are lost, e.g. loss of the heart border means that the shadow lies in the anterior half of the chest. Alternatively, loss of part of the diaphragm outline indicates disease of the pleura or of the lung in direct contact with the diaphragm, usually the lower lobes.
- The silhouette sign makes it possible, on occasion, to diagnose disorders such as pulmonary consolidation or collapse even when the presence of an opacity is uncertain. It is a surprising fact that a wedge- or lens-shaped opacity may be very difficult to see because of the way the shadow fades out at its margins, but if such a lesion is in contact with the mediastinum or diaphragm it causes loss of their normally sharp outlines.

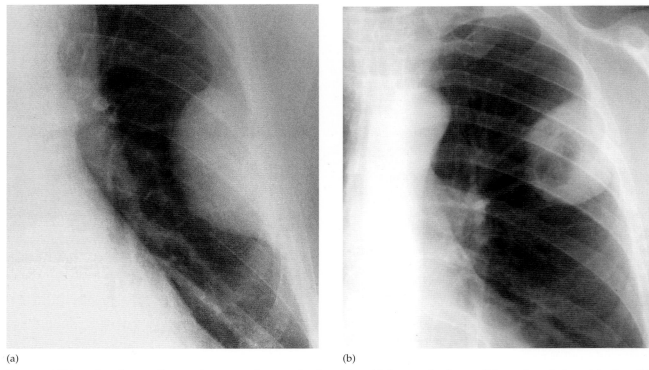

(a)   (b)

Fig. 2.11 (a) Extrapleural mass. The mass has a smooth convex border with a wide base on the chest wall (a myeloma lesion arising in a rib). This shape is quite different from a peripherally located pulmonary mass such as (b) a primary carcinoma of the lung.

Radiological signs of lung disease

It is helpful to try and place any abnormal intrapulmonary shadows into one or more of the following broad categories:

- air-space filling
- pulmonary collapse (atelectasis)
- spherical shadows
- line shadows
- widespread small shadows.

The presence of cavitation or calcification should be noted.

Air-space filling

Air-space filling means the replacement of air in the alveoli by fluid or, rarely, by other materials. 'Infiltrate' is a commonly used but less satisfactory term. The fluid can be either an exudate (often called 'consolidation') or a transudate (pulmonary oedema – a topic discussed in the section on heart disease on p. 102). The signs of consolidation are:

- A shadow with ill-defined borders (Fig. 2.13), except where the opacity is in contact with a fissure, in which case the shadow has a well-defined edge.
- An air bronchogram (Fig. 2.14). Normally, it is not possible to identify air in bronchi within normally aerated lung, because the walls of the normal bronchi are too thin and air-filled bronchi are surrounded by air in the alveoli, but if the alveoli are filled with fluid, the air in the bronchi contrasts with the fluid in the adjacent lung. This sign is seen to great advantage on CT.
- The silhouette sign, namely loss of visualization of the adjacent mediastinal or diaphragm outline (see p. 25 for explanation of this sign).

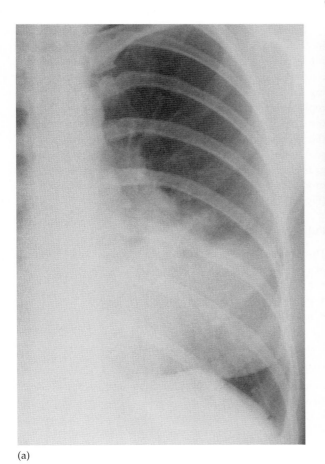

(a)

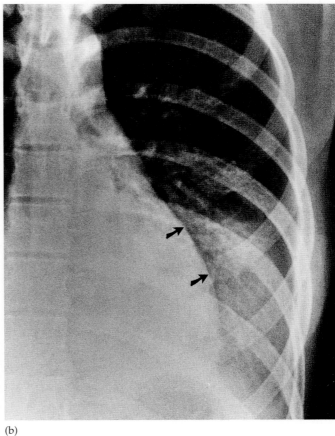

(b)

Fig. 2.12 The silhouette sign. (a) The left heart border is invisible because it is in contact with consolidation in the adjacent lingula. (b) The left heart border can be seen because the consolidation is in the left lower lobe and air in the lingula preserves the visibility of the cardiac silhouette (arrows). Note that now it is the diaphragm outline that is invisible. (c) The relationships of the lingula and lower lobes to the heart and diaphragm are explained by a diagram of the lung viewed from the side.

Consolidation in the lingula obliterates the left heart border but leaves the diaphragm visible

Consolidation in the left lower lobe obliterates the diaphragm but leaves the heart border visible

(c)

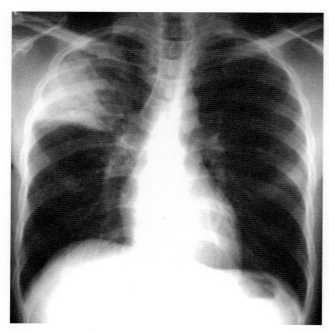

Fig. 2.13 Air-space filling. In this case, the consolidation in the right upper lobe is due to a pneumonia.

Consolidation of a whole lobe, or the majority of a lobe, is virtually diagnostic of bacterial pneumonia. The diagnosis of lobar consolidation requires an appreciation of the radiological anatomy of the lobes (Fig. 2.15). Lobar consolidation produces an opaque lobe, except for air bronchograms. Because of the silhouette sign, the boundary between the affected lung and the adjacent heart, mediastinum and diaphragm is invisible. Figure 2.16 shows an example of lobar consolidation.

Patchy consolidation, i.e. one or more patches of ill-defined shadowing (Fig. 2.17), is usually due to:

- pneumonia
- infarction
- contusion
- immunological disorders.

There is no reliable way of telling from either chest radiographs or CT which of these possibilities is the cause. In most instances the clinical and laboratory findings point to one or other cause.

Cavitation (abscess formation) within consolidated areas in the lung may occur with many bacterial and fungal infections (Fig. 2.18). Abscess formation is only recognizable once there is communication with the bronchial tree, allowing the liquid centre of the abscess to be coughed up and replaced by air. The air is then seen as a transradiancy within the consolidation and an air–fluid level may be present (Fig. 2.19). Cavitation is occasionally seen in other forms of pulmonary consolidation, e.g. infarction and Wegener's granulomatosis. Computed tomography is better and more sensitive than plain films for demonstrating cavitation (Fig. 2.20).

Pulmonary collapse (atelectasis)

The common causes of pulmonary collapse (loss of volume of a lobe or lung) are:

- bronchial obstruction
- pneumothorax or pleural effusion
- linear (discoid) atelectasis.

Collapse caused by bronchial obstruction

Collapse caused by bronchial obstruction occurs because air cannot get into the lung in sufficient quantities to replace the air absorbed from the alveoli. The signs of lobar collapse are:

- Displacement of structures.
- The shadow of the collapsed lobe – consolidation almost invariably accompanies lobar collapse, so the resulting shadow is usually obvious.
- The silhouette sign. The silhouette sign not only helps diagnose lobar collapse when the resulting shadow is difficult to appreciate, but also helps to decide which lobe is collapsed. Collapse of the anteriorly located lobes (upper and middle) obliterates portions of the mediastinal and heart outlines, whereas collapse of the lower lobes obscures the outline of the adjacent diaphragm and descending aorta.

The commoner causes of lobar collapse are:

- Bronchial wall lesions, usually primary carcinoma, but occasionally other bronchial tumours such as carcinoid tumours.
- Intraluminal occlusion, usually foreign body or retained mucus plugs, particularly in postoperative, asthmatic or unconscious patients, or in patients on artificial ventilation.
- Invasion or compression by an adjacent malignant tumour or, rarely by enlarged lymph nodes.

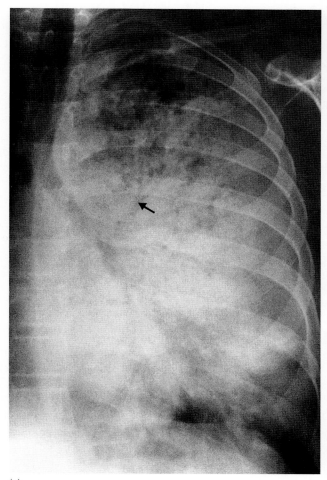

(a)

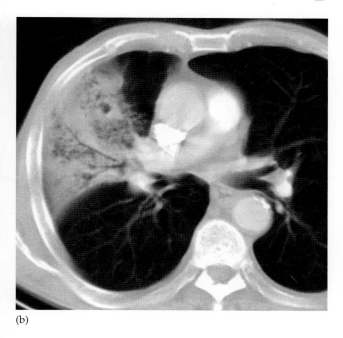

(b)

Fig. 2.14 The air bronchogram sign. (a) An extensive air bronchogram is seen in this patient with pneumonia. The arrow points to a bronchus that is particularly well seen.
(b) CT showing an air bronchogram in an area of pulmonary consolidation from pneumonia.

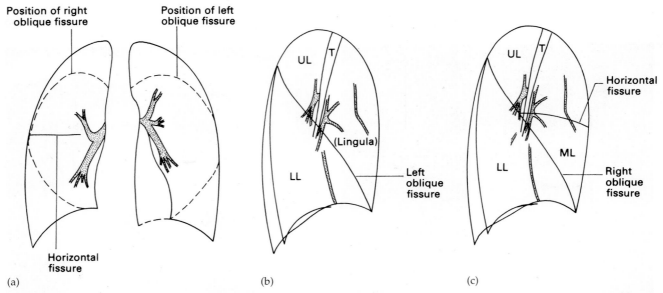

Fig. 2.15 Position of the lobes and fissures. (a) The oblique (major) fissure is similar on the two sides. The oblique fissures are not visible on the frontal view; their position is indicated by dotted lines. (b) In the left lung the oblique fissure separates the upper lobe (UL) and lower lobe (LL). (c) In the right lung, there is an extra fissure – the horizontal (minor) fissure, which separates the upper lobe (UL) and middle lobe (ML). (The lingular segments of the upper lobe are analogous to the segments of the middle lobe.) T, trachea.

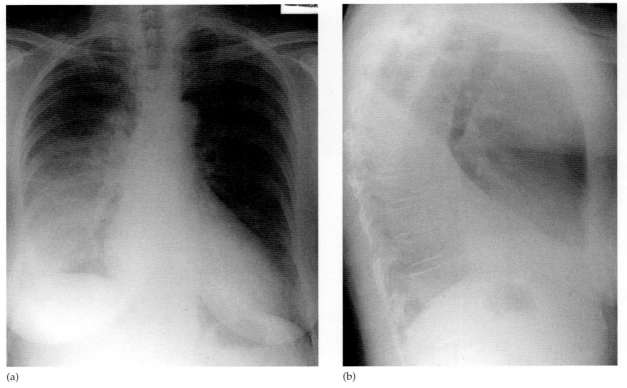

Fig. 2.16 Consolidation of the right lower lobe. Note the application of the silhouette sign here. (a) PA view. The heart border and the medial half of the right hemidiaphragm are visible, whereas the lateral half is invisible. On the lateral view (b), the oblique fissure forms a well-defined anterior boundary and the right hemidiaphragm is ill defined. Only the left hemidiaphragm is seen clearly.

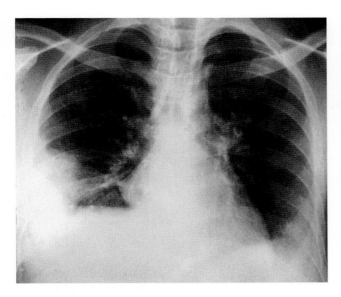

Fig. 2.17 Patchy consolidation in both lower lobes in a patient with bronchopneumonia.

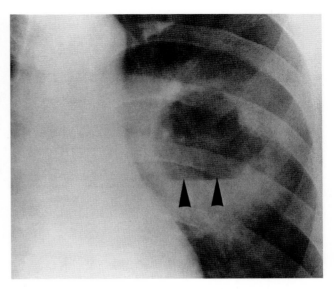

Fig. 2.19 Fluid level (arrows) in a lung abscess. Fluid levels are only visible if the chest radiograph is taken with a horizontal x-ray beam.

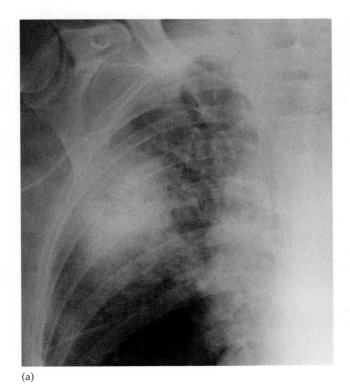

(a)

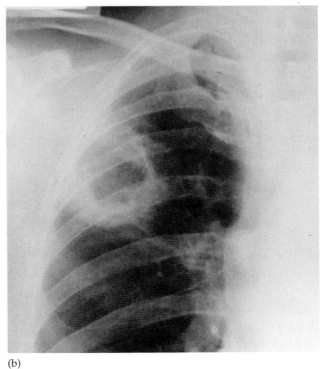

(b)

Fig. 2.18 Cavitation in staphylococcal pneumonia. (a) A round area of consolidation which, seven days later (b) shows central translucency due to the development of cavitation.

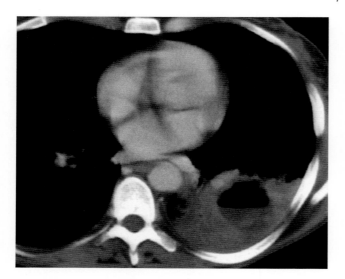

When a lobe collapses, the unobstructed lobe(s) on the side of the collapse undergoes compensatory expansion. The displaced fissure is seen as a well-defined boundary to an airless lobe in one or other view. The mediastinum and diaphragm may move towards the collapsed lobe.

As lobar collapse is such an important and often difficult diagnosis to make on chest radiographs, it is worth devoting time to study the appearance of collapse of each of the lobes (Figs 2.21–2.25). Computed tomography shows lobar collapse very well (Figs 2.25 and 2.26), but is rarely necessary simply to diagnose a collapsed lobe.

With collapse of the whole of one lung, the entire hemithorax is opaque and there is substantial mediastinal and tracheal shift (Fig. 2.27).

Fig. 2.20 Bacterial lung abscess shown by CT. Note the air–fluid level in a rounded cavity.

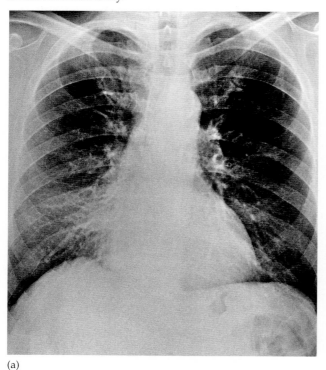

(a)

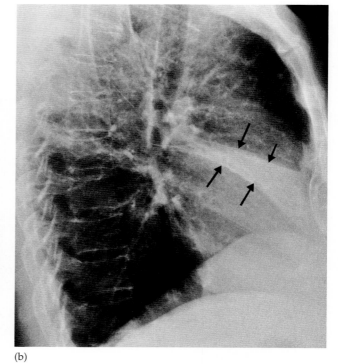

(b)

Fig. 2.21 Collapse of the middle lobe. The collapsed lobe is most obvious on the lateral view (arrows). Note the silhouette sign obliterating the lower right heart border.

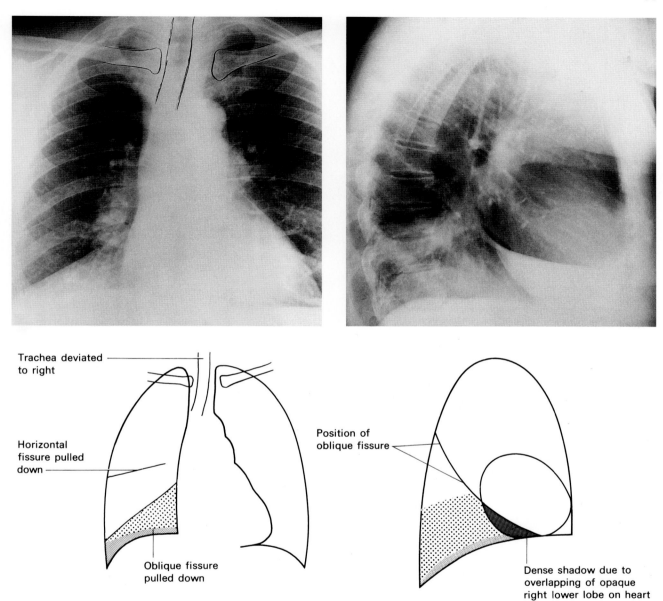

Fig. 2.22 Collapse of the right lower lobe. (In this example the apical segment is relatively well aerated.)

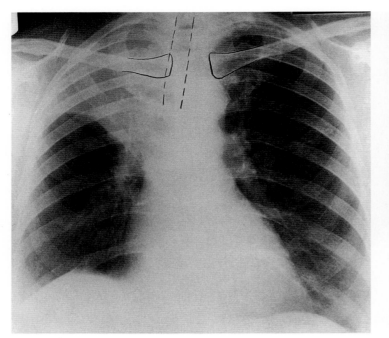
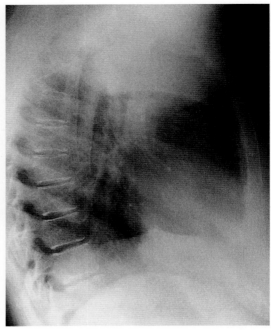

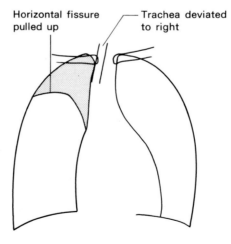
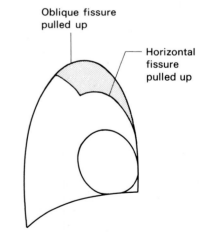

Horizontal fissure
pulled up

Trachea deviated
to right

Oblique fissure
pulled up

Horizontal
fissure
pulled up

Fig. 2.23 Collapse of the right upper lobe. Note the elevated horizontal fissure.

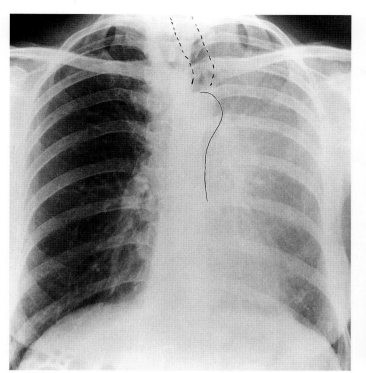

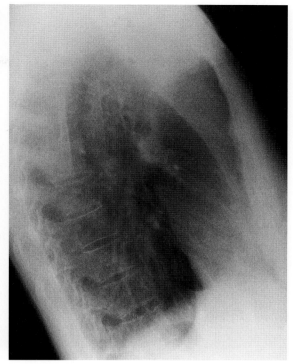

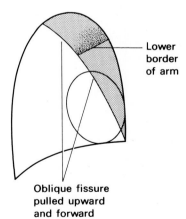

Fig. 2.24 Collapse of the left upper lobe. Note that the lower border of the collapsed lobe is ill defined on the posteroanterior view and that the upper two-thirds of the left mediastinal and heart borders are invisible, but that the aortic knuckle and descending aorta are identifiable. (The visible portions of the aorta have been drawn in for greater clarity.)

Lower border of arm

Oblique fissure pulled upward and forward

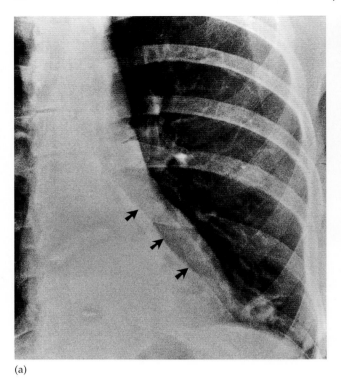

(a)

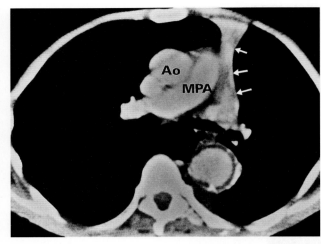

Fig. 2.26 CT of a severely collapsed left upper lobe. Note the smooth lateral border of the collapsed lobe formed by the displaced oblique (major) fissure (arrows). The scan shows compensatory overexpansion of the right upper lobe which has crossed the midline anterior to the ascending aorta (Ao) and main pulmonary artery (MPA).

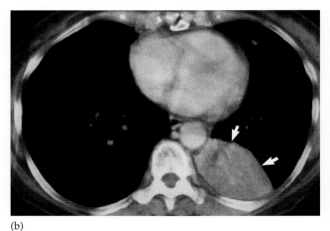

(b)

Fig. 2.25 Collapse of the left lower lobe. (a) Chest radiograph. The triangular shadow of the collapsed lobe is seen through the heart. Its lateral border is formed by the displaced oblique fissure (arrows). (b) CT. The collapsed lobe is seen lying posteriorly in the left thorax. The well-defined anterior margin is due to the displaced oblique fissure (arrows).

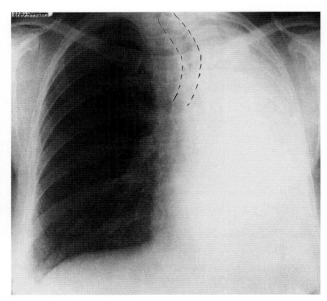

Fig. 2.27 Collapse of left lung showing tracheal and mediastinal displacement.

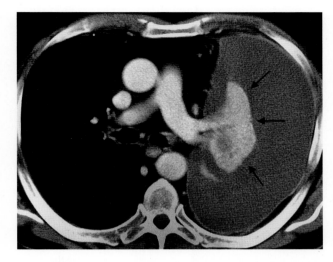

Fig. 2.28 CT showing pleural effusion and pulmonary collapse. The collapsed lobe (arrows) can be clearly seen beneath the large left pleural effusion.

Collapse in association with pneumothorax or pleural effusion

The presence of air or fluid in the pleural cavity allows the lung to collapse. In pneumothorax, the diagnosis is obvious but if there is a large pleural effusion with underlying pulmonary collapse it may be difficult to diagnose the presence of the collapse on a chest radiograph. This problem does not arise with CT where it is usually easy to recognize pulmonary collapse despite the presence of a pleural effusion (Fig. 2.28). If lobar collapse is identified, it can be difficult to tell whether the collapse is due to pleural fluid or whether both the collapse and the effusion are due to the same process, e.g. carcinoma of the bronchus.

Linear (discoid) atelectasis

Linear (discoid) atelectasis is not secondary to bronchial obstruction, it is due to hypoventilation – the commonest cause of which is postoperative or post-traumatic pain. The result is a horizontally orientated band or disc of collapse (see Fig. 2.37, p. 43).

Spherical shadows (lung mass, lung nodule)

The diagnosis of a solitary spherical shadow in the lung (solitary pulmonary nodule) (Fig. 2.29) is a common problem. The usual causes are:
- bronchial carcinoma/bronchial carcinoid
- benign tumour of the lung, hamartoma being the most common
- infective granuloma, tuberculoma being the most common in the UK and fungal granuloma the most frequent in the USA
- metastasis
- lung abscess
- rarely, spherical (round) pneumonia.

When a nodule is discovered in a patient who is over 50 and a smoker, bronchial carcinoma becomes the major consideration. In a patient less than 35 years old, primary carcinoma is highly unlikely. The patient's symptoms may be of help, e.g. obvious symptoms of chest infection in a patient with a lung abscess, but often there are no relevant symptoms even in patients with lung carcinoma. Metastasis is very unlikely in a patient without a known extrathoracic primary malignant tumour, but is an important consideration in those who are known to have such a tumour.

The possible diagnoses for a solitary pulmonary nodule listed above include lesions that require very different forms of management. Hamartomas and granulomas are best left alone, whereas bronchial carcinoma, active tuberculosis and lung abscess require specific treatment. If the nature of the nodule is not evident based on the clinical features and/or the plain chest radiograph, further investigation with CT, PET or biopsy may be necessary. Careful consideration of the following may help in making the diagnosis:

Comparison with previous films

Assessing the rate of growth of a spherical lesion in the lung is one of the most important factors in determining the correct management of the patient. Failure to grow over a period of 18 months or more is a strong pointer to either a benign tumour or an inactive granuloma. An

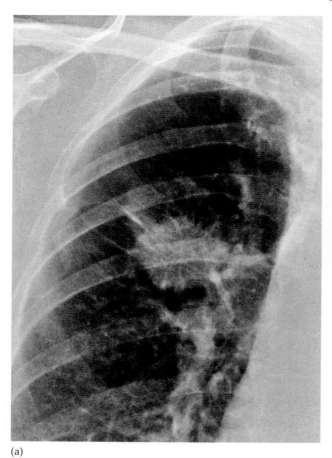

(a)

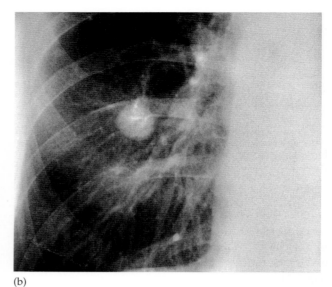

(b)

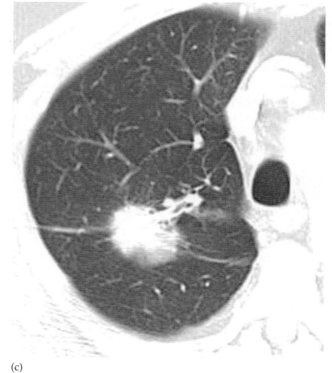

Fig. 2.29 Solitary spherical shadow. (a) The large size and the irregular infiltrating edge are important diagnostic features suggesting primary carcinoma of the lung. (b) The small size and relatively smooth border leads to a wider differential diagnosis. In this case the diagnosis was bronchial carcinoid. (c) Typical bronchial carcinoma on CT showing an infiltrating edge.

(c)

enlarging mass is highly likely to be a bronchial carcinoma or a metastasis.

Calcification

The presence of calcification is the other vital observation, because substantial calcification virtually rules out the diagnosis of a malignant lesion. Calcification is a common finding in hamartomas, tuberculomas and fungal granulomas. In hamartomas it is often of the 'popcorn' type (Fig. 2.30). Calcification can be difficult to recognize on plain chest radiography. Computed tomography is of great value in detecting calcification in a solitary pulmonary nodule. If benign patterns of calcification are seen at CT (uniform calcification throughout the nodule, concentric ring calcification, or popcorn calcifications) then carcinoma of the lung can be excluded from the differential diagnosis (Fig. 2.31).

Involvement of the adjacent chest wall

Destruction of the adjacent ribs is virtually diagnostic of invasion by carcinoma. Tumours of the lung apex are particularly liable to invade the chest wall and adjacent bones (Pancoast's tumour). Computed tomography or bone scan may be indicated to demonstrate this invasion (Fig. 2.32).

The shape of the shadow

Primary carcinomas are nearly always rounded with a lobulated, notched or infiltrating outline (Figs 2.29 and 2.33). Even if only one small portion of a round lesion has an irregular or lobular edge, the diagnosis of primary carcinoma should be seriously considered.

The shape may be obvious from plain films but CT can be used to confirm the rounded shape. Sometimes a lesion that is round and mass-like on chest radiographs is shown to be linear or band-like on CT, in which case the diagnosis is likely to be a focal pulmonary scar of no significance.

Cavitation

If the centre of the mass undergoes necrosis and is coughed up, air is seen within the mass. An air–fluid level may be visible on erect chest radiographs. These features, which may be difficult to appreciate on plain films, are seen particularly well at CT.

Cavitation almost always indicates a significant lesion. It is very common in lung abscesses (see Figs 2.18–2.20), relatively common in primary carcinomas (Fig. 2.34) and occasionally seen with metastases. It does not occur in benign tumours or inactive tuberculomas.

The distinction between cavitating neoplasms and lung abscesses can be very difficult and sometimes impossible, particularly if the walls are smooth. If, however, either the inner or outer walls are irregular, the diagnosis of carcinoma is highly likely.

Size

A solitary mass over 4 cm in diameter which does not contain calcium is nearly always either a primary carcinoma, a lung abscess or, rarely, spherical pneumonia. Lung abscesses of this size, however, virtually always show cavitation and spherical pneumonias cause obvious clinical features of acute pneumonia.

Other lesions

The rest of the film should be checked carefully after a single lung mass has been found. Metastases are the common cause of multiple nodules.

The role of CT

The role of CT in patients with a solitary pulmonary nodule is primarily to:
• Demonstrate calcification in the nodule, but CT is not worth doing if the nodule is clearly calcified on plain films.

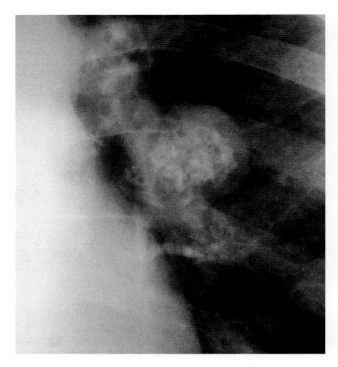

Fig. 2.30 Calcification in a pulmonary hamartoma. The central flocculant ('popcorn') calcification is typical of that seen in hamartomas.

As mentioned above, extensive calcification of a nodule effectively excludes primary carcinoma of the lung (see Fig. 2.31).

• Estimate the rate of growth of a very small asymptomatic nodule. Follow-up is a better option than resection for most nodules less than 1 cm in diameter, because of the high probability of such small nodules being incidentally discovered benign lesions.

• Stage the extent of disease in those cases where the nodule is likely to be a primary carcinoma.

• Localize the nodule accurately prior to bronchoscopic or percutaneous needle biopsy in cases where the position of the nodule is difficult to define on conventional films.

• Establish whether or not the nodule is solitary or multiple, when the lesion in question is likely to be a metastasis or when surgical resection of the mass is being considered.

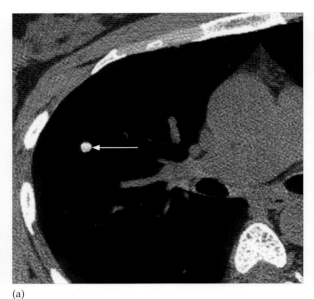

(a)

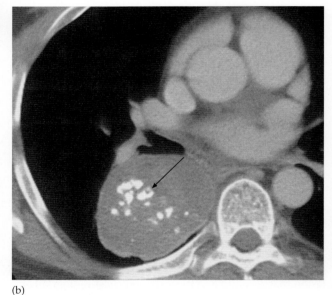

(b)

Fig. 2.31 Benign patterns of calcification. (a) A small calcified nodule (arrow). The calcific density of this fungal granuloma is clearly shown by CT. (b) Popcorn calcification (arrow) in an unusually large hamartoma. The calcification was difficult to appreciate on plain chest radiographs.

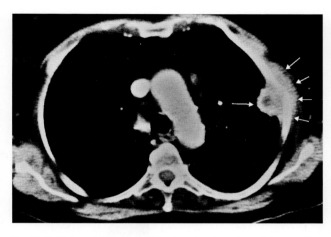

Fig. 2.32 Computed tomography showing invasion of chest wall by bronchial carcinoma (single arrow). The soft tissue mass within the chest wall (multiple arrows) is best appreciated by comparison with the normal opposite side.

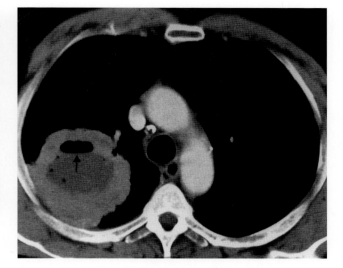

Fig. 2.34 Computed tomography of cavitating primary carcinoma of the lung. The variable thickness of the cavity wall is a striking feature. The air–fluid level is also well seen (arrow).

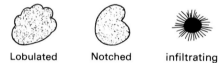

Lobulated   Notched   infiltrating

Fig. 2.33 Outline of primary carcinoma of the lung.

The role of needle biopsy

Transthoracic needle biopsy, using either fine needle aspiration or cutting needles to obtain samples is usually performed under CT control. If the sample yields lung cancer cells, then the diagnosis is established. However, failure to find malignant cells does not exclude the diagnosis of a malignant neoplasm, so the technique should only be used when establishing the diagnosis of malignancy will affect the management plan, e.g. ensuring a diagnosis of lung cancer prior to radiotherapy or chemotherapy.

Multiple pulmonary nodules

Multiple well-defined spherical shadows in the lungs are virtually diagnostic of metastases (see Figs 2.116 and 2.117, pp. 95 and 96). Occasionally, this pattern is seen with abscesses, other neoplasms or with granulomas caused by fungal infection, tuberculosis or collagen vascular disorders.

The role of PET

Most lung cancers concentrate the PET agent FDG (Fig. 2.35). Only a small proportion, notably very small tumours and slow-growing cancers do not show increased uptake. A negative PET scan is useful evidence in favour of a benign lesion or a very slow-growing tumour that can be reassessed after an interval. A positive PET scan is less reliable in diagnosing lung cancer, because active inflammatory disease causes increased uptake of FDG. But the combination of a mass on CT that has characteristics suggestive of lung cancer and a positive FDG uptake provides reasonable evidence of lung cancer.

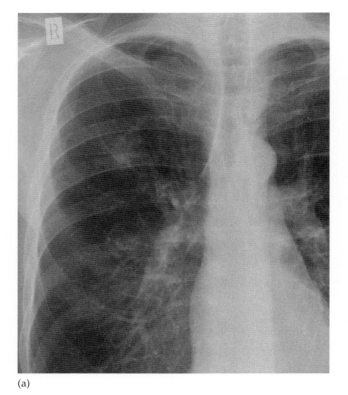

(a)

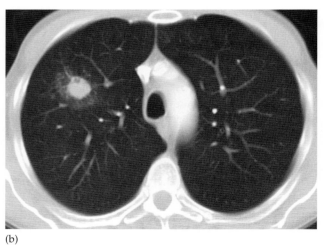

(b)

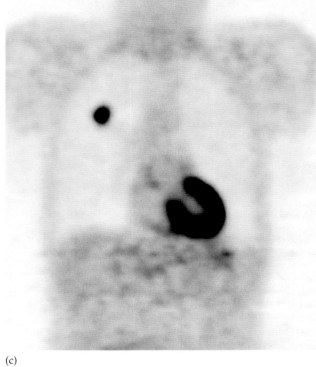

(c)

Fig. 2.35 FDG-PET imaging in solitary pulmonary nodule.
(a) The chest radiograph shows an ill-defined nodule.
(b) The CT shows a rounded nodule with a spiculated outline.
(c) The PET scan shows substantial activity in the nodule
(the myocardial activity is normal). The diagnosis was bronchial
carcinoma.

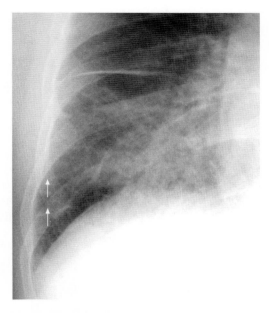

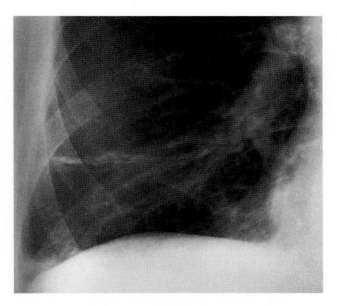

Fig. 2.36 Septal lines (Kerley B lines) in a patient with pulmonary oedema. The septal lines (arrows) are seen in the outer centimetre of lung where blood vessels are invisible or very difficult to identify. Note also thickening of the horizontal fissure, another manifestation of pulmonary oedema in this case.

Fig. 2.37 Band-like shadow in right lower lobe caused by discoid atelectasis.

Line or band-like shadows

All line shadows within the lungs, except fissures and the walls of the large central bronchi, are abnormal. Septal lines are by far the most important.

Septal lines

The interlobular septa within the lung are connective tissue planes containing lymph vessels. They are normally invisible. Only greatly thickened septa can be seen on a chest film. Septal lines are much thinner than the pulmonary blood vessels. On plain chest films, septal lines are seen as so-called Kerley B lines (Fig. 2.36), namely horizontal lines, never more than 2 cm in length, best seen at the periphery of the lung. Unlike the blood vessels they often reach the edge of the lung. On CT, even mild thickening of interlobular pulmonary septa can be readily identified. There are two important causes of thickened interlobular septa:
• pulmonary oedema
• lymphangitis carcinomatosa.

Pleuropulmonary scars and linear (discoid) atelectasis

These two conditions are common causes of line or band-like shadows and are somewhat similar in appearance. Neither are of clinical significance. Linear scars are due to previous infection or infarction; they usually reach the pleura and are often associated with visible pleural thickening. Linear (discoid) atelectasis results in horizontally orientated bands or discs of collapse (Fig. 2.37).

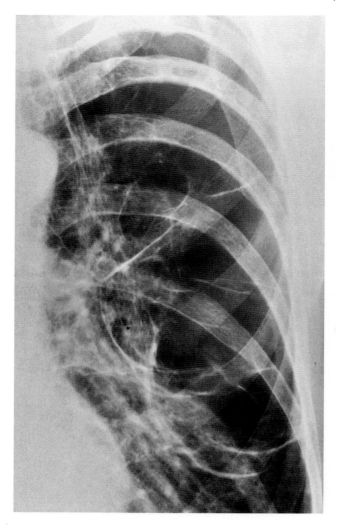

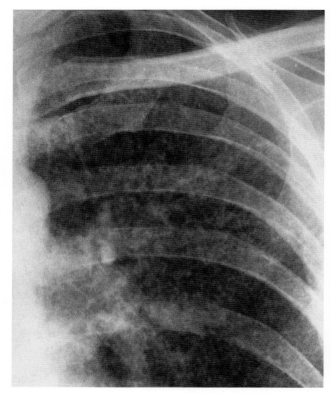

Fig. 2.39 Nodular shadowing in the lung of a patient with miliary tuberculosis.

Fig. 2.38 Line shadows caused by walls of bullae (blebs). The bullae are air spaces devoid of blood vessels.

Emphysematous bullae

Bullae (blebs) may be bounded and traversed by thin line shadows. Bullae have few, if any, normal vessels within them which makes the interpretation easy (Fig. 2.38).

The pleural edge in a pneumothorax

The pleural edge in a pneumothorax is seen as a line approximately parallel with the chest wall. No lung vessels can be seen beyond the pleural line. Once the line is spotted the diagnosis is rarely in doubt (see Fig. 2.53, p. 55).

Widespread small pulmonary shadows

Chest radiographs with widespread small (2–3 mm) pulmonary shadows often present a diagnostic problem. With few exceptions it is only possible to give a differential diagnosis when faced with such a film. A final diagnosis can rarely be made without an intimate knowledge of the patient's symptoms, signs and laboratory results.

Many descriptive terms have been applied to these shadows, the commonest being 'mottling', 'honeycomb', 'fine nodular', 'reticular' and 'reticulonodular' shadows. In this book we will use three basic terms: 'nodular', to signify discrete small round shadows (Fig. 2.39), 'reticular' to describe a net-like pattern of small lines, and 'reticulonodular' when both patterns are present (Fig. 2.40).

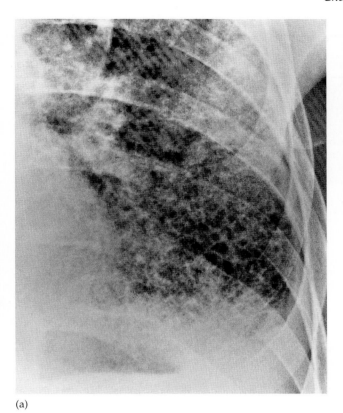

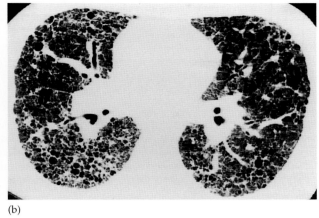

(b)

Fig. 2.40 (a) Reticulonodular shadowing in the lung in a patient with fibrosing alveolitis. (b) HRCT of a different patient with cryptogenic (idiopathic) fibrosing alveolitis showing the honeycomb pattern to advantage.

(a)

All three patterns are due to very small lesions in the lungs, no more than 1 or 2 mm in size. Individual lesions of this size are invisible on a chest film. That these very small lesions are seen at all is explained by the phenomenon of superimposition; when myriads of tiny lesions are present in the lungs it is inevitable that many will lie in line with one another.

How to decide whether or not multiple small pulmonary shadows are present on a plain chest film

Often, the greatest problem is to decide whether widespread abnormal shadowing is present at all, as normal blood vessels can appear as nodules and interconnecting lines. To be confident involves looking carefully at many hundreds of normal films to establish the range of normal in one's mind. Look particularly at the areas between the ribs where the lungs are free of overlying shadows. The normal vessel pattern is a branching system which connects up in an orderly way. The vessels are larger centrally and become smaller as they travel to the periphery. Vessels seen end-on appear as small nodules, but these nodules are no bigger than vessels seen in the immediate vicinity and their number corresponds to the expected number of vessels in that area. There are no visible vessels in the outer 1–2 cm of the lung. An important sign is that the abnormal shadows obscure the adjacent vessels and the borders of the mediastinum and diaphragm may be less sharp than normal.

Table 2.1 Commoner causes of nodular and reticular shadowing on chest radiographs and HRCT

Diagnosis	Radiographic/HRCT pattern	Distribution of shadows	Other features which may be seen	Value of HRCT
Miliary tuberculosis	Small nodules of uniform size	Uniform	Mediastinal/hilar lymph nodes. One or more patches of consolidation	Only necessary in cases of clinical uncertainty
Sarcoidosis	Usually reticulonodular, but may show small nodules of uniform size very similar to miliary tuberculosis	Usual reticulonodular pattern radiates from hila (military pattern is usually uniform in distribution)	Hilar and middle mediastinal lymph node enlargement	Usually unnecessary. Characteristic pattern of pulmonary involvement and shows lymphadenopathy when doubtful on chest radiograph
Asbestosis	Fine reticulonodular	Predominant in peripheral portions of lungs, notably in lower zones	Pleural plaques which may be calcified. Pleural thickening which may be extensive (diffuse pleural thickening)	HRCT very useful to quantify interstitial lung fibrosis and diffuse pleural thickening
Interstitial pulmonary fibrosis (usual interstitial pneumonia, UIP)	Reticulonodular	Usually predominant in periphery of lobes and in lower zones	Diaphragm often high and indistinct	HRCT very useful to quantify interstitial pulmonary fibrosis and to assess potential responsiveness to steroids
Lymphangitis carcinomatosa	Reticulonodular Septal lines	No predominant distribution	Bronchial wall thickening hilar adenopathy Other signs of carcinoma	HRCT very useful in any doubtful cases as the HRCT features are usually reasonably characteristic

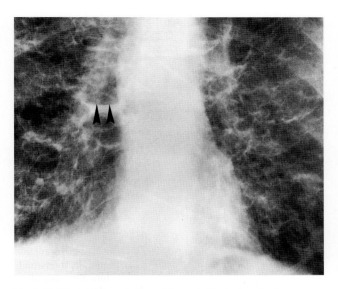

Fig. 2.41 Ring shadows in bronchiectasis. Each ring shadow represents a dilated bronchus. A fluid level in one of the dilated bronchi is arrowed.

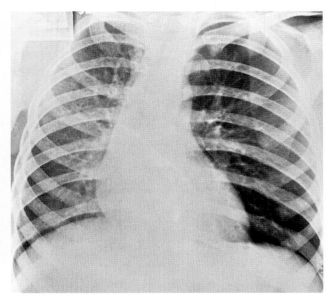

Fig. 2.42 Inhaled foreign body causing check valve obstruction of the left main bronchus. Note the increased transradiancy of the left lung, and the slight displacement of the heart to the right. (The film was exposed in expiration.)

HRCT

When abnormal diffuse shadowing is present or suspected, the next step is to obtain a high resolution CT (HRCT) to determine the precise pattern and distribution: particularly whether the disease process is distributed uniformly, whether it is more severe in one or other zone, and whether it extends outward from the hila or is peripherally predominant. Other abnormalities within the chest should then be sought. Once these observations have been made it is possible to produce the differential diagnosis shown in Table 2.1. A few conditions have quite specific appearances, e.g. lymphangitis carcinomatosa (see p. 94) and interstitial pulmonary fibrosis, although the precise cause of pulmonary fibrosis cannot be ascertained by CT.

Multiple ring shadows of 1 cm or larger

Multiple ring shadows larger than 1 cm are diagnostic of

bronchiectasis (Fig. 2.41). The shadows represent dilated thick-walled bronchi.

Widespread small pulmonary calcifications

Widespread small pulmonary calcifications may occur following pulmonary infection with tuberculosis, histoplasmosis or chickenpox.

Increased transradiancy of the lungs

Generalized increased transradiancy of the lungs is one of the signs of emphysema. The other signs are discussed on p. 81.

When only one hemithorax appears more transradiant than normal the following should be considered:
• Compensatory emphysema occurs when a lobe or lung is collapsed or has been excised and the remaining lung expands to fill the space.

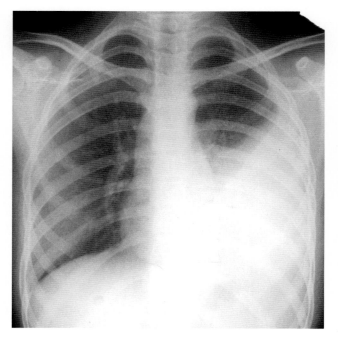

Fig. 2.43 Large left pleural effusion. The shadow of the pleural fluid is entirely homogeneous and lies outside the lung edge. The fluid appears higher laterally than medially, a point that can be useful in differentiating pleural fluid from pulmonary shadows. The trachea and heart are slightly displaced to the right.

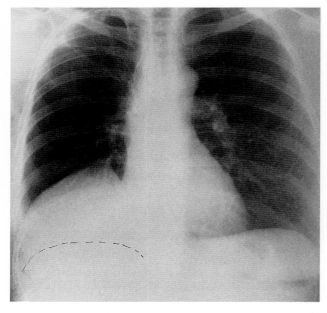

Fig. 2.44 Large right subpulmonary effusion (the patient has had a right mastectomy). Almost all the fluid is between the lung and the diaphragm. The right hemidiaphragm cannot be seen, but its estimated position has been pencilled in.

• Pneumothorax. The diagnosis of pneumothorax depends on visualization of the lung edge with air peripheral to it, and checking that the space in question does not contain any vessels (see Figs 2.53 and 2.54, p. 55).
• Reduction in the chest wall soft tissues, e.g. mastectomy.
• Air-trapping due to central obstruction (Fig. 2.42). Most obstructing lesions in a major bronchus lead to lobar collapse. Occasionally, particularly with an inhaled foreign body, a check-valve mechanism may lead to air-trapping. Inhaled foreign bodies are commonest in children; they usually lodge in a major bronchus. Often the chest radiograph is normal, but sometimes the affected lung becomes abnormally transradiant and the heart is displaced to the opposite side on expiration.

THE PLEURA

Pleural effusion

Pleural effusions may lie free within the pleural cavity, in which case the fluid falls to the most dependent portion of the pleura and assumes a shape dependent on the thoracic cage and the shape of the underlying lung (Figs 2.43–2.46), or it may become loculated by pleural adhesions (Figs 2.47–2.49). Although loculation occurs in all types of effusion, it is a particular feature of empyema. Such loculations may either be at the periphery of the lung or within the fissures between the lobes. A loculated effusion may simulate a lung tumour on chest radiographs.

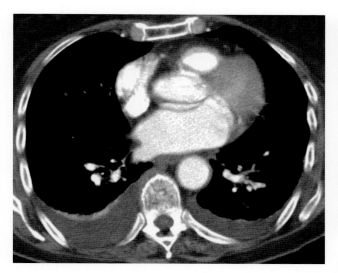

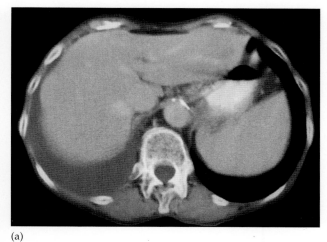

(a)

Fig. 2.45 CT of pleural fluid. The bilateral pleural effusions are of homogeneous density, with a CT number between zero and soft tissue. The well-defined meniscus-shaped border with the adjacent lung is typical. The right-sided effusion is causing a little compression collapse of the underlying lung (which shows contrast enhancement).

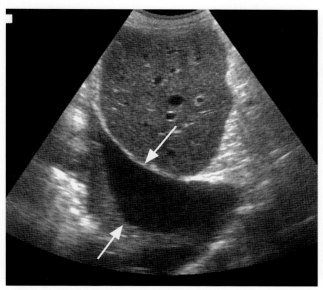

Fig. 2.46 CT and ultrasound of pleural effusion.
(a) CT. The section is taken through the lowermost portion of the pleural cavity and at this level the distinction from ascites is a potential problem because the diaphragm itself is not visible. Pleural fluid, as here, is not affected by the peritoneal reflections of the bare area (see Fig. 8.1, p. 272). (b) Ultrasound – sagittal image. The pleural effusion (PE) is seen as a transonic area between the diaphragm (downward pointing arrow) and adjacent lung (upward pointing arrow).

(b)

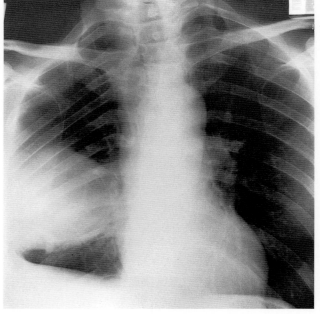

(a)

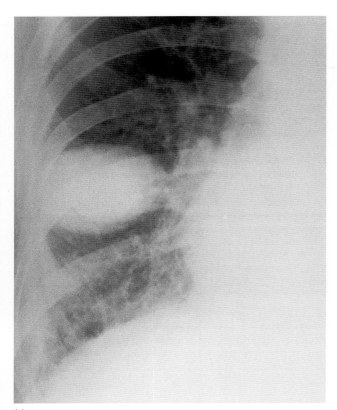

(c)

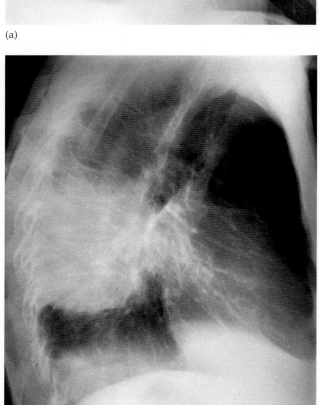

(b)

Fig. 2.47 Loculated pleural fluid. (a) Posteroanterior and (b) lateral views show an empyema loculated against the posterior chest wall. (c) Fluid loculated in the horizontal (minor) fissure in another patient. Both these fluid collections could be confused with an intrapulmonary mass.

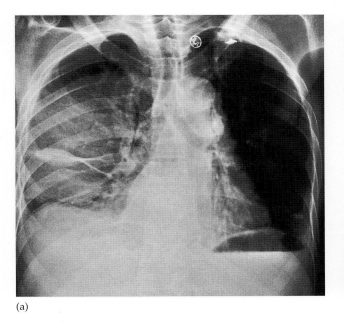

(a)

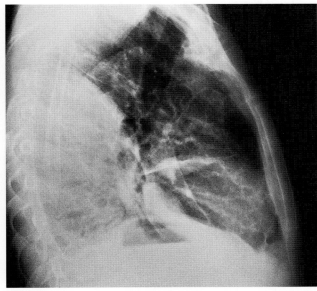

(b)

Fig. 2.48 Loculated pleural fluid (empyema). The fluid is loculated behind the right lower lobe and in the horizontal (minor) fissure. On the plain chest films (a) and (b) the large posterior collection resembles right lower lobe consolidation. (c) CT scan in a similar patient clearly shows the characteristic shape and location of two loculated pleural fluid collections [larger one posteriorly and a smaller one anteriorly (arrow)].

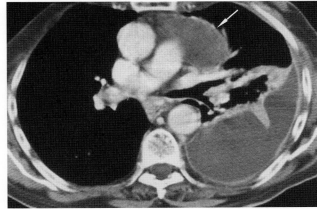

(c)

There are a number of causes of pleural effusion, notably:

• *Infection*. Pleural effusions due to pneumonia are, on the whole small, and the pneumonia is usually the dominant feature on the chest film. Large loculated effusions in association with pneumonia often indicate empyema formation (Figs 2.47–2.49). In some cases of tuberculosis the effusion is the only visible abnormality and the effusion may be large.

• *Subphrenic abscess*, which is nearly always accompanied by a pleural effusion.

• *Malignant neoplasm*. Effusions occur with pleural metastases, but it is unusual to see the pleural deposits themselves on plain chest radiographs. Pleural metastases are occasionally seen on CT, MRI or ultrasound as nodular or mass-like pleural thickening. Malignant effusions are frequently large. If the effusion is due to bronchogenic carcinoma or

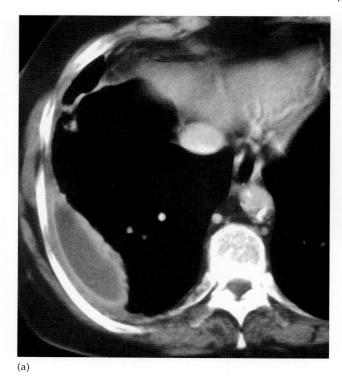

(a)

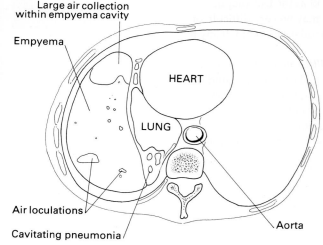

(b)

Large air collection
within empyema cavity

Empyema

HEART

LUNG

Air loculations

Cavitating pneumonia

Aorta

Fig. 2.49 Empyema. (a) CT showing a typical lens-shaped pleural fluid collection with a clearly marginated wall consisting of thickened pleura. (b) CT showing multiple loculated air collections within the pus.

malignant mesothelioma, other signs of the primary tumour are usually, but not always, evident.

• *Cardiac failure*. Small bilateral pleural effusions are seen frequently in acute left ventricular failure. Larger pleural effusions may be present in longstanding congestive cardiac failure. The effusions are usually bilateral, often larger on the right than the left. Other signs of cardiac failure, such as alteration in the size or shape of the heart, pulmonary oedema or the signs of pulmonary venous hypertension, are usually visible.

• *Pulmonary infarction*. Pulmonary emboli which result in pulmonary infarction may cause pleural effusion. Such effusions are usually small and accompanied by a lung shadow caused by the pulmonary infarct.

• *Collagen vascular diseases*. Pleural effusions, either unilateral or bilateral, are relatively common in various collagen vascular diseases. They may be the only abnormal features on chest imaging.

• *Nephrotic syndrome*, *renal failure* and *ascites* are all associated with pleural effusion.

Plain radiographic findings (Figs 2.43, 2.44, 2.47 and 2.48). The radiographic appearances of fluid in the pleural cavity are the same regardless of whether the fluid is a transudate, an exudate, pus or blood. Free fluid collects in the most dependent portion of the pleural cavity and always fills in the costophrenic angles. Usually the fluid surrounds the lung and is higher laterally than medially. Very large effusions run over the top of the lung. The smooth edge between the lung and the fluid can be recognized on an adequately penetrated film, providing the underlying lung is aerated. It is worth remembering that a large effusion may hide an abnormality in the underlying lung.

Sometimes, even with a large effusion, little or no fluid is seen running up the chest wall. The fluid is then known as a 'subpulmonary effusion' (Fig. 2.44). The upper border of the fluid is much the same shape as the normal diaphragm, and as the true diaphragm shadow is obscured by the fluid it may be very difficult, or even impossible, to tell from the standard erect film if any fluid is present at all.

Ultrasound. Ultrasound is a simple method of determining whether pleural fluid is present. Pleural fluid can be recognized as a transonic area between the lung and diaphragm or between the chest wall and the lung (Fig. 2.46b). It is only rarely possible to determine the nature of the fluid e.g. in empyema, multiple echoes may be seen due to the pus in the fluid. Ultrasound is particularly useful in defining the presence, size and shape of any pleural collection loculated against the chest wall or diaphragm and is a convenient method of imaging control for pleural fluid aspiration or drainage.

Computed tomography. Pleural effusions are usually seen as homogeneous fluid density between the chest wall and lung (Figs 2.45 and 2.46). Computed tomography is particularly useful for showing loculated pleural effusions (Fig. 2.48). If the fluid is due to recent haemorrhage it will show the high density of blood, otherwise it is not possible to determine the nature of the fluid. Free pleural fluid moves to the dependent portion of the chest. Surprisingly, it is sometimes difficult to determine from CT whether fluid is pleural effusion or ascites. The distinction is made by noting the relationship of the fluid to the diaphragm. Pleural fluid collects outside the diaphragmatic dome and can be seen posterior to the portion of diaphragm that covers the bare

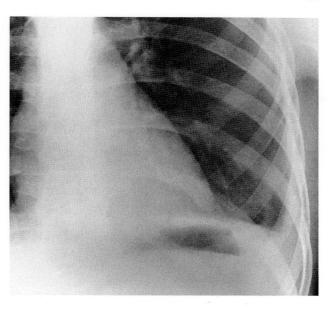

Fig. 2.50 Pleural thickening at the left base. This patient had been treated for a tuberculous pleural effusion, which had resolved leaving pleural thickening, which obliterated the left costophrenic angle.

area of the liver (Fig. 2.46a). Computed tomography can be used to distinguish between lung abscess and empyema (Figs 2.48 and 2.49). Like ultrasound, CT can be used to direct the placement of drainage tubes.

Pleural thickening (pleural fibrosis) (Fig. 2.50)

Fibrotic pleural thickening (scarring), especially in the costophrenic angles, may follow resolution of a pleural effusion, particularly following pleural infection or haemorrhage, or following an asbestos-related pleural effusion. Pleural scarring is nearly always much smaller in volume than the original pleural effusion.

It is sometimes impossible to distinguish pleural fluid from pleural thickening on conventional radiographic projections, especially if comparison with previous films is not possible. Ultrasound or CT can usually resolve the problem.

Localized plaques of pleural thickening along the lateral chest wall commonly indicate asbestos exposure. Such plaques may show irregular calcification.

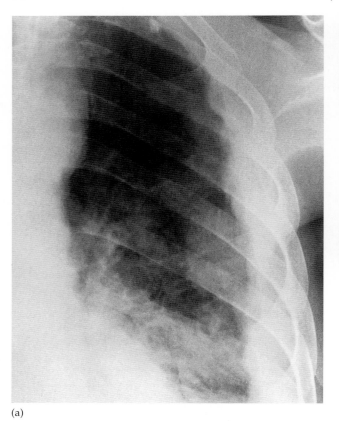

(a)

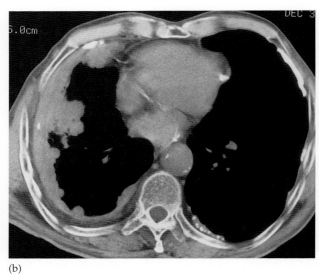

(b)

Fig. 2.51 (a) Lobulated pleural thickening caused by malignant neoplasm. The tumour in this instance was a malignant mesothelioma of the pleura. (b) CT of mesothelioma of the pleura. Note also the calcified pleural plaques following asbestos exposure.

Pleural tumours (Fig. 2.51)

The commonest pleural tumours are metastatic carcinomas. Primary pleural tumours, such as mesothelioma, are relatively uncommon. Many patients with malignant mesotheliomas give a history of asbestos exposure and may show the other features of asbestos-related disease.

Pleural tumours produce lobulated masses based on the pleura. Malignant pleural tumours, both primary (malignant mesothelioma) and secondary, frequently cause pleural effusions which may obscure the tumour itself. The predominant feature of metastatic pleural tumours and some malignant mesotheliomas is a pleural effusion with no visible mass on imaging examinations.

Pleural calcification

Irregular plaques of calcium may be seen with or without accompanying pleural thickening. When unilateral they are likely to be due to either an old empyema, usually tuberculous (Fig. 2.52), or an old haemothorax. Bilateral pleural calcification is often related to asbestos exposure (see Fig. 2.93, p. 81). Sometimes no cause for pleural calcification can be found.

Pneumothorax (Fig. 2.53)

The majority of pneumothoraces occur in young people with no recognizable lung disease. These patients have

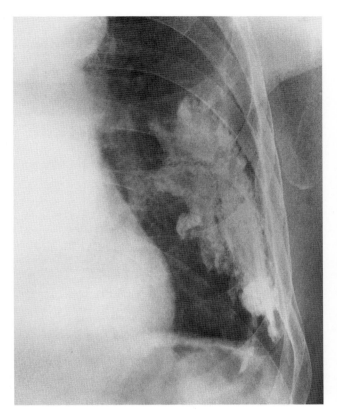

Fig. 2.52 Unilateral pleural calcifications from old tuberculous empyema.

small blebs or bullae at the periphery of their lungs which burst. Occasionally pneumothorax is due to:

- emphysema
- trauma
- certain forms of interstitial pulmonary disease
- *pneumocystis carinii* pneumonia
- metastases, rarely.

The diagnosis of pneumothorax depends on recognizing:

- A line of pleura due to the lung edge being separated from the chest wall, mediastinum or diaphragm by air.
- Absence of vessel shadows outside this line. Lack of vessel shadows alone is insufficient evidence on which to make the diagnosis, as there may be few, or no, visible vessels in emphysematous bullae.

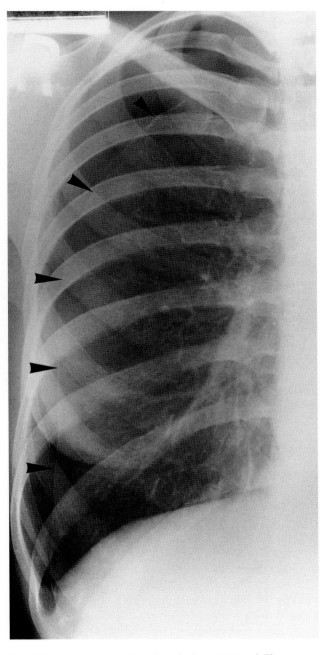

Fig. 2.53 Pneumothorax. The pleural edge is arrowed. The diagnosis of pneumothorax requires the identification of this edge and a clear space beyond it.

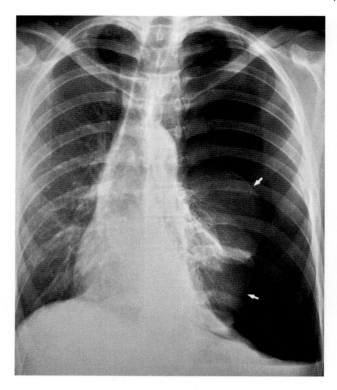

Fig. 2.54 Tension pneumothorax. The left hemidiaphragm is depressed and the mediastinum is shifted to the right. The left lung (arrows) is substantially collapsed.

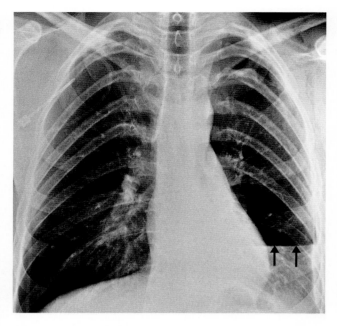

Fig. 2.55 Hydropneumothorax. The arrows point to the air–fluid level in the pleural space. In this case, the edge of the lung is difficult to see on the posteroanterior view; most of the fluid and air were loculated posteriorly.

- If the pneumothorax is very large, there may an appreciable increase in the density of the underlying lung.

The detection of a small pneumothorax can be very difficult. The ribs may take a similar course to the line of the pleural edge, so the abnormality may not strike the casual observer. Sometimes a pneumothorax is more obvious on a film taken in expiration.

Once the presence of a pneumothorax has been noted, the next step is to decide whether or not it is under tension. This is easy if there is mediastinal shift and flattening or inversion of the hemidiaphragm (Fig. 2.54). Most tension pneumothoraces are large because the underlying lung collapses due to increased pressure in the pleural space, but small pneumothoraces can cause serious symptoms if the underlying pulmonary reserve is poor.

Hydropneumothorax, haemopneumothorax and pyopneumothorax

Fluid in the pleural cavity, whether it be a pleural effusion, blood or pus, assumes a different shape in the presence of a pneumothorax. The diagnostic feature is the air–fluid level (Fig. 2.55).

Some fluid is present in the pleural cavity in most patients with pneumothorax. In spontaneous pneumothorax, the amount is usually small.

The mediastinum

The mediastinum is divided into anterior, middle and posterior divisions for descriptive purposes (Fig. 2.56). However, masses often cross from one compartment to the other. Mediastinal widening can be due to many different pathological processes. These are usually classified according to

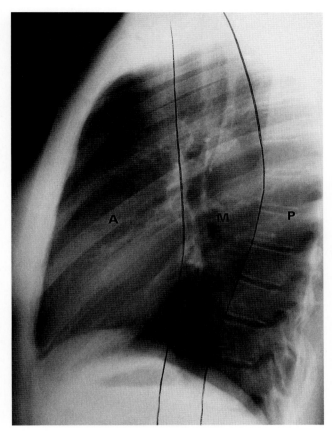

Fig. 2.56 The anterior (A), middle (M) and posterior (P) compartments of the mediastinum. The divisions are arbitrary and do not correspond to those used by anatomists. The anterior mediastinum refers to the structures anterior to the trachea and the major bronchi. The posterior mediastinum refers to structures posterior to a line joining the anterior boundary of the vertebral bodies.

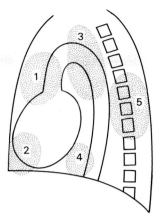

ANTERIOR
1. Thyroid tumour
   Thymic tumour or cyst
   Teratoma/Dermoid cyst
   Lymphadenopathy
   Aortic aneurysm

2. Pericardial cyst
   Fat pad
   Morgagni hernia

MIDDLE
3. Thyroid tumour
   Lymphadenopathy
   Bronchogenic cyst
   Aortic aneurysm

4. Hiatus hernia

POSTERIOR
5. Neurogenic tumours
   Soft tissue mass of vertebral infection or neoplasm
   Lymphadenopathy
   Aortic aneurysm

Fig. 2.57 The causes of mediastinal masses divided according to location. Note that both lymphadenopathy and aortic aneurysms occur in all three major compartments.

their position in the mediastinum (Fig. 2.57); so if a mediastinal mass is identified on the frontal chest radiograph, the next step should be to attempt to localize it in the lateral view or on CT (Fig. 2.58).

CT and MRI of the normal mediastinum

Computed tomography is the standard method for imaging the mediastinum. Magnetic resonance imaging is used only occasionally. The cross-sectional display and the ability to distinguish between fat, various soft tissues and blood vessels are major advantages of both techniques. The normal appearances are illustrated in Figs 2.59 and 2.60. The features to note while viewing these images are:

1 The bulk of the mediastinum is due to blood vessels. For CT they are often enhanced using intravenous contrast medium. At MRI, the larger vessels are readily seen without contrast agent.

2 The only other normal structures of appreciable size are the thymus, oesophagus, trachea and bronchi.

3 Normal lymph nodes are small, usually less than 6 mm in diameter (maximum 10 mm), and many are not visible.

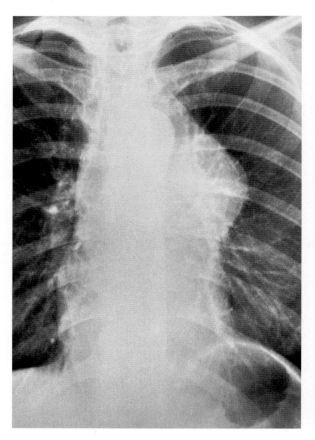 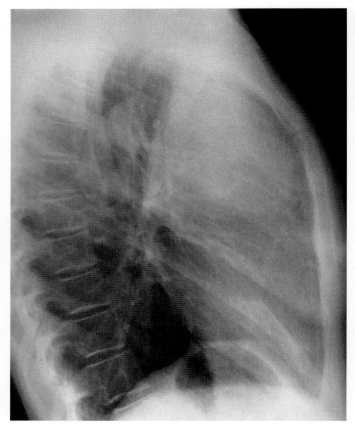

Fig. 2.58 Anterior mediastinal mass. There is a large mass situated anteriorly in the mediastinum projecting to the left side which was due to a mass of lymph nodes involved by malignant lymphoma. Diagnosing the anterior location of the mass depends on noting the density of the retrosternal areas. This area should normally have the same density as the retrocardiac area.

4 The mediastinal structures are surrounded by fat. The sites listed below normally contain nothing but fat or small lymph nodes. They are, therefore, areas in which small masses, particularly enlarged lymph nodes, can be readily recognized:

 • Between the right tracheal wall and the adjacent lung (the one exception being the azygos vein which lies in the right tracheobronchial angle).
 • Between the right wall of the oesophagus and the adjacent lung all the way down the chest, an anatomical region known as the azygo-oesophageal recess.

 • Anterior and to the left of the aorta and main pulmonary artery (other than the thymus and the left brachiocephalic vein).

Mediastinal masses

Plain chest films in mediastinal masses

 • Intrathoracic thyroid masses (goitres) are the most frequent cause of a superior mediastinal mass (Figs 2.61 and 2.62). The characteristic feature is that the mass extends

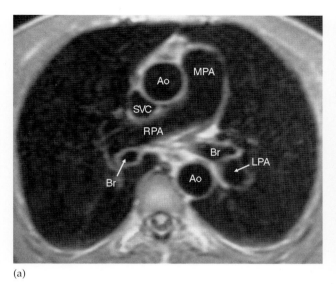

(a)

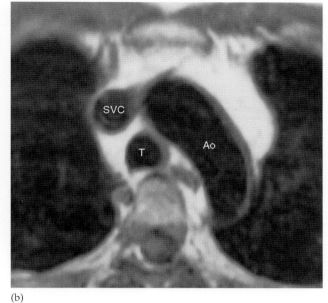

(b)

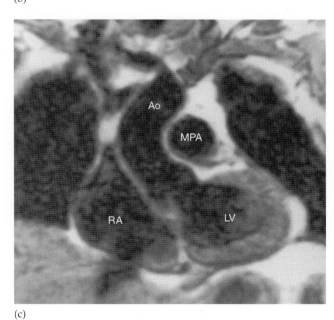

Fig. 2.59 MRI of normal mediastinum (T1-weighted, cardiac gated). (a) Axial scan through the level of the pulmonary hila. (b) Higher axial section through the level of the aortic arch. (c) Coronal scan. Ao, aorta; Br, bronchi; LPA, left pulmonary artery; LV, left ventricle; MPA, main pulmonary artery; RA, right atrium; RPA, right pulmonary artery; RV, right ventricle; SVC, superior vena cava; T, trachea.

(c)

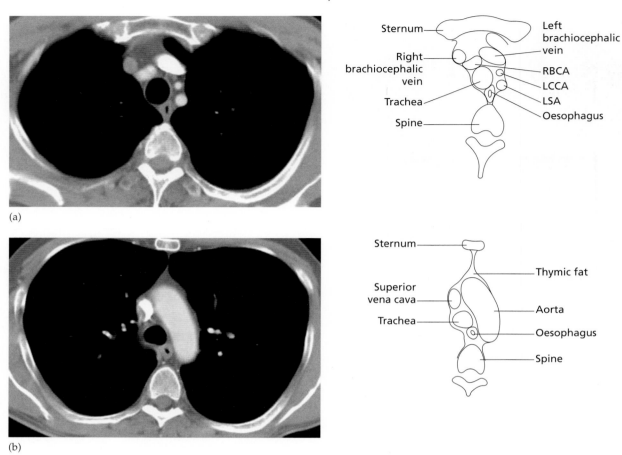

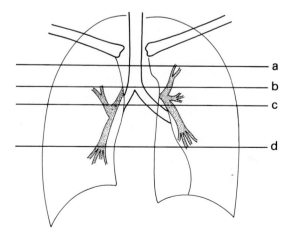

Fig. 2.60 Computed tomography of normal mediastinum. The levels at which the four selected levels were taken is shown right. Intravenous contrast has been given; it is particularly concentrated in the right brachiocephalic vein and superior vena cava. Air is present in the oesophagus; this can be a normal finding. LCCA, left common carotid artery; LMB, left main bronchus; LSA, left subclavian artery; RBCA, right brachiocephalic (innominate) artery; RMB, right main bronchus.

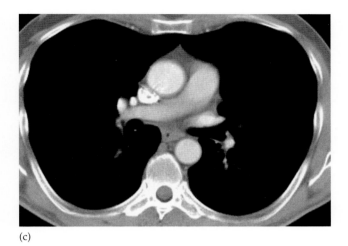

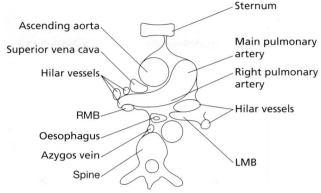

(c)

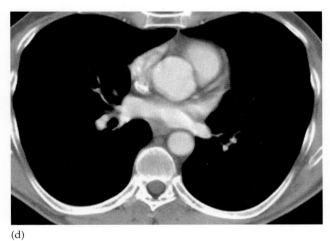

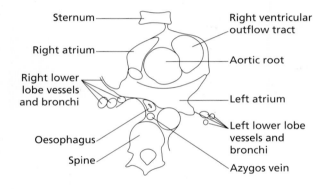

(d)

Fig. 2.60 *Continued*

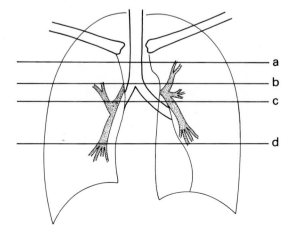

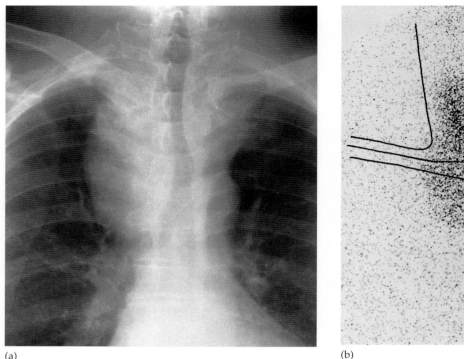

(a)   (b)

Fig. 2.61 Retrosternal goitre. (a) The plain chest film shows a large superior mediastinal mass narrowing the trachea. (b) A radionuclide scan in the same patient shows uptake of the ^{123}I below the level of the clavicles on the right, confirming that the mass is due to thyroid tissue.

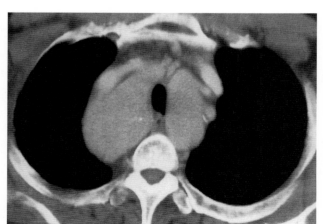

Fig. 2.62 Retrosternal goitre. CT showing a bilateral superior mediastinal mass that was shown on adjacent sections to be contiguous with the thyroid gland in the neck and to have the same density as thyroid tissue. Note the compression of the trachea.

from the superior mediastinum into the neck and almost invariably compresses or displaces the trachea.

• Lymphadenopathy is the next most frequent cause of a mediastinal swelling. Lymphadenopathy may occur in any of the three compartments and it is often possible to diagnose enlarged lymph nodes from their lobulated outlines and the multiple locations involved (Fig. 2.63).

• Neurogenic tumours are by far the commonest cause of posterior mediastinal masses. Pressure deformity of the adjacent ribs and thoracic spine is often visible.

• Certain tumours, such as dermoid cysts and thymomas, are, for practical purposes, confined to the anterior mediastinum.

• Calcification occurs in many conditions, but almost never in malignant lymphadenopathy. Occasionally, the calcification is characteristic in appearance, e.g. in aneurysms of the aorta.

• A mediastinal mass due to a hiatus hernia is usually easy to diagnose on plain films because it often contains

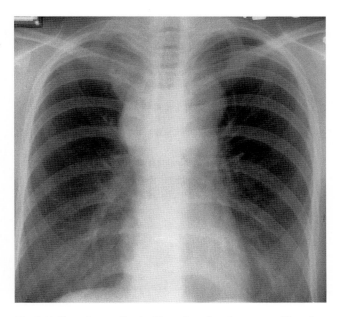

Fig. 2.63 Superior mediastinal lymph node enlargement. Note the bilateral lobular masses.

air and may have a fluid level, best seen on the lateral view (Fig. 2.64).

• Masses in the right cardiophrenic angle anteriorly are virtually never of clinical significance. They are nearly all either large fat pads, benign pericardial cysts or hernias through the foramen of Morgagni (Fig. 2.65).

Computed tomography of mediastinal masses

Computed tomography provides much more information than plain chest radiographs; occasionally, a specific diagnosis can be made. Magnetic resonance imaging is used only in highly selected cases, e.g. where CT contrast agents are contraindicated or in demonstrating the relationship of a posterior mass to the spinal canal (Fig. 2.66). The advantages of CT are:

1 Abnormalities can be accurately localized. Knowledge of the precise shape, position and size of a mediastinal mass frequently narrows the differential diagnosis. For instance, contiguity of the mass with the thyroid in the neck suggests

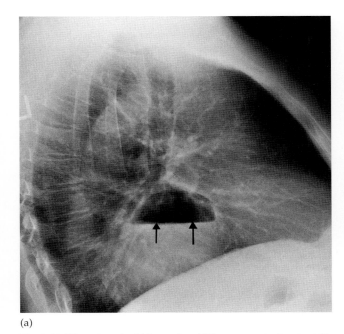

(a)

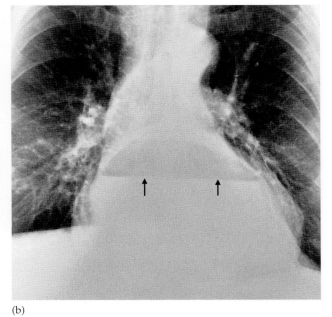

(b)

Fig. 2.64 Hiatus hernia. (a) Lateral and (b) posteroanterior chest films show the characteristic retrocardiac density containing an air–fluid level (arrows).

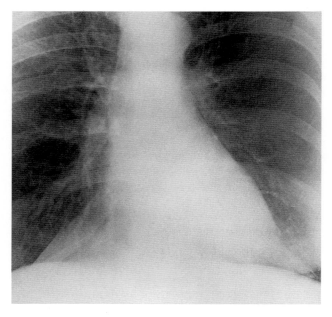

Fig. 2.65 Fat pads in both cardiophrenic angles. Note the loss of clarity of the adjacent cardiac outline – an example of the silhouette sign. The anterior location was confirmed on the lateral view.

a goitre (see Fig. 2.61), and multiple oval-shaped masses suggest lymphadenopathy (Fig. 2.67). Solid masses in the anterior mediastinum (Fig. 2.68) have a limited number of possibilities.

2 Occasionally, the density of the abnormality reveals its nature:

- Fat can be recognized as such, which is useful in distinguishing large cardiophrenic angle fat pads or unusual mediastinal fat collections from tumours, e.g. in Cushing's disease. Cystic teratomas (dermoid cysts) may contain recognizable fat.
- Because of its high iodine content, thyroid tissue is of higher attenuation than muscle prior to contrast medium administration. After contrast, it enhances brightly (Fig. 2.62). (A radio-iodine scan is a highly specific alternative to CT for confirming that an intrathoracic mass is a goitre – see Fig. 2.61).
- Intravenous contrast enhancement permits ready differentiation of aneurysms (see below) and anomalous blood vessels from other masses.
- Calcification is readily seen. The presence of calcification in a mass effectively excludes untreated malignant neoplastic adenopathy.

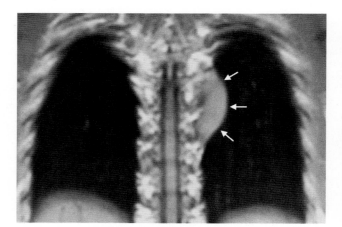

Fig. 2.66 Neurofibroma in posterior mediastinum. Magnetic resonance imaging showing the neurofibroma (arrows) lying against the spine, but not growing into the spinal canal.

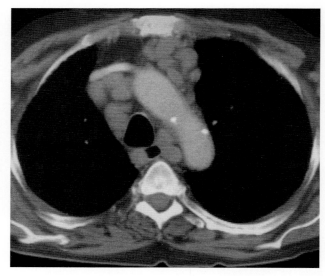

Fig. 2.67 Extensive mediastinal lymphadenopathy (caused by lymphoma) shown by CT.

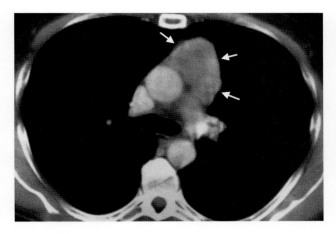

Fig. 2.68 Thymoma. CT showing a lobular mass (arrows) in the left side of the thymus.

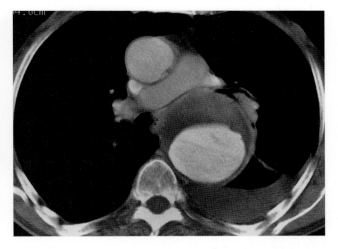

Fig. 2.69 CT showing an aneurysm of the descending aorta. The lumen has been opacified by intravenous contrast enhancement. The unopacified component is clot lining the aneurysm.

• Cysts containing clear fluid, e.g. pericardial cysts and some bronchogenic cysts, can be recognized as such by a CT number close to water (0 Hounsfield units).

Aortic aneurysm

Dilatation of the *ascending aorta* may be due to aneurysm formation or secondary to aortic regurgitation, aortic stenosis or systemic hypertension. Substantial dilatation of the ascending aorta is needed before a bulge of the right mediastinal border can be recognized; aortic unfolding is a commoner cause of a bulge of the right superior mediastinum than ascending aortic aneurysm.

The two common causes of aneurysm of the *descending aorta* are atheroma and aortic dissection. A rarer cause is previous trauma, usually following a severe deceleration injury. Descending aortic aneurysms are often visible on plain chest radiographs and atheromatous aneurysms usually show calcification in their walls.

Computed tomography with intravenous contrast enhancement and/or echocardiography is very useful when aortic aneurysms are assessed (Figs 2.69–2.71). It is important to know the extent of aortic dissections because those involving the ascending aorta are treated surgically, while those confined to the descending aorta are usually treated

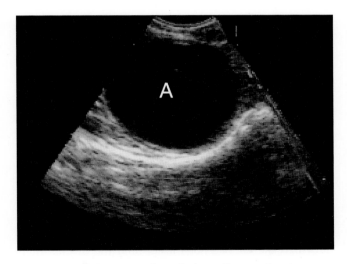

Fig. 2.70 Normal transoesophageal echocardiogram showing normal descending aorta.

conservatively with hypotensive drugs. Standard echocardiography shows dissection of the aortic root, but transoesophageal echocardiography shows dissections distal to the aortic root and in the descending aorta as well. Aortic dissections can also be shown with CT (and MRI) and these

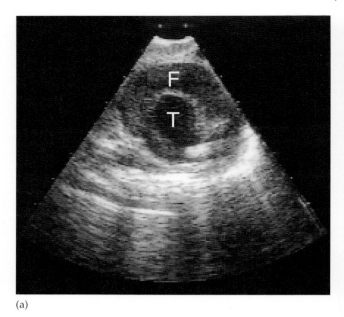

(a)

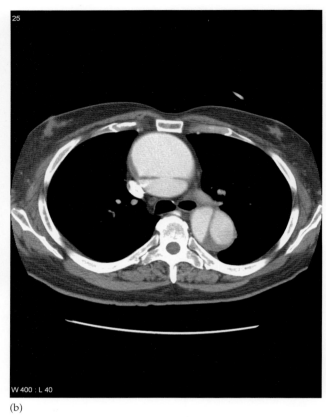

(b)

Fig. 2.71 (a) Transoesophageal echocardiogram showing the true (T) and false (F) lumina in the descending aorta. (b) CT showing the displaced intima separating the true and false lumina in the ascending and descending aorta.

non-invasive techniques have, in practice, replaced aortography, which is only performed in selected cases.

Pneumomediastinum

Provided the air has not tracked into the mediastinum from the root of the neck, adjacent chest wall or retroperitoneum, air in the mediastinum indicates a tear in the oesophagus or an air leak from bronchi in the mediastinum or lung. These tears may be spontaneous or follow trauma, including barotrauma and trauma from endoscopy or swallowed foreign bodies.

Spontaneous leakage from small bronchi in the lungs is most commonly seen in patients with asthma or following severe vomiting. The air, which tracks through the interstitial tissues of the lung into the mediastinum, is seen as fine streaks of transradiancy within the mediastinum, often extending upward into the neck (Fig. 2.72).

Hilar enlargement

The normal hilar shadows are composed of pulmonary arteries and veins. The main lower lobe arteries are the thickness of an adult's little finger (9–16 mm). Hilar lymph nodes cannot be identified as separate shadows on plain chest radiographs and the walls of the central bronchi are too thin to contribute to any extent to the bulk of the hilar shadows.

Hilar enlargement (Fig. 2.73) raises two questions. Firstly, is the enlarged hilum due entirely to large blood vessels or

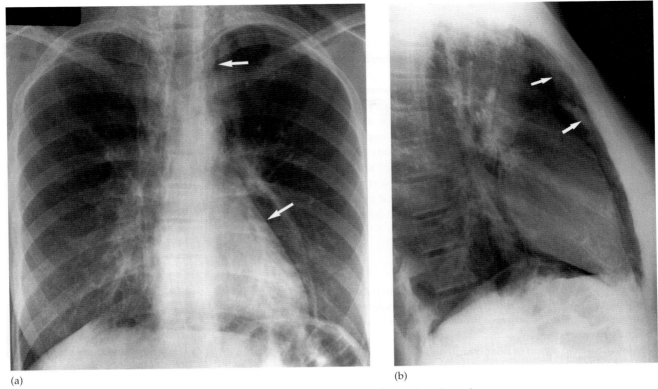

(a)

(b)

Fig. 2.72 Pneumomediastinum showing air (arrows) in the mediastinum extending up into the neck.

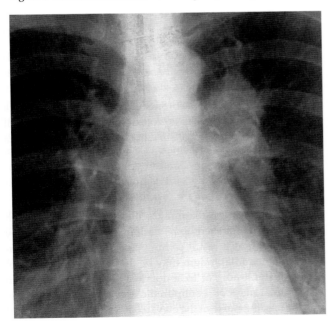

Fig. 2.73 Lobulated mass at left hilum from enlarged lymph nodes. The right hilum is normal. The lymphadenopathy in this case was due to metastases from a bronchial carcinoma (not visible on this image) in the left lower lobe.

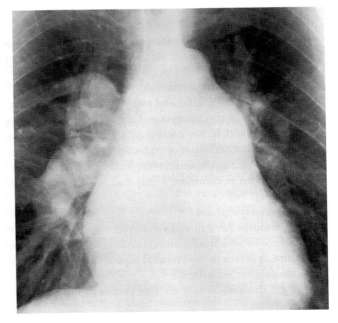

Fig. 2.74 Enlargement of the hilar arteries in a patient with severe pulmonary hypertension. Note that the heart and the main pulmonary artery are also enlarged and that the hilar shadows branch in the manner expected of arteries.

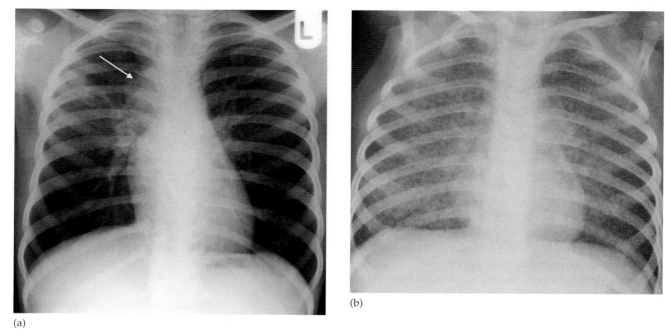

(a)

(b)

Fig. 2.80 Tuberculosis. (a) The primary complex. This 7-year-old child shows ill-defined consolidation in the right lung together with enlargement of the draining lymph nodes (arrow). (b) Miliary tuberculosis. The innumerable small nodular shadows uniformly distributed throughout the lungs in this young child are typical of miliary tuberculosis. In this instance, no primary focus of infection is visible.

nodules are difficult to appreciate. A pleural effusion may be present. It is important to note that the chest film may be normal in the early stages of miliary tuberculosis.

Primary tuberculosis may present with a pleural effusion. Occasionally the primary complex is also visible, but more often the effusion is the only visible abnormality.

Postprimary tuberculosis

Postprimary tuberculosis usually presents with cough, haemoptysis, weight loss, night sweats or malaise. Occasionally, the disease is discovered on a routine chest film. Postprimary tuberculosis is usually confined to the upper posterior portions of the chest, namely the apical and posterior segments of the upper lobes and the apical segments of the lower lobes. The initial lesions are multiple small areas

of consolidation (Fig. 2.81a) and are often bilateral. Occasionally, the disease takes the form of lower or middle lobe bronchopneumonia. Pleural effusions are frequent and may be the only radiographic abnormality. The predominant or sole feature, particularly in non-Caucasians, may be mediastinal and/or hilar lymphadenopathy (Fig. 2.82).

If the infection progresses, any areas of consolidation may enlarge and frequently undergo cavitation. Cavities are seen as rounded air spaces (translucencies) completely surrounded by pulmonary shadowing (Fig. 2.81b). The diagnosis of cavitation can be difficult. As with the primary form, postprimary tuberculosis may spread to give widespread bronchopneumonia or miliary tuberculosis.

The infection may undergo partial or complete healing at any stage. Healing occurs by fibrosis, often with calcification (Fig. 2.83), but both fibrosis and calcification may be

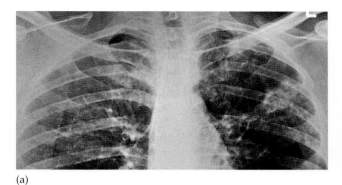

(a)

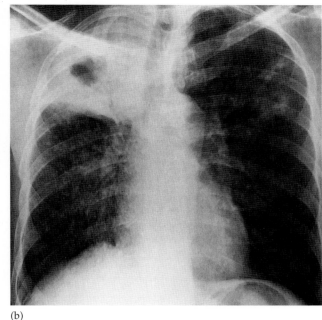

(b)

Fig. 2.81 Postprimary tuberculosis. (a) There are ill-defined consolidations scattered in both upper lobes; their size and distribution should suggest the diagnosis of postprimary tuberculosis. (b) The right upper lobe is consolidated and contains a large central cavity. Patchy consolidation from tuberculous bronchopneumonia is seen in the right mid and lower zones and in the left upper zone.

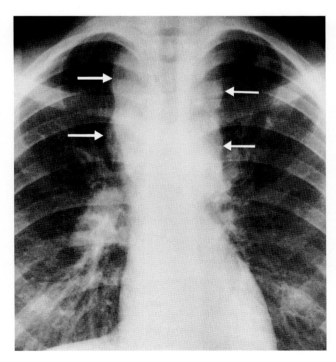

Fig. 2.82 Mediastinal lymphadenopathy (arrows) caused by tuberculosis.

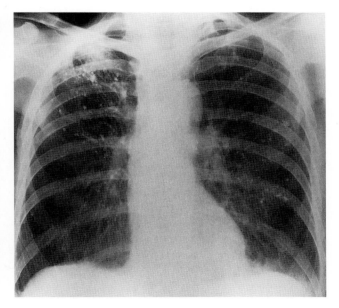

Fig. 2.83 Old calcified tuberculous disease. There are numerous foci of calcification in both lungs. The right upper lobe shows extensive fibrosis and bullae. There was no evidence in this patient that active infection was present. However, given this film in isolation, active disease could not be excluded.

seen in the presence of continuing activity. Pleural effusions often leave permanent pleural thickening which may, on occasion, calcify.

Tuberculoma. The term tuberculoma refers to a tuberculous granuloma in the form of a spherical mass, usually less than a centimetre or two in diameter, and mostly much smaller. The edge is usually sharply defined and the lesions are often partly calcified. Computed tomography may be needed to demonstrate the calcification. Tuberculomas are almost invariably inactive even though viable tubercle bacilli may be present deep within the lesions.

Mycetoma (Fig. 2.84). The fungus *Aspergillus fumigatus* may colonize old tuberculous cavities to produce a ball of fungus (mycetoma) lying free within the cavity. Air is seen between the mycetoma and the wall of the cavity. Cavities

containing mycetomas are usually surrounded by other evidence of old tuberculous infection, particularly fibrosis and calcification of the adjacent lung. Computed tomography often allows a specific diagnosis of mycetoma to be made.

Is the tuberculosis active? Valuable diagnostic signs of activity are:
• development of new lesions on serial films
• demonstration of cavities.

Lack of change over a period of years is useful evidence against activity, but the progression on serial chest films may be subtle, even with active disease. Many routine chest films in asymptomatic patients show evidence of tuberculosis. In a few, the diagnosis of active disease is readily apparent by the presence of cavities or by comparison with previous films. In the remainder it can be a considerable

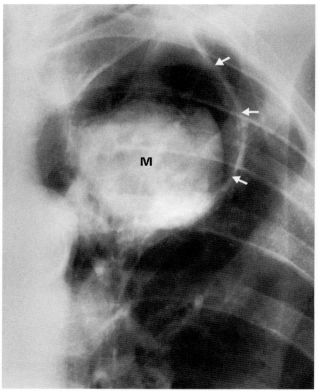

(a)

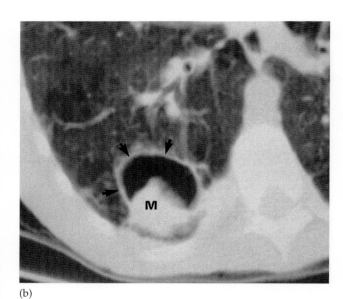

(b)

Fig. 2.84 Mycetoma (M) in pre-existing, old tuberculous cavity, the wall of which is arrowed. (a) Plain film. The fungus ball moved around the cavity when the patient was placed on his side. (b) CT of a different patient showing a mycetoma in a pre-existing old tuberculous cavity.

problem to decide which patients to investigate further and which to accept as having old inactive disease. The better defined the shadows and the greater the degree of calcification, the less the likelihood of activity. The presence of ill-defined shadows, even if partially calcified, is suggestive of active disease. However, the decision is often largely based on the clinical findings and the results of sputum examination for tubercle bacilli. It is important to realize that there is no way of excluding activity radiologically unless serial films show no change in the appearances over a prolonged period of time.

Fungal and parasitic diseases

When fungi are inhaled they may produce lung infection. The radiological appearances vary with the particular fungus, but two broad divisions can be made:

• Infection of an otherwise normal patient. Organisms such as histoplasmosis, coccidioidomycosis and blastomycosis (Fig. 2.85), which are found chiefly in North America, produce lung lesions that are very similar and often identical to tuberculosis. Cavitation is a particular feature. Healing by fibrosis and calcification is frequent.

• Infection in an immunocompromised host. With impaired immunity, fungi such as *Candida albicans* and *Aspergillus fumigatus*, as well as several of the fungi native to North America, may cause widespread pneumonia. It is not possible to predict the infecting organism from the chest film. Indeed, it is usually not possible to distinguish fungal infection from infection with bacteria, viruses and parasites.

Aspergillus fumigatus affects the lung in three ways: it may colonize a pre-existing cavity forming a fungus ball (mycetoma) (see Fig. 2.84); it may infect the lung in an immunocompromised patient causing severe pneumonia (see below); or it may be responsible for allergic bronchopulmonary aspergillosis, a condition discussed on p. 80.

Hydatid disease

Pulmonary infection with *Echinococcus granulosus* may result in cysts in the lung or pleural cavity. These cysts may be solitary or multiple and are seen as spherical shadows with very well-defined borders. Hydatid cysts occasionally rupture to produce complex cavities.

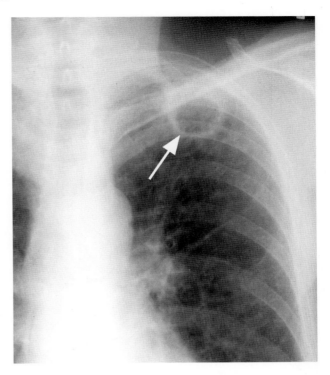

Fig. 2.85 Fungus infection. The cavity (arrow) in this patient from southeast USA was due to North American blastomycosis. Note the similarity to tuberculosis. Other fungi, e.g. histoplasmosis, can give an identical appearance.

Pneumonia in the immunocompromised host

Patients who are immunocompromised are not only more susceptible to pulmonary infection, often with unusual organisms, but also the pattern of the resulting pneumonia frequently shows an atypical radiographic appearance. Pneumonia in these patients may be due to the usual pathogens, but often it is due to opportunistic fungi, tuberculosis or *Pneumocystis carinii*.

Pneumonia in immunocompromised patients usually causes widespread non-specific pulmonary shadowing. It may not even be possible to say whether the shadowing is due to infection or to such conditions as pulmonary oedema, pulmonary haemorrhage or neoplastic disease.

The predilection of people with AIDS to develop *Pneumocystis carinii* pneumonia means that widespread, uniformly distributed pulmonary shadowing in a patient with AIDS

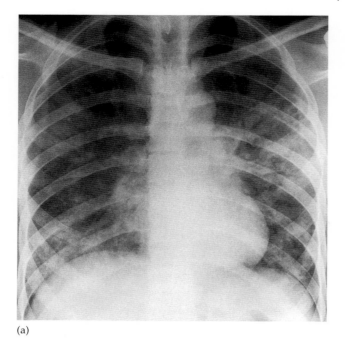

(a)

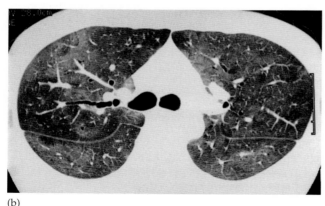

(b)

Fig. 2.86 *Pneumocystis carinii* pneumonia in a patient with AIDS showing (a) typical widespread low-density air space shadowing on chest x-ray. (b) HRCT in another patient with similar but less advanced changes.

is usually due to this organism (Fig. 2.86), though AIDS patients are also prone to tuberculous infection and the development of extensive Kaposi's sarcoma, both of which can appear similar to *Pneumocystis carinii* pneumonia on plain chest radiography.

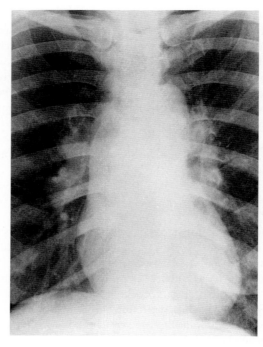

Fig. 2.87 Sarcoidosis. The lobular outline to the hila is characteristic of lymph node enlargement. In this case the paratracheal nodes are not visibly enlarged. This patient had no symptoms or signs, the abnormality being discovered on a routine chest film.

Sarcoidosis

Sarcoidosis is characterized pathologically by non-caseating granulomas in many organs including lung, liver, spleen, lymph nodes, skin and bone. The aetiology is unknown and the diagnosis depends on correlating the clinical, pathological and radiological manifestations.

The radiological manifestations are largely confined to the chest. The features on plain chest radiograph and CT are:
• Hilar and paratracheal lymphadenopathy. When hilar lymphadenopathy is present it is almost invariably bilateral and is usually symmetrical (Fig. 2.87). Mediastinal adenopathy is common and the nodes are large enough to be visible on a plain chest radiograph in about half the patients. The mediastinal lymphadenopathy is most readily recognized in the right paratracheal region. On chest CT, the widespread distribution of the mediastinal lymphadenopathy is readily

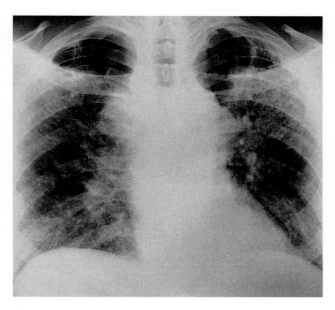

Fig. 2.88 Late fibrotic stage of sarcoidosis. The dense reticulonodular shadowing radiates outwards from the hila, maximally in the mid and upper zones. Enlarged lymph nodes are still visible at the hila and in the right paratracheal region. Many patients with this degree of pulmonary fibrosis from sarcoidosis do not have visibly enlarged lymph nodes.

apparent. Unlike lymphoma, the lymph node enlargement is never predominant in the anterior mediastinum.
• Reticulonodular shadowing in the lungs. The pattern varies from uniform small nodular shadows, which may clear on steroid therapy, to coarse reticular shadows maximal in the mid and upper zones, which represent pulmonary fibrosis (Fig. 2.88). At this stage, the pulmonary disease is often irreversible.

The majority of patients with sarcoidosis of the chest have lymphadenopathy only, which clears without treatment and does not progress to pulmonary involvement. Many are discovered on routine chest x-ray and have no symptoms. Some present with iridocyclitis, some with erythema nodosum and fever, and a few with polyarthritis.

Approximately 10% of patients with sarcoidosis develop a significant degree of lung involvement; some have visibly enlarged lymph nodes at this stage. Often the lymph nodes get smaller and may return to normal, even though the lung changes persist.

Computed tomography, which can demonstrate the hilar/mediastinal adenopathy and the lung shadowing to advantage, does not provide useful extra information and is rarely indicated in sarcoidosis.

Diffuse interstitial pulmonary fibrosis

The known causes of diffuse interstitial pulmonary fibrosis include: extrinsic allergic alveolitis, collagen vascular diseases (notably rheumatoid arthritis), drug-induced fibrosis, pneumoconiosis and sarcoidosis, but a substantial proportion of cases are idiopathic in origin. Several names are given to the most common idiopathic form of diffuse interstitial fibrosis, notably usual interstitial pneumonia (UIP), idiopathic pulmonary fibrosis (IPF) and idiopathic or cryptogenic fibrosing alveolitis (CFA).

Usual interstitial pneumonia (cryptogenic fibrosing alveolitis, idiopathic pulmonary fibrosis)

In UIP there is thickening of the alveolar walls with fibrosis and desquamation. As the disease progresses, the alveolar walls break down and small, rounded air spaces develop. At this stage, the appearances are known by the descriptive term 'honeycomb lung'. It causes a restrictive ventilation defect with severe reduction in gas transfer across the alveolar walls. The imaging features are:
• Hazy shadowing at the lung bases leading to a lack of clarity of the vessel outlines. Later, ill-defined nodules with connecting lines become discernible, which may contain circular lucencies (honeycomb lung) (Fig. 2.89).
• Decreased lung volume, often marked (Fig. 2.89).
• Eventually, the heart and pulmonary arteries enlarge due to increasingly severe pulmonary hypertension.

These signs are seen on both plain chest radiographs and high resolution CT. High resolution CT is more sensitive for detecting the changes, particularly areas of ground glass shadowing and honeycombing, and demonstrates the distribution and severity of disease (Fig. 2.89b).

Determining the cause of diffuse pulmonary fibrosis

The distribution of pulmonary shadowing may give a clue to its aetiology. In UIP, the lung shadowing is often maximal at the bases and at the lung periphery, although it may be

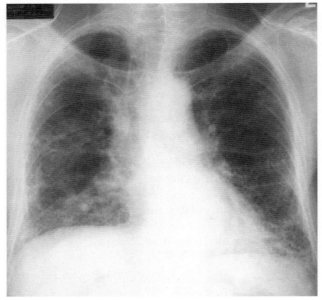

(a)

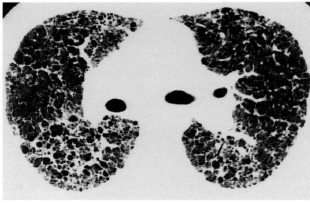

(b)

Fig. 2.89 Idiopathic usual interstitial pneumonia [Idiopathic (cryptogenic) fibrosing alveolitis]. (a) In this example there is reticulonodular shadowing (honeycomb lung) with basal predominance. Scleroderma, rheumatoid arthritis and drug-induced interstitial fibrosis give a similar picture. Notice the reduction in lung volume and that the left hemidiaphragm is indistinct because of the changes in the adjacent lung.
(b) HRCT of a different patient showing the honeycomb pattern in the lungs.

fairly uniformly distributed in advanced cases (Fig. 2.89). Scleroderma and rheumatoid arthritis give an identical picture.

The combination of pulmonary fibrosis with certain other signs may lead to a specific diagnosis:

• substantial past or present hilar/mediastinal adenopathy suggests sarcoidosis (Fig. 2.88)
• coexistent conglomerate masses in the mid and upper zones are virtually diagnostic of silicosis or coal miners' pneumoconiosis (Fig. 2.92, p. 80)
• coexistent bilateral pleural thickening and calcification are highly suggestive of asbestosis
• past or present pleural effusions are highly suggestive of rheumatoid arthritis.

Radiation pneumonitis (Figs 2.90 and 2.91)

Radiation pneumonitis may occur following x-ray therapy for intrathoracic neoplasms and breast carcinoma. The response of the lung to radiation varies from patient to patient. Initially, there is no radiological change, but within a few weeks ill-defined small shadows, indistinguishable from infective consolidation, are seen within the radiation field. If the inflammatory change goes on to fibrosis, there is dense coarse shadowing that may be sharply demarcated from the normal lung in a geometric fashion, conforming to the field of radiation but ignoring the lobar boundaries of the lung. There is loss of volume of the fibrosed areas. Extensive pleural thickening is also sometimes seen.

Collagen vascular diseases

This group of diseases includes rheumatoid arthritis, systemic lupus erythematosus, polyarteritis nodosa, systemic sclerosis, dermatomyositis and Wegener's granulomatosis. Various radiological signs occur:

Rheumatoid lung

The most common finding in the chest is pleural effusion. Pulmonary fibrosis, indistinguishable from that seen in idiopathic pulmonary fibrosis, is another important feature.

An interesting sign of pulmonary involvement in rheumatoid arthritis is the development of rounded granulomas

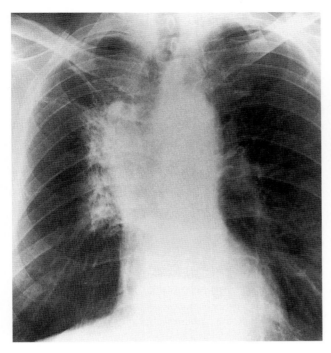

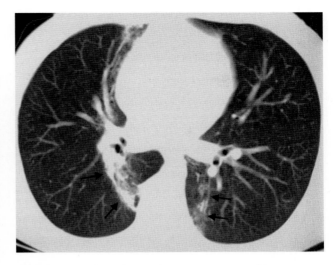

Fig. 2.91 Computed tomography in a patient treated for lymphoma. Note the linear fibrosis (arrows) in the lungs on either side of the mediastinum.

Fig. 2.90 Postradiation fibrosis. The patient had received radiation therapy for a carcinoma in the right upper lobe. Notice the geometric outline to the shadowing corresponding to the radiation field, the resulting mediastinal deviation and distortion of the pulmonary vessels.

in the periphery of the lung, histologically similar to the subcutaneous nodules seen in this disease. These spherical nodules, which may be single or multiple, rarely exceed 3 cm in size. Eventually, many cavitate and then go on to resolve.

Systemic lupus erythematosus

The chest radiograph is usually normal. The commonest abnormalities are pleural effusion and cardiac enlargement due to pericardial effusion. Patchy consolidation in the lungs is occasionally seen.

Scleroderma and dermatomyositis

The cardinal feature is basal reticulonodular shadows from pulmonary fibrosis, similar to that seen in idiopathic pulmonary fibrosis. Pleural effusion is rare.

Wegener's granulomatosis

The lungs may show one or more well-defined consolidations or masses, usually in the mid zones, which may cavitate. These lesions are often difficult to distinguish from bronchogenic carcinoma, when single, or metastases, when multiple, on radiographic grounds alone.

Pneumoconiosis

The pneumoconioses consist of a group of conditions caused by the inhalation of a variety of dusts related to people's work.

Coal workers' pneumoconiosis

Coal workers' pneumoconiosis is now very uncommon, following the introduction of preventative measures. Simple pneumoconiosis is due to dust retention in the lungs with minor fibrosis. It does not give rise to symptoms, but radiologically it causes many small nodules similar in appearance to military tuberculosis. For reasons that are not entirely clear, progressive massive fibrosis (PMF) may supervene. Progressive massive fibrosis causes homogeneous rounded shadows in the upper halves of

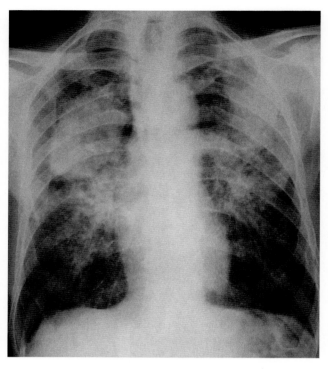

Fig. 2.92 Progressive massive fibrosis (PMF). Note the large oval shadows in the upper halves of both lungs. A nodular pattern is present elsewhere in the lung fields.

the lungs. The shadows may be unilateral or bilateral and there is usually nodular shadowing in the rest of the lungs (Fig. 2.92). Progressive massive fibrosis is usually associated with breathlessness.

Asbestos-related disease (Fig. 2.93)

Inhalation of asbestos fibres may lead to:

1 *Pleural plaques.* Localized plaques of pleural thickening, some of which are calcified, are seen along the lateral chest wall and diaphragm. The plaques in themselves are harmless, but they are a useful pointer to previous asbestos exposure.

2 *Diffuse pleural thickening*, which may encase one or both lungs, and cause restrictive reduction in pulmonary function.

3 *Pulmonary fibrosis.* Unlike the pleural plaques, which may be seen following minor exposure to asbestos, pulmo-

nary fibrosis (asbestosis) only follows significant exposure. Pulmonary fibrosis in asbestosis is symmetrically bilateral and maximal at the bases, similar to cryptogenic fibrosing alveolitis.

4 *The development of malignant neoplasms.* Malignant mesothelioma (see Fig. 2.51, p. 54) and bronchial carcinoma are both seen with far higher frequency in asbestos-exposed patients than in the general population.

Diseases of the airways

Asthma

The chest film in asthma is usually normal or shows only air trapping with flattening of the diaphragm. Bronchial wall thickening may be seen. The main purpose of the chest x-ray in asthma is:

• to determine complications, e.g. atelectasis
• to detect associated pneumonia
• to exclude other causes of acute dyspnoea, e.g. pulmonary oedema, pneumothorax or, rarely, tracheal obstruction.

A chest x-ray should only be undertaken when one or more of the above conditions are a realistic possibility.

Allergic bronchopulmonary aspergillosis results from hypersensitivity to *Aspergillus fumigatus*. Asthma is the cardinal clinical feature of this disease. The radiological signs are allergic consolidations in the lung and bronchiectasis, particularly in the mid and upper zones. The thickened walls of the dilated bronchi may be visible on a plain chest film.

Bronchiolitis

Severe bronchiolitis in young children, even when life-threatening, may show surprisingly little change on plain chest radiographs. The major sign is overinflation of the lungs leading to a low position of the diaphragm. Some children show widespread small ill-defined areas of consolidation, but in many the lungs are clear.

Acute bronchitis

Acute bronchitis in adults and older children does not produce any radiological abnormality unless complicated by pneumonia.

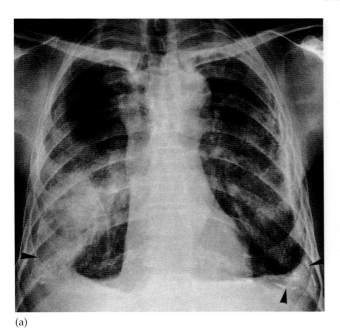

(a)

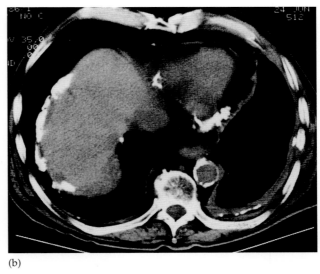

(b)

Fig. 2.93 Asbestos-related pleural disease. (a) There is extensive bilateral pleural thickening and pleural calcification (arrows) best appreciated along the lateral chest wall. (b) CT showing numerous calcified pleural plaques in the right hemithorax, predominantly over the right hemidiaphragm, and diffuse pleural thickening circumferentially around the left lower lobe.

Chronic obstructive airway disease

Chronic obstructive airway disease is an imprecise, but convenient, term that includes several common diseases, including chronic bronchitis and emphysema, and bronchiectasis.

Chronic bronchitis and emphysema. Chronic bronchitis and emphysema often coexist though pure forms of each are seen.

Chronic bronchitis is a clinical diagnosis based on productive cough for at least three consecutive months in two successive years. Pathologically, there is hypertrophy of the mucous glands throughout the bronchial tree. The chest film in uncomplicated chronic bronchitis is normal. If the film is abnormal, a complication such as emphysema, pneumonia or cor pulmonale has occurred, and the radiological features are then those of the complication in question.

Emphysema is defined pathologically as an increase beyond normal size of air spaces distal to the terminal bron-

chiole with destructive changes in their walls. The radiological signs of emphysema are (Fig. 2.94):
• Increased lung volume. The lungs increase in volume because of the combined effect of airways obstruction on abnormally compliant lungs. The diaphragm is pushed down and becomes low and flat. The heart is elongated and narrowed. The ribs are widely spaced and more lung lies in front of the heart and mediastinum. (Overinflation of the lungs can be said to be present if the hemidiaphragms at their midpoint are below the seventh rib anteriorly or the twelfth rib posteriorly.)
• Attenuation of the vessels. The reduction in size and number of the pulmonary blood vessels can be generalized or localized. If severe, the involved area is called a bulla. The edge of a bulla is usually sharply demarcated. In some cases, the normal lung adjacent to the bulla is compressed and appears opaque.

Bronchiectasis is defined as irreversible dilatation of the bronchi often accompanied by impairment of drainage of bronchial secretions leading to persistent infection.

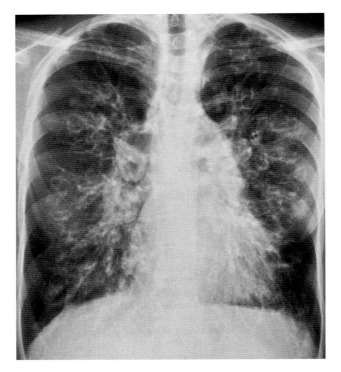

Fig. 2.97 Cystic fibrosis in a 14-year-old child. There is bronchial wall thickening, ring shadows of bronchiectasis and widespread ill-defined shadowing. All these phenomena tend to be maximal in the mid and upper zones. The diaphragm is somewhat low from obstructive airways disease.

• Evidence of airway obstruction. The diaphragm is low and flat and the heart is narrow and vertical, until cor pulmonale develops when cardiac enlargement may occur.

Respiratory distress in the newborn

There are many causes of respiratory distress in the first few days of life. Abnormalities are visible on the chest x-ray in the majority; only two conditions are discussed here.

Hyaline membrane disease is one of the commonest abnormalities. It is a disease of the premature infant and is due to deficiency of surfactant in the lungs. Consequently, the alveoli collapse, so preventing gas exchange. The chest radiographic appearance is one of the most important criteria in making the diagnosis.

The basic signs are widespread very small pulmonary opacities and visible air bronchograms (Fig. 2.98). Air bronchograms are visible because the bronchi are surrounded by airless alveoli. In the milder forms, the nodules are small and the air bronchograms may be the most obvious and easily recognized sign. In the more severe forms, the pulmonary opacities become more obvious and may be confluent; the lungs then appear almost opaque, except for air bronchograms. The changes are nearly always uniform in distribution.

Meconium aspiration (Fig. 2.99). In meconium aspiration, the pulmonary shadowing is usually patchy and distinctly streaky. Air bronchograms are not an obvious feature. The diaphragm is often lower than normal due to airways obstruction associated with sticky meconium in the bronchi.

Complications of therapy. In addition to establishing the initial diagnosis in neonates with various causes of respiratory distress, the plain chest film is vital in detecting complications of therapy. These include pneumothorax, lobar collapse and pneumomediastinum.

Adult respiratory distress syndrome

Adult respiratory distress syndrome (ARDS) is the name given to a syndrome in which the pulmonary capillaries leak proteinaceous fluid into the surrounding pulmonary interstitium and alveoli. The condition is also known as 'non-cardiogenic pulmonary oedema'. There are many precipitating causes including severe trauma, significant hypotension, septicaemia and fat embolism. It is believed that these insults produce a cascade of events, the nature of which has yet to be fully elucidated, leading to capillary damage, and, hence, to increased capillary permeability. The patients become increasingly short of breath and hypoxic, requiring mechanical ventilation to stay alive. The mortality, even with intense therapy and assisted ventilation, can be high. There is no specific treatment.

Chest radiographs (Fig. 2.100) show widespread pulmonary shadowing resembling cardiogenic pulmonary oedema at first, but the pulmonary shadowing becomes more widespread and more uniform over the ensuing 24–48 hours. The radiological abnormality may only develop 12–24 hours after the onset of tachypnoea, dyspnoea or hypoxaemia. As patients with ARDS require assisted ventilation, the chest film is used to detect the complications of

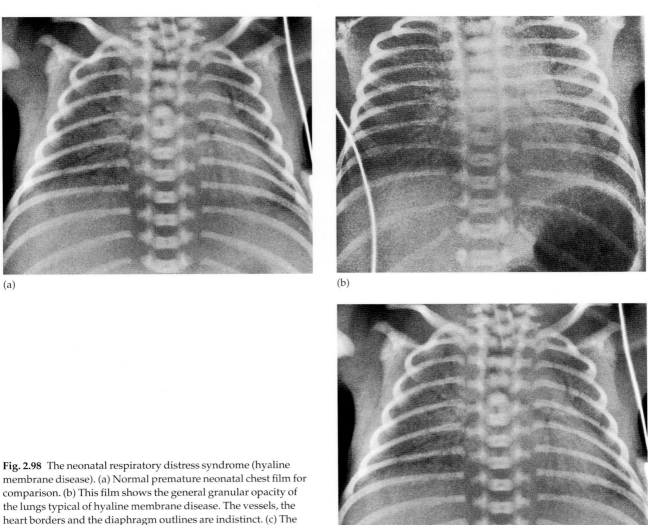

(a)

(b)

Fig. 2.98 The neonatal respiratory distress syndrome (hyaline membrane disease). (a) Normal premature neonatal chest film for comparison. (b) This film shows the general granular opacity of the lungs typical of hyaline membrane disease. The vessels, the heart borders and the diaphragm outlines are indistinct. (c) The air bronchogram sign in another baby with hyaline membrane disease. Note the uniformity of distribution of the changes in the lungs – an important diagnostic feature of hyaline membrane disease.

(c)

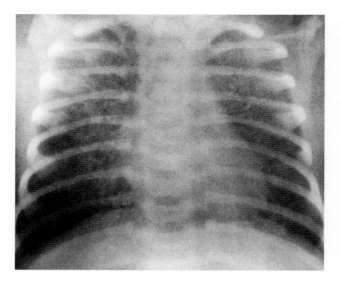

Fig. 2.99 Meconium aspiration. This baby born at term had fetal distress during delivery and was born through meconium-stained liquor. The film shows patchy consolidations rather than the uniform changes seen in hyaline membrane disease. The diaphragm is lower than normal in position, which is another differentiation from hyaline membrane disease.

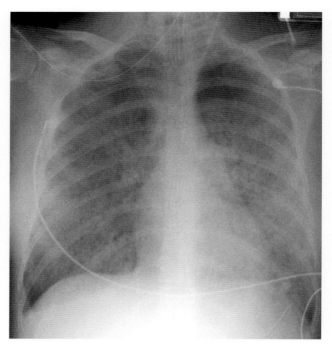

Fig. 2.100 Adult respiratory distress syndrome (ARDS). There is widespread air space shadowing in the lungs.

ventilator therapy, notably pneumothorax and pneumomediastinum.

Pulmonary emboli and infarction

Pulmonary emboli from thrombi originating in the veins of the legs and pelvis are very common in patients confined to bed, particularly those with heart disease and those who have had major surgery. Small emboli occurring over a long period of time may cause pulmonary hypertension. (See p. 101 for a discussion of pulmonary hypertension.) Radionuclide lung scans can be performed to confirm or exclude the diagnosis of pulmonary emboli, but CT pulmonary angiography has become the investigation of choice.

Plain film abnormalities

In most cases, even with massive pulmonary embolism, plain chest radiographs show no abnormalities due to the emboli. However, in some patients, particularly those with heart disease, infarction occurs. Radiologically, infarcts cause one or more areas of consolidation based on the pleura and the diaphragm. They often affect both lungs and are indistinguishable from pneumonia. The differentiation between pneumonia and pulmonary infarction depends on clinical rather than radiological factors.

Radionuclide lung scans

Radionuclide lung scans for diagnosing pulmonary embolism have largely been replaced by CT angiography. The diagnosis on radionuclide lung scanning depends on observing the distribution of radionuclide particles in the lungs following intravenous injection. The radionuclide particles do not reach the underperfused portions of the lungs, and, therefore, one or more defects are seen in the perfusion scan. A normal perfusion scan for practical purposes excludes pulmonary embolism.

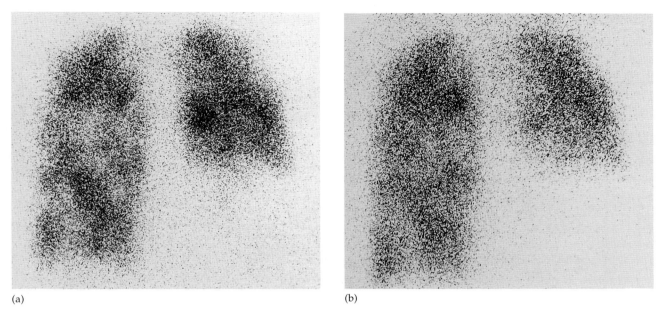

(a) (b)

Fig. 2.101 Matched ventilation/perfusion defects. ^{99m}Tc macroaggregate perfusion scan (a) showing matched defects when compared to the ^{81m}Kr ventilation scan (b). Both are anterior scans. The patient had widespread emphysema.

A ventilation scan is also required in patients with perfusion defects in order to differentiate between the various other causes of perfusion defects, which include pneumonia, pulmonary oedema, tumours, bronchiectasis and emphysema. The ventilation and perfusion scans are compared. If similar defects of the same size and position are present on both scans, they are regarded as matched (Fig. 2.101), and, therefore, due to pneumonia, pulmonary oedema or airways disease; if not, the defects are mismatched (Fig. 2.102) and are likely to be due to pulmonary emboli. Unfortunately, many radionuclide scans are indeterminate and, therefore, unhelpful.

CT pulmonary angiography

Computed tomography pulmonary angiography involves imaging the pulmonary arteries during a rapid injection of intravenous contrast agent (Fig. 2.103 and see Fig. 2.7, p. 22). It shows the emboli as filling defects within the lumen of the opacified pulmonary arteries. The technique can demonstrate emboli in large and medium-sized pulmonary vessels, but is less reliable for excluding pulmonary emboli in the more distal, smaller pulmonary arteries.

Trauma to the chest

In major trauma CT is often needed, but a chest radiograph is usually sufficient following minor trauma. A rib fracture can be diagnosed by noting a break or step in the cortex of a rib. Special views of the ribs may be necessary, as rib fractures are often invisible in the standard projections, particularly if the fracture lies below the diaphragm. Extrapleural soft tissue swelling from bruising, or frank haematoma may be visible and guide the observer toward the site of the fracture. Rib fractures are frequently multiple and may result in a flail segment. Pleural effusion often accompanies rib fractures, the fluid frequently being blood.

Pneumothorax may occur if the lung is punctured by direct injury or by the sharp edge of a rib fracture. An air–fluid level in the pleural cavity due to the associated haemorrhage is common in such situations.

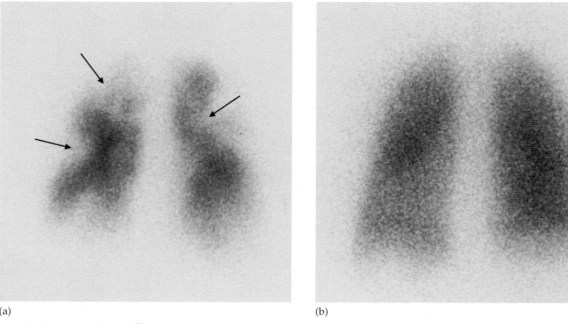

(a)   (b)

Fig. 2.102 Pulmonary emboli. (a) ^{99m}Tc macroaggregate perfusion scan (posterior view) showing multiple wedge-shaped defects. The more obvious ones have been arrowed. (b) The ventilation scan, using ^{81m}Kr (also a posterior view), is normal.

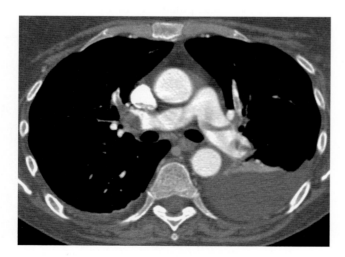

Fig. 2.103 Pulmonary emboli demonstrated by CT pulmonary angiography. The emboli have resulted in pulmonary infarction which has caused a large left and a small right pleural effusion.

Surgical emphysema of the chest wall may indicate the escape of air from the lungs. The presence of mediastinal emphysema in the absence of chest wall emphysema may indicate the unusual phenomenon of rupture of a bronchus.

Pulmonary contusion. Localized traumatic alveolar haemorrhage and oedema (Fig. 2.104) may be seen whether or not a rib fracture can be identified. The resulting pulmonary shadow is indistinguishable from other forms of pulmonary consolidation, the relationship to the injury being important in establishing the diagnosis.

Adult respiratory distress syndrome may follow severe trauma to any part of the body. Fat embolism is a specific subtype of ARDS, but its radiographic manifestations are identical to those of the other causes of ARDS (see p. 84).

Rupture of the diaphragm is due to penetrating injury or compression of the abdomen and may permit herniation of the stomach or intestines into the chest. Such herniation is much commoner on the left than the right. Gas shadows

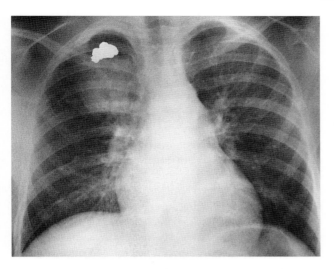

Fig. 2.104 Pulmonary contusion from a gunshot wound. The ill-defined consolidation represents haemorrhage and oedema in the right upper lobe. The deformed metallic fragments of the bullet are clearly visible.

of the stomach or intestines are seen above the presumed position of the diaphragm, the diaphragm itself often being invisible, because of an associated pleural effusion. Barium meal and follow-through may be indicated to establish the diagnosis. The only technique that can demonstrate the tear itself is ultrasound, but even when an expert performs the ultrasound examination, it may be difficult to make the diagnosis.

Rupture of the aorta is a particularly serious consequence of rapid deceleration injuries. In patients that survive, the injury to the aorta is usually at the level of the ligamentum arteriosum. Ruptured aorta is a surgical emergency and is best diagnosed by angiography, either catheter aortography or high quality CT angiography using multidetector CT.

Mediastinal widening due to bleeding, with or without pleural fluid, is the plain film sign of ruptured aorta, but mediastinal widening is a difficult sign to assess. It may be due to excess mediastinal fat, or it may be artefactual due to the portable AP films that are often the only films that can be taken in these severely injured patients. Computed tomography may be used to confirm or exclude blood in the mediastinum. When blood is identified, it may be due

to bleeding from the aortic rupture or to bleeding from other vessels – either arterial or venous. Although fractures of the ribs or sternum are usually present, there are many cases of aortic rupture on record without visible damage to the thoracic cage.

In some patients the diagnosis of aortic rupture is only made several months or years after the injury, when the development of an aneurysm is noted.

Rupture of the tracheobronchial tree only occurs with major chest trauma. The cardinal signs are pneumomediastinum, or pneumothorax that does not respond to chest tube suction. The main complication is subsequent bronchostenosis.

Carcinoma of the bronchus

Carcinoma of the bronchus is one of the most common primary malignant tumours. It has a clear association with cigarette smoking. It is convenient to consider the radiological features of central and peripheral tumours separately.

Signs of a central tumour

• The tumour itself may present as a hilar mass (Fig. 2.105) with or without narrowing of the adjacent major bronchus.
• Collapse and/or consolidation of lung beyond the tumour (see Fig. 2.111, p. 93). Lung collapse occurs because air is absorbed beyond the obstructed bronchus and cannot be replaced, whereas consolidation is the consequence of retained secretions and secondary infection.

Signs of a peripheral tumour

A peripheral tumour (Fig. 2.106) usually presents as a solitary pulmonary nodule/mass on plain films or chest CT. It is very unusual to see a lung carcinoma of less than 1 cm in diameter on plain chest radiographs. Much smaller cancers, some even as small as a few millimetres may be discovered on CT (Fig. 2.107).

The signs of a peripheral primary carcinoma are:
• A rounded shadow with an irregular border. Lobulation, notching and infiltrating edges are the common patterns.

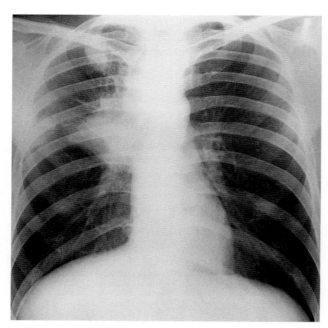

Fig. 2.105 Right hilar mass due to carcinoma of the bronchus. There is also a patch of consolidation in the right upper lobe laterally, from the central obstruction.

• Cavitation within the mass. The walls of the cavity are classically thick and irregular, but thin-walled smooth cavities due to carcinoma do occur.

Spread of bronchial carcinoma

Evidence of spread of bronchial carcinoma may be visible on plain chest radiography, but CT has made a major contribution to the staging of lung cancer. PET scanning is being used increasingly to stage potentially operable tumours. Magnetic resonance imaging is only used for highly specific indications. The features to look for are:

Hilar and mediastinal lymph node enlargement due to lymphatic spread of tumour. Only greatly enlarged lymph nodes can be recognized on plain chest radiography. Computed tomography, on the other hand, has the ability to show even mildly enlarged nodes, that are not identifiable on plain film.

But, enlargement of lymph nodes does not necessarily mean metastatic involvement, because reactive hyperplasia to the tumour or associated infection can be responsible for nodal enlargement, as can pre-existing disease – notably previous granulomatous infection. PET imaging can be a great help. The PET imaging agent FDG is taken up by metastatic neoplastic tissue, but not by normal lymph nodes. Unfortunately, the uptake is not entirely specific for malignancy. False-positive PET scans are obtained in patients with incidental and often unimportant inflammatory changes in the lymph nodes. In practice, therefore, the roles of CT and PET are to decide which patients need preoperative lymph node biopsy, and to tell the surgeon which nodes to biopsy. Nodes below 1 cm in diameter on CT and PET negative need not be biopsied. Nodes above 1 cm in diameter and/or PET-positive (Fig. 2.108) should be biopsied prior to surgical resection of the primary tumour. It should be borne in mind, however, that nodes of 2 cm or greater in short-axis diameter (Figs 2.109 and 2.110), which are PET-positive in a patient with a bronchial carcinoma, almost invariably contain metastatic neoplasm.

Pleural effusion in a patient with lung cancer is usually due to malignant involvement of the pleura, but it may be secondary to associated infection of the lung or coincidental, as in heart failure.

Invasion of the mediastinum is best assessed by CT, because the neoplasm is directly visualized and the detailed anatomy is displayed (Fig. 2.111).

Invasion of the chest wall. Destruction of a rib immediately adjacent to a pulmonary shadow is virtually diagnostic of bronchial carcinoma with chest wall invasion (Fig. 2.112). Recognizing the rib destruction can be difficult. It is important, therefore, to make a conscious effort to look directly at the ribs adjacent to the tumour. Computed tomography (and MRI) can demonstrate rib and soft tissue invasion when the bone is not visibly eroded on plain films (Fig. 2.113). Imaging techniques, even CT and MRI, may not always be reliable for determining chest wall invasion, and local chest wall pain remains an important indication that the tumour has crossed the pleura.

Rib metastases. Carcinoma of the lung frequently metastasizes to the ribs, where it produces bone destruction. Sclerotic secondary deposits from lung carcinoma are rare.

Pulmonary metastases. Primary lung carcinoma may metastasize to other parts of the lungs. The rounded shadows that

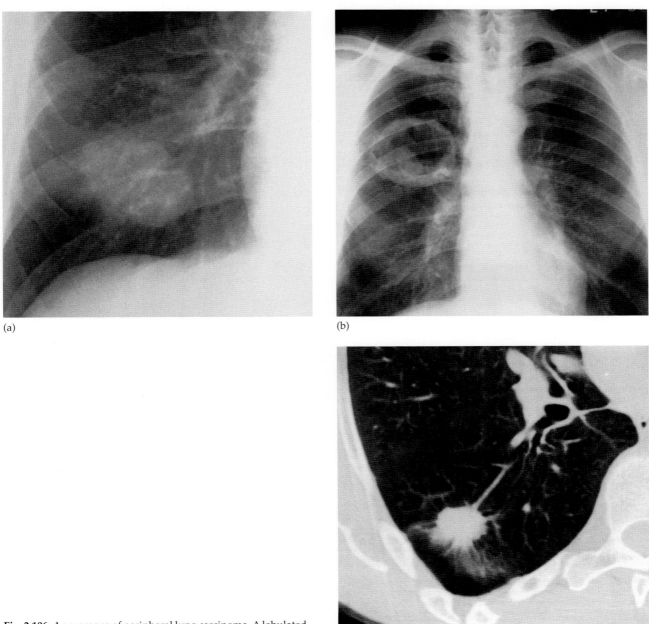

(a)

(b)

(c)

Fig. 2.106 Appearance of peripheral lung carcinoma. A lobulated (a) and a cavitating (b) mass are shown on plain films. (c) A spiculated mass is shown on CT.

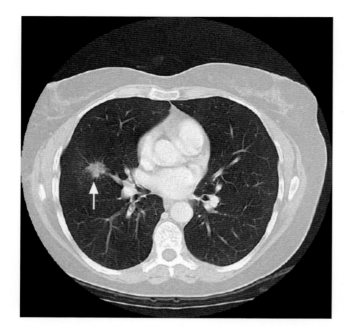

Fig. 2.107 Typical appearance and small size of a carcinoma of the bronchus discovered incidentally at CT.

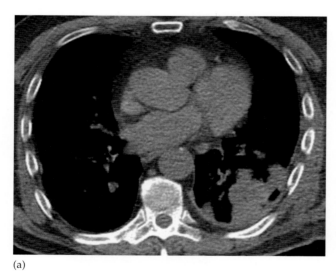

(a)

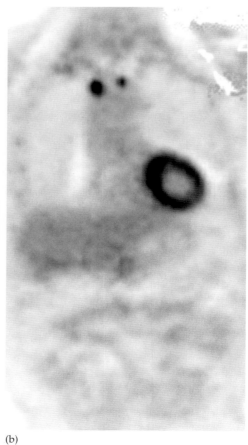

(b)

Fig. 2.108 PET scan demonstrating spread of lung cancer to mediastinal lymph nodes. (a) CT showing large primary lung carcinoma in the left lower lobe. (b) Coronal PET scan in the same patient showing high uptake of the PET agent in lymph nodes in the upper mediastinum. The uptake in the myocardium is normal. (The primary tumour shown is not visible in this particular section.) Fused PET-CT images of this patient are shown in Plate 2.

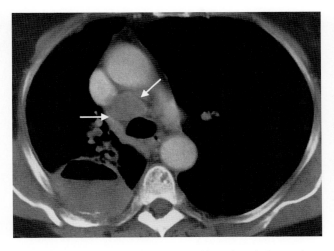

Fig. 2.109 (a) CT scan of greatly enlarged lymph node (arrows). Note that the primary tumour lying posteriorly in the right lung has invaded the chest wall and partially destroyed the adjacent rib.

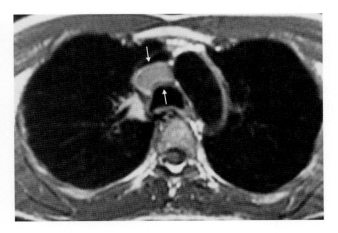

Fig. 2.110 MRI (T1-weighted) shows enlarged node (arrow) which stands out clearly against the background of no signal in lung, trachea or aorta.

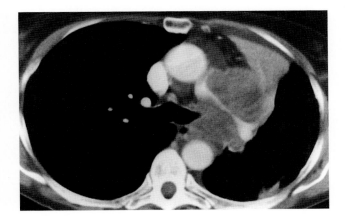

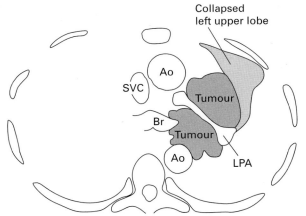

Fig. 2.111 Mediastinal invasion. Contrast-enhanced CT shows extensive tumour in mediastinum compressing the left pulmonary artery and causing left upper lobe collapse. Ao, aorta; Br, bronchus; LPA, left pulmonary artery; SVC, superior vena cava.

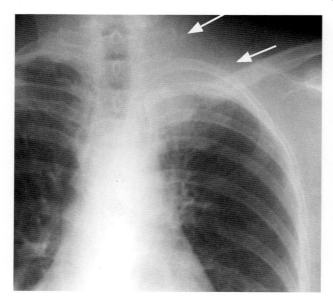

Fig. 2.112 Pancoast's tumour. The carcinoma arising at the apex of the left lung has invaded and destroyed the adjacent ribs and spine. Note that no bone is visible within the area indicated by the arrows.

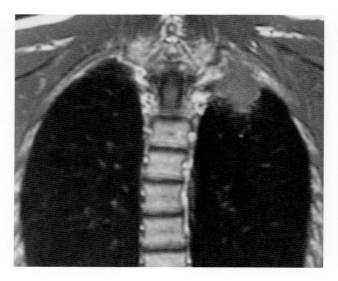

Fig. 2.113 Pancoast's tumour. The carcinoma of the lung can be seen invading the root of the neck on this coronal MRI scan (T1-weighted).

result are similar to secondary deposits from other primary tumours.

Lymphangitis carcinomatosa is the term applied to blockage of the pulmonary lymphatics by carcinomatous tissue. Lymphangitis carcinomatosa can be due to spread from abdominal and breast cancers as well as from carcinoma of the lung. The lymphatic vessels become grossly distended and the lungs become oedematous. The signs (Fig. 2.114) can be identical to those seen in interstitial pulmonary oedema (septal lines, loss of vessel clarity and peribronchial thickening), but if the heart is normal in size and there is hilar adenopathy and/or lobar consolidation, the diagnosis of lymphangitis carcinomatosa becomes more certain. The clinical story is very helpful, as if the changes are due to pulmonary oedema, the patient usually complains of sudden onset of breathlessness, whereas the patient with lymphangitis carcinomatosa gives a story of slowly increasing dyspnoea over the preceding weeks or months. Computed tomography, particularly HRCT, has proven very valuable in demonstrating lymphangitis carcinomatosa, because the appearances, in the correct clinical circum-

stances, are specific enough to obviate the need for biopsy (Fig. 2.115).

Metastatic neoplasms

Metastases from extrathoracic primary tumours may be seen in the lungs, the pleura or the bones of the thoracic cage or, very rarely, in hilar and mediastinal lymph nodes.

Pulmonary metastases

Pulmonary metastases are, typically, spherical and well defined (Figs 2.116 and 2.117), although irregular borders are occasionally seen. Usually, they are multiple and vary in size. Metastases have to be almost a centimetre in diameter, or larger, to be visible on plain chest radiographs. Computed tomography can demonstrate metastases as small as 3–6 mm. There is, however, a disadvantage attached to the excellent sensitivity of CT. Some small nodules are not metastases, but are benign processes such as tuberculomas or fungal granulomas. This is a major diagnostic problem in many parts of the United States, where fungal granulomas are very common.

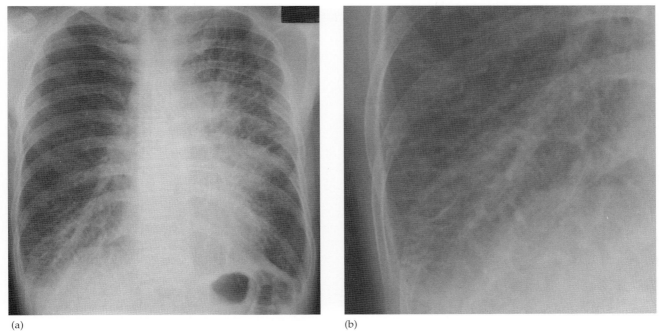

(a)   (b)

Fig. 2.114 Lymphangitis carcinomatosa. (a) There is widespread ill-defined pulmonary shadowing with numerous septal lines. (b) The magnified view of the right lung base shows the septal (Kerley B) lines to advantage.

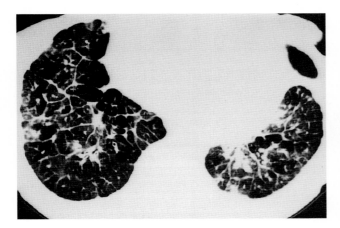

Fig. 2.115 Lymphangitis carcinomatosa. The widespread connecting lines representing irregularly thickened interlobular septa are very well shown by HRCT. This appearance is virtually pathognomonic of lymphangitis carcinomatosa.

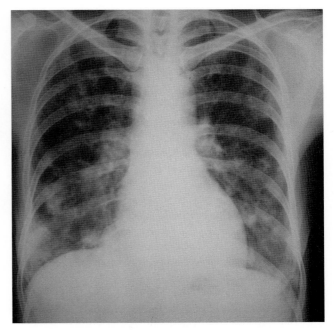

Fig. 2.116 Pulmonary metastases. There are numerous ill-defined irregular rounded shadows of varying sizes in both lungs.

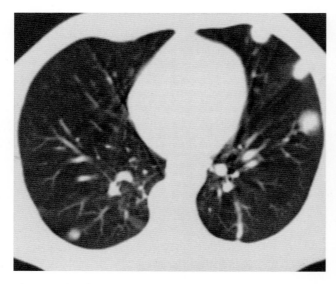

Fig. 2.117 CT of pulmonary metastases (malignant teratoma of testis). The peripheral location shown here is typical.

Pleural metastases

Pleural metastases usually give rise to pleural effusion; individual pleural metastases are rarely seen.

Metastases to ribs

Rib metastases are common with those primary tumours that metastasize to bone, notably bronchus, breast, kidney, thyroid and prostate. All except prostatic and breast cancers produce mainly or exclusively lytic metastases.

With lytic metastases, the most reliable sign is destruction of the cortex, particularly of the upper border of a rib. One should be wary of diagnosing destruction of the lower borders of the posterior portions of the ribs, as these regions are often ill defined even under normal conditions. When in doubt, it is always wise to compare with the opposite side. Another pitfall in the diagnosis of rib metastases is that blood vessels in the lungs may cause confusing shadows. This confusion cannot arise at the edges of the chest where there is no lung projected over the ribs, so the extreme edge of the chest is a useful place to look for rib destruction. Soft tissue swelling is frequently seen adjacent to the rib deposit, so it is a good rule to look at the outer margin of the lung for

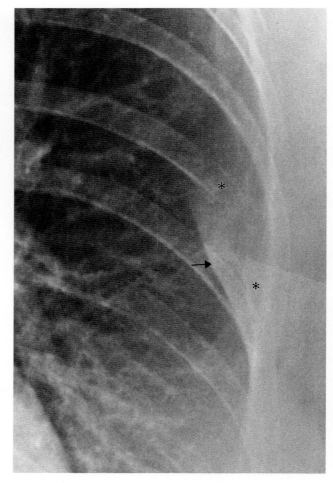

Fig. 2.118 Lytic metastasis. The soft tissue mass (arrow) is more obvious than the underlying bone destruction shown between the two asterisks.

soft tissue swelling as a clue to the presence of rib metastases (Fig. 2.118).

Lymphoma

The common manifestations of intrathoracic malignant lymphoma are mediastinal and hilar adenopathy, and pleural effusion. These features can often be seen on plain films, but CT is much the best method of confirming or excluding intrathoracic lymph node enlargement. Pulmo-

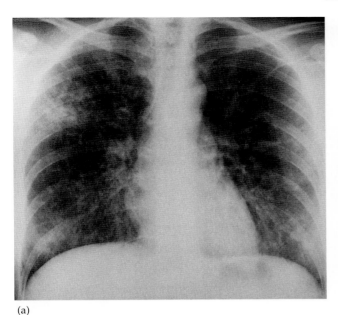

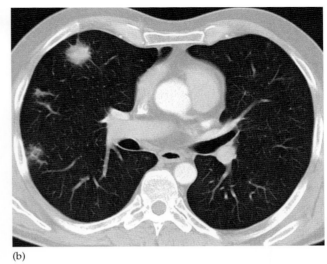

(b)

(a)

Fig. 2.119 (a) Lymphoma involving the lung. The extensive pulmonary consolidations were due to neoplastic involvement. Pneumonia can give a similar appearance. (b) CT in a patient with primary pulmonary lymphoma showing more nodular opacities.

nary involvement by lymphoma is unusual. It may take the form of large areas of infiltration of the lung parenchyma, resembling pulmonary pneumonia (Fig. 2.119a). As pulmonary infection is a common complication in patients with malignant lymphoma, it may be impossible to decide on radiological grounds whether the pulmonary consolidation is due to lymphomatous tissue or to infection. Occasionally, pulmonary lymphoma is seen as one or more mass lesions (Fig. 2.119b), which may cavitate. Pleural masses are a rare feature.

Cardiac disorders

Cardiac imaging has become highly specialized and only a brief introduction is provided. Posteroanterior chest radiographs, sometimes supplemented by lateral chest films, are useful for assessing the effects of cardiac disease on the lungs and pleural cavities and measuring overall heart size, but the evaluation of the size of specific chambers is unreliable. Echocardiography is the major imaging technique for morphological, as well as functional, information about the heart. It is excellent for looking at the

heart valves, assessing chamber morphology and volume, determining the thickness of the ventricular wall and diagnosing intraluminal masses. Doppler ultrasound is used to determine the velocity and direction of blood flow through the heart valves and within cardiac chambers. Radionuclide examinations are used to assess myocardial blood flow and ventricular contractility, but provide little anatomical detail. Magnetic resonance imaging provides both functional and anatomical information, but is only available at specialized centres and is used only for specific reasons.

Plain chest radiography

Plain chest radiographic evidence of heart disease may be given by the size and shape of the heart together with any cardiac calcification, and by the size of pulmonary vessels and the presence of pulmonary oedema.

Heart size and shape on plain chest radiography

The standard plain films for the evaluation of cardiac disease are the PA view and a lateral chest film (Fig. 2.120).

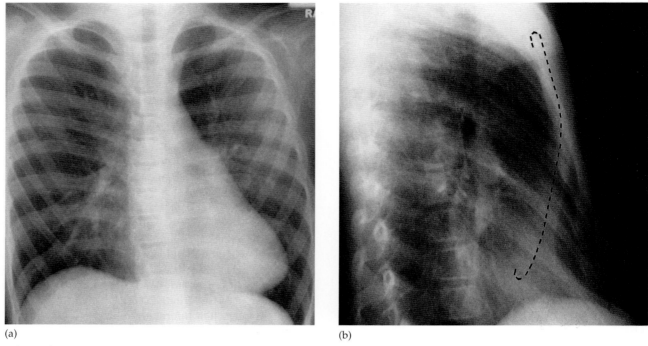

(a)   (b)

Fig. 2.122 Pectus excavatum. (a) Posteroanterior view. Note how the heart is displaced and altered in shape by the depressed sternum. (b) Lateral film. The edge of the sternum has been traced in on this film. There was no cardiac disease in this patient.

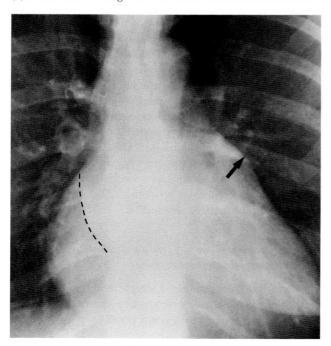

Fig. 2.123 Left atrial enlargement in a patient with mitral valve disease showing the 'double contour sign' (the left atrial border has been drawn in) and dilatation of the left atrial appendage (LAA) (arrow).

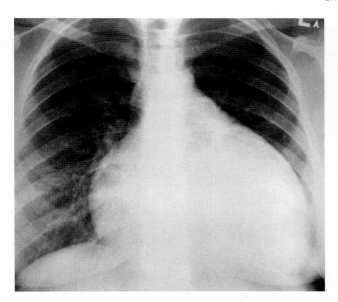

Fig. 2.124 Pericardial effusion. The heart is greatly enlarged. (Three weeks before, the heart had been normal in shape and size.) The outline is well defined and the shape globular. The lungs are normal. The cause in this case was a viral pericarditis. This appearance of the heart, though highly suggestive of, is not specific to, pericardial effusion – a similar appearance can be seen with other causes of cardiac enlargement, e.g. cardiomyopathy.

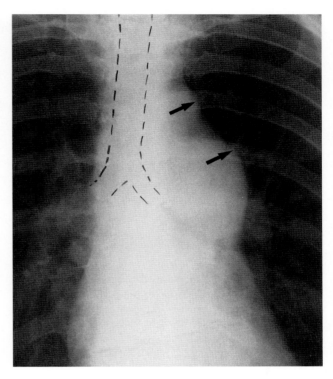

Fig. 2.125 Enlarged main pulmonary artery in a patient with pulmonary valve stenosis. The bulge of the main pulmonary artery (lower arrow) is clearly greater than normal and at first glance one might be deceived into diagnosing enlargement of the aorta. However, the aortic knuckle is the first 'bump' on the left mediastinal border (upper arrow). It projects 2.5–3 cm lateral to the trachea. The pulmonary artery forms the segment immediately below the aortic knuckle.

true diameter of the main pulmonary artery on plain film, there are degrees of bulging that permit one to say that it is indeed enlarged (Fig. 2.125). The assessment of the hilar vessels can be more objective since the diameter of the right lower lobe artery can be measured: the diameter at its midpoint is normally between 9 and 16 mm. The size of the vessels within the lungs reflects pulmonary blood flow. There are no generally accepted measurements of normality, so the diagnosis is based on experience with normal films. By observing the size of these various vessels it may be possible to diagnose one of the following haemodynamic patterns.

Increased pulmonary blood flow due to left to right shunts (Fig. 2.126)

Atrial septal defect, ventricular septal defect and patent ductus arteriosus are the common anomalies in which there is shunting of blood from the systemic to the pulmonary

circuits (so-called left to right shunts), thereby increasing pulmonary blood flow. In patients with a haemodynamically significant left to right shunt (2:1 or more), all the vessels from the main pulmonary artery to the periphery of the lungs are large. This radiographic appearance is sometimes called *pulmonary plethora*.

Pulmonary arterial hypertension (Figs 2.127)

The conditions that cause significant pulmonary arterial hypertension all increase the resistance of blood flow through the lungs. There are many such conditions including:

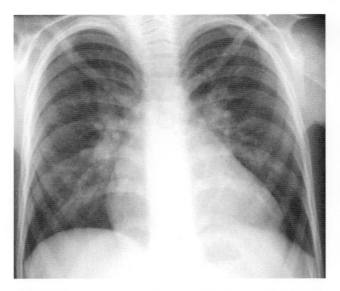

Fig. 2.126 Ventricular septal defect in a child. The heart is enlarged and there is obvious enlargement of the pulmonary vessels. The left to right shunt in this case was 3:1.

- various lung diseases (cor pulmonale)
- pulmonary emboli
- mitral valve disease
- left to right shunts
- idiopathic pulmonary hypertension.

Pulmonary arterial hypertension has to be severe before it can be diagnosed on plain films, and is difficult to quantify in most cases. The plain chest film features are enlargement of the pulmonary artery and hilar arteries, the vessels within the lung being normal or small. The reason for pulmonary arterial hypertension may be visible on the chest film; in cor pulmonale the lung disease is often radiologically obvious, and in mitral valve disease the echocardiographic features described on p. 107 will be seen.

Pulmonary venous hypertension (Fig. 2.128)

Mitral valve disease and left ventricular failure are the common causes of elevated pulmonary venous pressure. In the normal upright person, the lower zone vessels are larger than those in the upper zones. In raised pulmonary venous pressure, the upper zone vessels enlarge and in severe cases

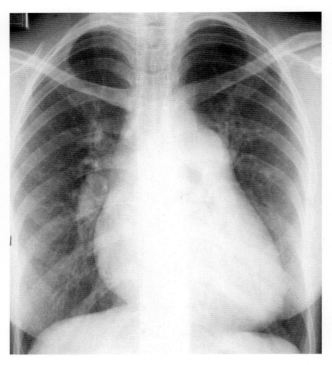

Fig. 2.127 Right ventricular enlargement in an adult with primary pulmonary hypertension. The heart is enlarged with the apex of the heart somewhat lifted off the diaphragm. Note also the features of pulmonary arterial hypertension – enlargement of the main pulmonary artery and hilar arteries with normal vessels within the lungs.

become larger than those in the lower zones. Eventually, pulmonary oedema will supervene and may obscure the blood vessels.

Pulmonary oedema

There are two radiographic patterns of cardiogenic pulmonary oedema: alveolar and interstitial. As oedema initially collects in the interstitial tissues of the lungs, all patients with alveolar oedema also have interstitial oedema.

Interstitial oedema (Fig. 2.129). There are many septa in the lungs which are invisible on the normal chest film because they consist of little more than a sheet of connective tissue

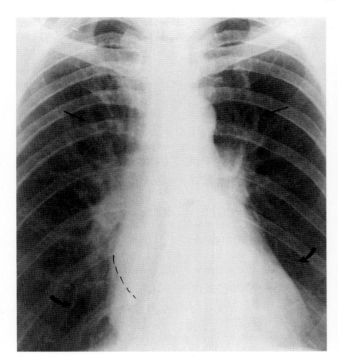

Fig. 2.128 Pulmonary venous hypertension in a patient with mitral valve disease. The upper zone vessels (straight arrows) are larger than the equivalent vessels in the lower zones (curved arrows). This is the reverse of the normal situation. (The left atrial border has been drawn in.)

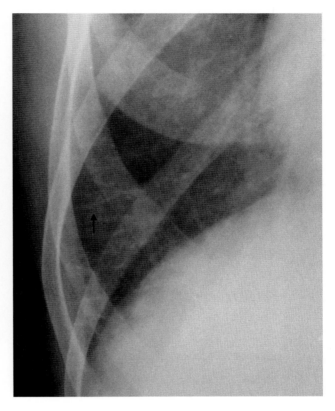

Fig. 2.129 Septal lines known as Kerley B lines in a patient with mitral stenosis. Note that these oedematous septa are horizontal non-branching lines which reach the pleura. One such line in the right costophrenic angle is arrowed.

containing very small blood and lymph vessels. When thickened by oedema, the peripherally located septa may be seen as line shadows. These lines, known as Kerley B lines, named after the radiologist who first described them, are horizontal lines never more than 2 cm long seen laterally in the lower zones. They reach the lung edge and are, therefore, readily distinguished from blood vessels, which never extend into the outer centimetre of the lung. Another sign of interstitial oedema is that the outline of the blood vessels may become indistinct owing to oedema collecting around them. This loss of clarity is a difficult sign to evaluate and it may only be recognized by looking at follow-up films after the oedema has cleared. Fissures may appear thickened because oedema may collect against them.

Alveolar oedema (Fig. 2.130) is a more severe form of oedema in which the fluid collects in the alveoli. It is always acute and almost always bilateral, involving all the lobes bilaterally. The pulmonary shadowing is usually maximal close to the hila and fades out peripherally, leaving a relatively clear zone that may contain septal lines around the edge of the lobes. This pattern of oedema is sometimes referred to as the 'butterfly' or 'bat's wing' pattern. Later on, the shadowing becomes more widespread, but is often most obvious in the lower zones.

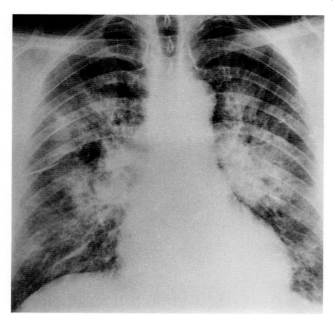

Fig. 2.130 Alveolar oedema in a patient with acute left ventricular failure following a myocardial infarction. The oedema fluid is concentrated in the more central portion of the lungs leaving a relatively clear zone peripherally. Note that all the lobes are fairly equally involved.

Echocardiography

Standard two-dimensional echocardiography (Fig. 2.131) demonstrates fan-shaped sections of the pericardial space, and individual cardiac chambers and valves in motion, by placing the transducer on the anterior chest wall in an intercostal or subcostal position to provide orthogonal projections (Fig. 2.132). It is also possible to place the ultrasound probe in the oesophagus or stomach to look at the cardiac structures from behind the heart.

Normally, all parts of the ventricular wall show equal movement and the left ventricular ejection fraction should be greater than 50%. Segments of ventricular wall with reduced movement or aneurysm formation can be demonstrated. Increased contractility of the left ventricle indicates hypertrophy, which can be primary (hypertrophic cardiomyopathy) or secondary to conditions such as aortic stenosis or systemic hypertension. The dimensions of each chamber can be readily assessed. For example, the internal diameter of the left ventricle should not exceed 5.7 cm, and that of the left atrium in the parasternal view should be less than 4.0 cm. Echocardiography also provides accurate estimates of wall thickness. Valve motion can be observed. Normally, the leaflets of all the valves are thin and give rise to clearly defined echoes with characteristic opening and closing motions. Valve stenosis causes thickening of the valve leaflets, restriction of movement and narrowing of the orifice. Calcification is often present and is seen as a multiplicity of bright echoes arising within the leaflets.

Echocardiography can be performed after exercise on a treadmill or bicycle or with a pharmacologically induced tachycardia to demonstrate dyskinetic areas of ventricular muscle due to underlying coronary artery disease. Fluids containing tiny bubbles which reflect ultrasound can be injected intravenously and act as intravascular contrast agents.

Doppler echocardiography

As discussed on p. 6, when sound waves are reflected from a moving object, the frequency of the reflected waves is altered, depending on the velocity of the reflecting surface. With the Doppler technique, red blood cells can be used as reflecting surfaces and the velocity of blood flow in a given direction can be calculated and/or colour coded. The accuracy of the technique depends on the angle of flow with respect to the ultrasound beam, flow directly in line with the beam being the most accurately measured.

Doppler flow measurements/colour coding are used to:
• Quantify pressure gradients across stenotic valves (derived from formulae that convert velocity across a valve into a pressure gradient).
• Detect and quantify flow, notably valvular regurgitation (see Plate 4), cardiac output and left to right shunts (see Plate 6).

Radionuclide studies

Nuclear medicine techniques are simpler to perform than angiocardiography, are non-invasive and can be readily repeated. They give information on cardiac

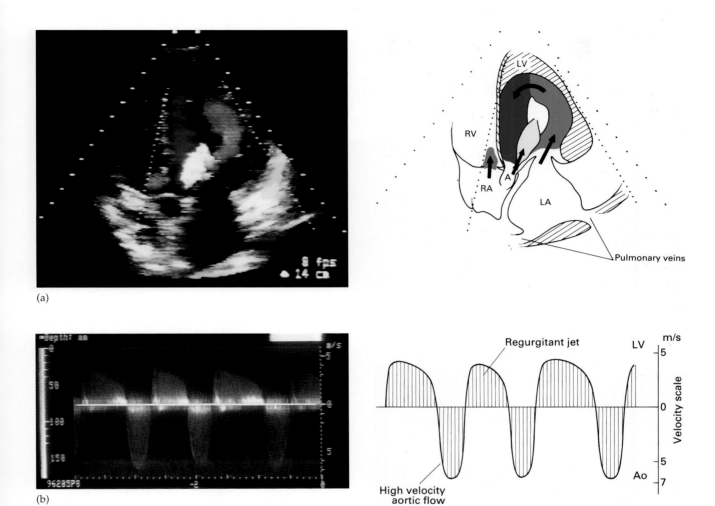

(a)

(b)

Plate 4 Aortic valve disease. (a) Colour flow Doppler in a patient with aortic regurgitation. Apical four-chamber view showing turbulent jet (white) of regurgitant blood impinging on anterior leaflet of mitral valve to mix with the stream (red) passing from left atrium to left ventricle. Note change in colour to blue as the stream is directed by the ventricular apex towards the aortic valve. A small portion of right atrial to right ventricular flow is depicted in red. (b) Continuous wave Doppler from the apical position in a patient with aortic stenosis and regurgitation showing a high velocity (7 m/s) jet into the aorta. There is immediate diastolic flow back into the left ventricle representing aortic regurgitation.

(Facing p. 104)

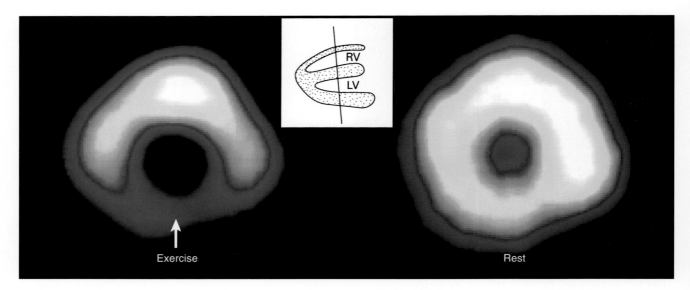

Plate 5 Thallium-201 myocardial perfusion scans. On the exercise scan there is a large area of very reduced uptake in the inferior wall of the left ventricle (arrow) with normal redistribution of the thallium on the rest scan indicating an area of ischaemia. Only the left ventricular wall is demonstrated as there is too little uptake of thallium by the normal right ventricle.

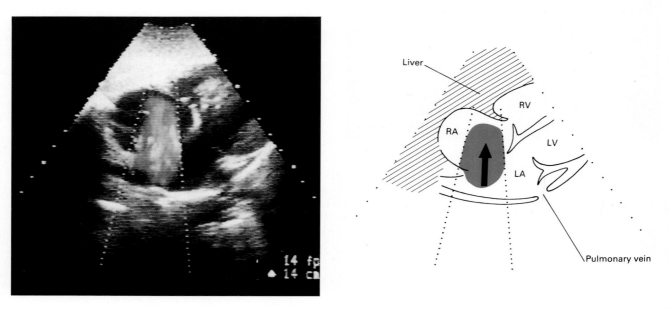

Plate 6 Atrial septal defect. Colour flow Doppler in the subcostal four-chamber view showing substantial flow (red) passing from left to right atrium.

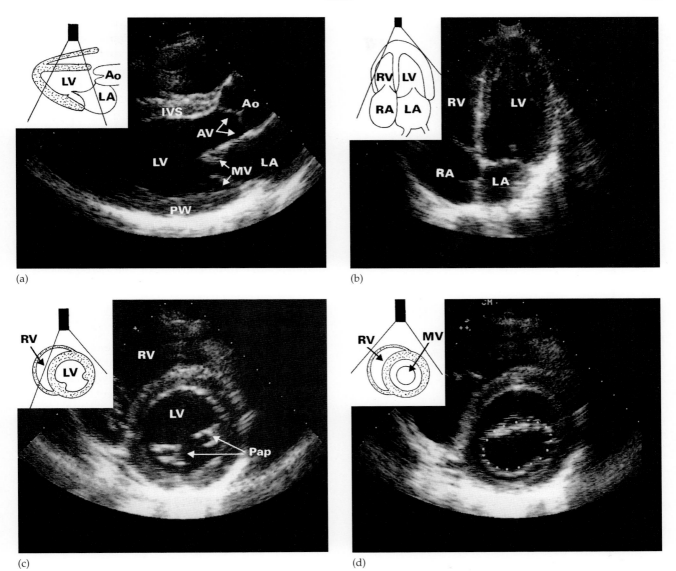

Fig. 2.131 Normal two-dimensional echocardiogram. (a) Parasternal long axis view. (b) Apical four-chamber view. (c) Parasternal short axis view at the level of papillary muscles. (d) Similar view to (c) but at the level of the mitral valve. The dots indicate the area of the open valve. Ao, aorta; AV, aortic valve; IVS, interventricular septum; LA, left atrium; LV, left ventricle; MV, mitral valve; Pap, papillary muscles; PW, posterior wall of LV; RA, right atrium; RV, right ventricle. Courtesy of Andrew A. McLeod and Mark J. Monaghan.

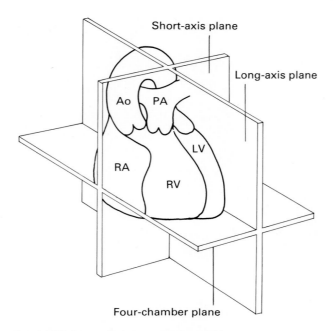

Short-axis plane

Long-axis plane

Ao   PA

LV

RA

RV

Four-chamber plane

Fig. 2.132 Diagram illustrating the three orthogonal imaging planes used to demonstrate the heart with two-dimensional echocardiography. Ao, aorta; PA, pulmonary artery; RA, right atrium; RV, right ventricle; LV, left ventricle.

function, but provide only limited anatomical detail. The two main radionuclide investigations in cardiology are myocardial perfusion scintigraphy and radionuclide angiocardiography.

Myocardial perfusion scintigraphy

Myocardial perfusion scintigraphy uses agents now including PET agents, which are taken up by the myocardium in proportion to blood flow, so regions of reduced perfusion appear as areas of reduced uptake. Myocardial perfusion imaging is used in patients with known or suspected ischaemic chest pain. As many patients only show impaired myocardial perfusion on exercise, the radionuclide is injected during actual or pharmacologically induced exercise. The images are repeated after the patient has rested for 3–4 hours. The sites and sizes of ischaemic areas can be assessed and a distinction between ischaemic and infarcted regions can be made by compar-

ing peak exercise and resting images (see p. 111 and Plate 5). The investigation should only be performed under medical supervision with full resuscitation equipment available.

Radionuclide angiography

Radionuclide angiocardiography is also known as 'multiple gated equilibrium blood pool imaging', sometimes abbreviated to MUGA (multiple gated) scanning. It uses technetium-99m (^{99m}Tc) attached to red blood cells to image the blood pool. Because insufficient radioactive counts are collected from each cardiac cycle, images from successive cardiac cycles are combined with the use of electronic gating. Radionuclide angiograms are used to calculate the *ventricular ejection fraction* in patients with valvular disease and myocardial disorders, and for *wall motion analysis* in patients with ischaemic heart disease.

Computed tomography

Standard CT plays little part in the management of intracardiac disorders. Pericardial effusions and cardiac tumours are recognizable, but they are usually equally well or better seen at ultrasound. Screening for coronary artery calcification is being undertaken in some centres in order to determine who should receive prophylactic treatment for atheroma in the hope of preventing future cardiac events. Modern 64-slice CT scanners can produce specialized images of the coronary arteries (see p. 113).

Magnetic resonance imaging

Electronic gating of the standard MRI sequences using an electrocardiogram is capable of providing an immense amount of information, but currently its role is relatively limited because the technique is expensive and the specialized equipment and expertise are only available in a few centres. Magnetic resonance imaging can, however, provide unique information, notably:
• details of complex congenital heart disease
• details of myocardial thickness and disease
• pericardial disease
• intracardiac tumours, which can be shown with great precision, better in many cases than with ultrasound.

Cardiac catheterization and angiography

Contrast can be injected through catheters which have been introduced under fluoroscopic control into the various chambers of the heart and into vessels that lead in and out of these chambers. Cardiac angiography is a specialized topic which will not be discussed further.

Coronary angiography (see Fig. 2.139, p. 112), which provides detailed information about coronary artery stenoses, occlusions and collateral or anomalous vessels, is widely practised in patients being considered for cardiac surgery, particularly for coronary artery revascularization. Catheters are usually introduced into the femoral artery and passed selectively into the orifices of each coronary artery.

Specific cardiac disorders

Heart failure

One or more of the following signs of heart failure may be seen on plain chest radiographs (Fig. 2.133):
- Cardiac enlargement, with or without specific chamber enlargement.
- Evidence of raised pulmonary venous pressure, namely enlargement of the vessels in the upper zones of the lung.
- Evidence of pulmonary oedema.
- Pleural effusions, which are usually bilateral, often larger on the right than the left, and if unilateral are almost always right-sided. (In acute left ventricular failure, small effusions are seen in the costophrenic angles running up the lateral chest wall. This fluid may, in fact, be oedema in the lungs rather than true pleural effusions.)

Cardiac ultrasound allows ventricular volumes and ejection fractions to be measured with considerable accuracy, as well as enabling valve gradients and degrees of regurgitation to be assessed. It is, therefore, an excellent diagnostic tool in evaluating heart failure.

Pericardial effusion

Pericardial effusion is recognized on echocardiography as an echo-free space between the walls of the cardiac chambers and the pericardium (Fig. 2.134a). Even quantities as small as 20–50 ml of pericardial fluid can be diagnosed by ultrasound. Computed tomography also readily demon-

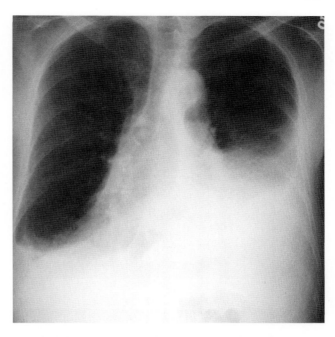

Fig. 2.133 Congestive cardiac failure. There are large bilateral pleural effusions. The heart is enlarged although it is difficult to measure it precisely because the pleural fluid obscures its borders.

strates pericardial fluid (Fig. 2.134b). The nature of the fluid cannot usually be ascertained, and needle aspiration of the fluid may be necessary; such aspiration is best performed under ultrasound control.

Valvular heart disease

Valve stenosis and incompetence are readily diagnosed and quantified by echocardiography. The role of the plain chest radiograph (see Fig. 2.123) is minor. It can reveal the size of the heart and show left atrial enlargement and severe calcification of the mitral or aortic valves. It can also show evidence of raised pulmonary venous pressure and any pulmonary oedema.

The important echocardiographic features of mitral stenosis are enlargement of the left atrium, thickening and calcification of the valve leaflets, and restriction of valve movement (Fig. 2.135). The gradient across the mitral valve can be calculated and orifice of the mitral valve during diastole can be measured; a valve area of less than 1 cm^2

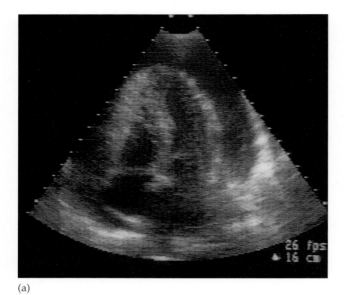

(a)

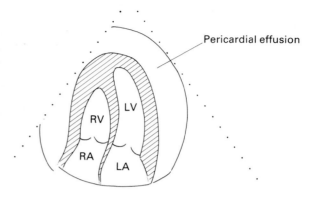

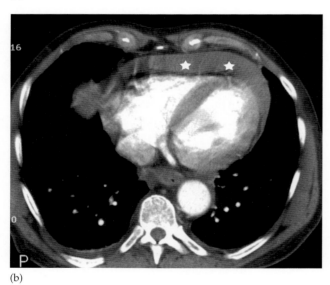

(b)

Fig. 2.134 (a) Large pericardial effusion on an apical four-chamber view echocardiogram. (b) CT scan showing fluid density (asterisks) in pericardium.

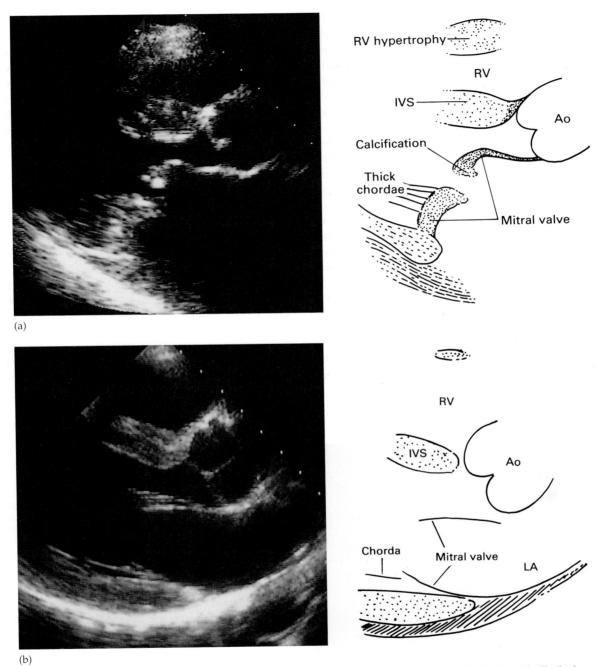

Fig. 2.135 Mitral stenosis. Two-dimensional echocardiogram – parasternal long axis view. (a) The mitral valve is markedly thickened and shows calcification. The image is during diastole when the valve should be open, but in this case the orifice is narrowed and opening is impaired. (b) Normal image for comparison. Ao, aorta; IVS, interventricular septum; LA, left atrium; RV, right ventricle. Courtesy of Andrew A. McLeod and Mark J. Managhan.

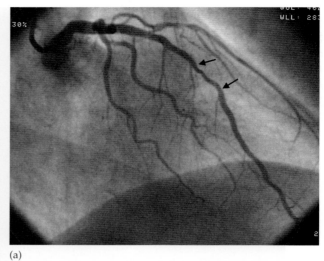

(a)

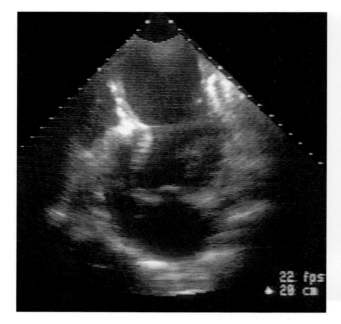

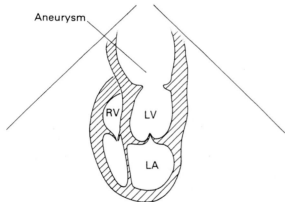

Fig. 2.138 Left ventricular aneurysm. Apical four-chamber view echocardiogram of a left ventricular aneurysm.

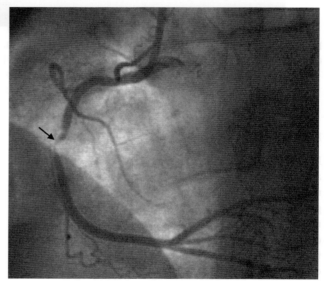

(b)

Fig. 2.139 Coronary artery disease. (a) Left coronary artery injection showing a moderate stenosis between the arrows in the mid left anterior descending artery. (b) Right coronary artery injection showing tight stenosis (arrow) of the mid right coronary artery.

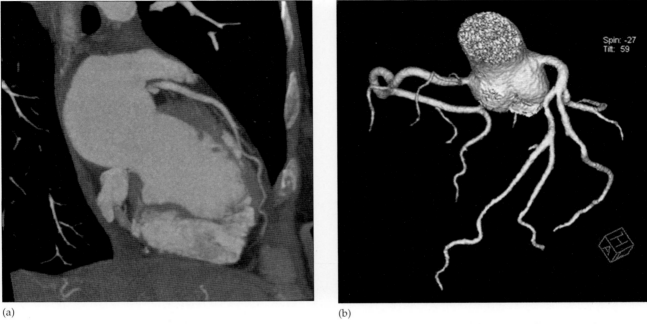

(a)   (b)

Fig. 2.140 CT coronary angiography – haemodynamically insignificant coronary artery disease. (a) Oblique coronal reconstruction showing the left coronary artery on the posterior surface of the heart. (b) Three-dimensional reconstruction of the aortic root and both coronary arteries.

this information, the appropriate treatment can be decided; this may be bypass surgery or balloon dilatation of the artery. Coronary arteriography is usually combined with a left ventricular angiogram which shows the contractility of the left ventricle and any concomitant mitral regurgitation. Computed tomography coronary angiography is making rapid progress, but its use is limited to specialist centres (Fig. 2.140).

Hypertensive heart disease and other myocardial problems

Ventricular hypertrophy without dilatation does not cause recognizable abnormality on plain chest films. Therefore, in systemic hypertension and various forms of cardiomyopathy, the chest x-ray only becomes abnor-

mal once ventricular dilatation has taken place. If there is a rise in left ventricular end-diastolic pressure, moderate left atrial enlargement and the signs of elevation of the pulmonary venous pressure may be seen. The shape of the heart is the same regardless of the cause of the myocardial disorder. The aorta is, however, large only in systemic hypertension.

Echocardiography in systemic hypertension shows symmetrical increase in the thickness of the left ventricular wall with a normal aortic valve. Once decompensation occurs, the cavity will enlarge. The pattern of hypertrophy may be difficult to differentiate from that of idiopathic hypertrophic cardiomyopathy (also known as hypertrophic obstructive cardiomyopathy – HOCM). In HOCM the hypertrophy is much greater in the ventricular septum than in the free wall. This asymmetrical septal hypertrophy is diagnostic of the condition (Fig. 2.141).

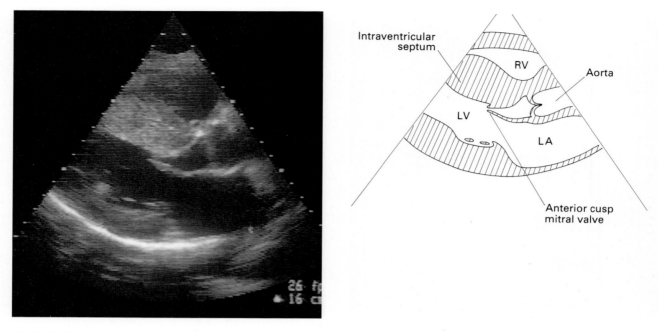

Fig. 2.141 Hypertrophic cardiomyopathy, parasternal long axis view echocardiogram. Note very thickened septum (almost 3 cm) and thickened ventricular walls. The anterior cusp of the mitral valve contacts the septum during diastole – a diagnostic feature of this condition. LA, left atrium; LV, left ventricle; RV, right ventricle.

Congenital heart disease

There are a large number of congenital malformations of the heart and great vessels. Frequently, they are multiple. Some conditions may be detected antenatally. Echocardiography, MRI, angiocardiography and, to a much lesser extent, plain chest radiography (see p. 101) are usually necessary for their elucidation. The topic is beyond the scope of this book.

Mammography

X-ray examination of the breast is carried out with dedicated equipment designed to demonstrate the soft tissues of the breast to advantage. A normal mammogram shows ductal and connective tissue in a background of fat. With increasing age, glandular tissue atrophies and cancers become easier to identify. The mammographic appearances of the normal breast vary greatly from one patient to another.

Mammography is used to screen women for breast cancer, and can also be helpful in patients presenting with a lump or lumpy areas in the breast. Magnetic resonance mammography is a developing subject with, at present, highly specific indications.

Mammographic signs

The cardinal mammographic signs of *carcinoma* are:
- A mass with ill-defined or spiculated borders (Fig. 2.142).
- Clustered, fine linear or irregular calcifications – so-called malignant microcalcifications (Fig. 2.143), which can on occasion be the only sign of breast cancer even in the absence of a visible mass.

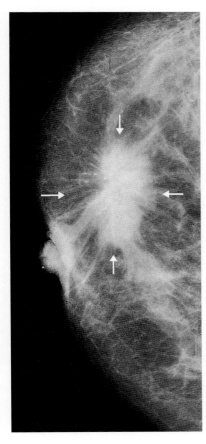

Fig. 2.142 Carcinoma of the breast. Mammogram showing irregular soft tissue mass (arrows) behind the nipple. Microcalcifications are present but difficult to see in reproduction.

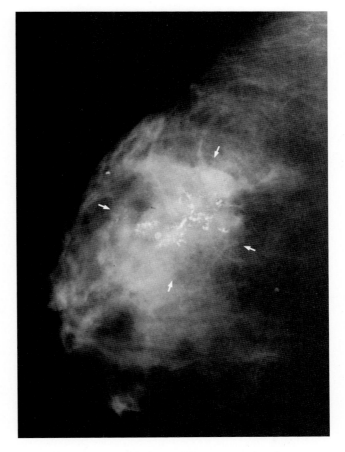

Fig. 2.143 Carcinoma of the breast. Mammogram showing ill-defined mass (arrows) containing numerous malignant linear and branching microcalcifications.

• Other signs that may point to the diagnosis of carcinoma are distortion of adjacent breast stroma and skin thickening.

Benign masses tend to be spherical with well-defined borders (Fig. 2.144a) and not infrequently contain calcification. The calcifications differ from malignant microcalcification in that they are larger, coarser and often ring-like in configuration (Fig. 2.145).

Ultrasound can be very helpful in determining whether a mass is a simple cyst (Fig. 2.144b), and, therefore, benign, or solid and, therefore, possibly a carcinoma.

Breast screening

Mammography can detect breast cancer in asymptomatic women even before the tumour is palpable (Fig. 2.146). There is evidence from large-scale trials that early detection by mammography can reduce the mortality from breast cancer in women over the age of 50. Though the degree of improved survival varies from country to country, in some series, reductions in mortality have been found to be as high as 30% of those screened.

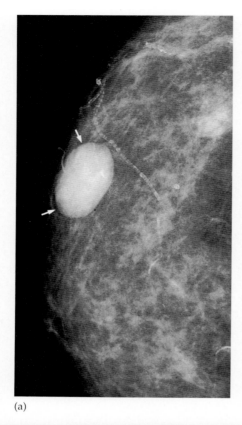

(a)

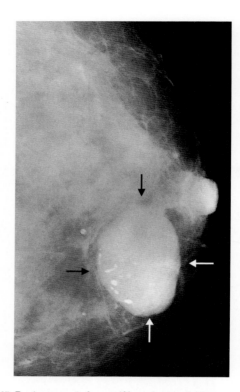

Fig. 2.145 Benign mass in breast (fibroadenoma). Mammogram showing mass (arrows) with very well-defined borders and coarse-structured calcification.

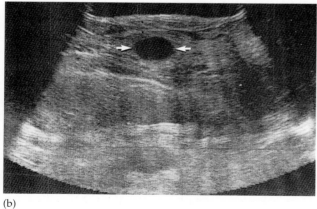

(b)

Fig. 2.144 Benign cyst of breast. (a) Mammogram showing oval, very well-defined mass without calcifications (arrows).
(b) The mass (arrows) was shown to be cystic on ultrasound; cyst aspiration was undertaken.

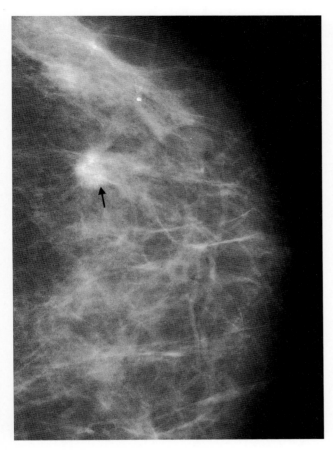

Fig. 2.146 Small (7 mm) primary breast carcinoma (arrow) detected by screening mammography. This tumour was asymptomatic and was not palpable.

Breast cancer is the most frequent cancer in women, affecting one woman in 12. In an attempt to reduce mortality, the UK government has decided to invite all women aged 50–69 years to attend a regular screening programme, currently consisting of a mammogram every three years.

It is expected that at least 50 cancers will be detected by mammography for every 10 000 women screened, but inevitably a number of breast carcinomas will escape detection.

Conversely, as with all screening tests, there are false-positive interpretations. For this reason, all patients with an abnormal mammogram are asked to attend an assessment clinic at which they undergo a physical examination, and further mammographic views, ultrasound, or needle biopsy as necessary. In some instances, follow-up mammography after a short interval is advised.

3

Plain Abdomen

The standard plain films of the abdomen are supine (Fig. 3.1) and erect anteroposterior (AP) views. An alternative to the erect AP view in patients unable to sit or stand is a lateral decubitus view (i.e. an AP film with the patient lying on his or her side). This view, like the erect view, uses a horizontal x-ray beam. The main purpose of horizontal beam films is to detect air–fluid levels and free intraperitoneal air.

How to look at a plain abdominal film

- Analyze the intestinal gas pattern and identify any dilated portion of the gastrointestinal tract.
- Look for gas outside the lumen of the bowel.
- Look for ascites and soft tissue masses in the abdomen and pelvis.
- If there are any calcifications, try to locate exactly where they lie.
- Assess the size of the liver and spleen.

Intestinal gas pattern

Relatively large amounts of gas are usually present in the stomach and colon in a normal patient. The stomach can be readily identified by its location above the transverse colon, by the band-like shadows of the gastric rugae in the supine view, and by the air–fluid level beneath the left hemidiaphragm in the erect view. The duodenum often contains air and shows a fluid level. There may be some gas in the normal small bowel, but it is rarely sufficient to outline the whole of a loop. Short fluid levels in the small and large bowel are

Diagnostic Imaging, 6th Edition. By Peter Armstrong, Martin Wastie and Andrea Rockall. Published 2009 by Blackwell Publishing. ISBN: 978-1-4051-7039.

normal. Fluid levels become abnormal when they are seen in dilated loops of bowel or when they are very numerous. If the bowel is dilated it is important to try and decide which portion is involved.

Dilatation of the bowel

The initial diagnosis of *intestinal obstruction* is usually made on clinical examination with the help of plain abdominal films. Dilatation of the bowel is the cardinal plain film sign of intestinal obstruction, and the pattern of dilatation is the key to the radiological distinction between small and large bowel obstruction. In small bowel obstruction, the small intestine is dilated down to the point of obstruction and the bowel beyond this point is either empty or of reduced caliber. In large bowel obstruction, the large, as well as the small, bowel is dilated down to the level of obstruction. Making this distinction depends on the ability to recognize which portions of bowel are dilated.

Dilated small bowel usually lies in the centre of the abdomen within the 'frame' of the large bowel (but the sigmoid and transverse colon may be redundant and may also lie in the centre of the abdomen, particularly when dilated). When the proximal and mid small intestine are dilated, the valvulae conniventes (plica circulares) can be identified. The valvulae conniventes are always closer together than the colonic haustra and cross the width of the bowel, often giving rise to the appearance known as 'a stack of coins' (Fig. 3.2). The distal small intestine has a relatively smooth outline and it may be difficult to distinguish the lower ileum and the sigmoid colon because both may be smooth in outline. The radius of curvature of the loops is sometimes helpful: the tighter the curve, the more likely the loop is to be dilated small bowel.

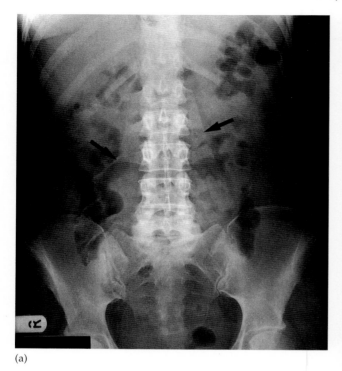

(a)

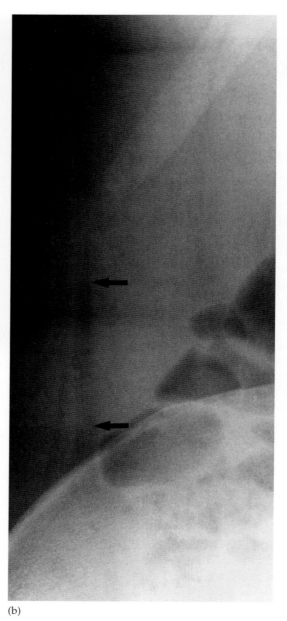

(b)

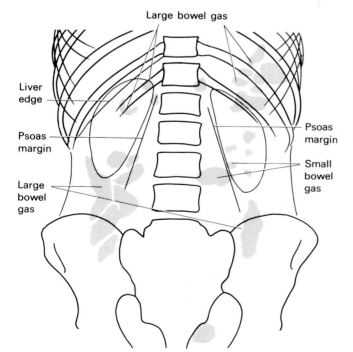

Fig. 3.1 Normal plain abdominal film. (a) Normal abdomen. The arrows point to the lateral borders of the psoas muscles. The renal outlines are obscured by the overlying colon. (b) Normal extraperitoneal fat stripe. Part of the right flank showing the layer of extraperitoneal fat (arrows), which indicates the position of the peritoneum.

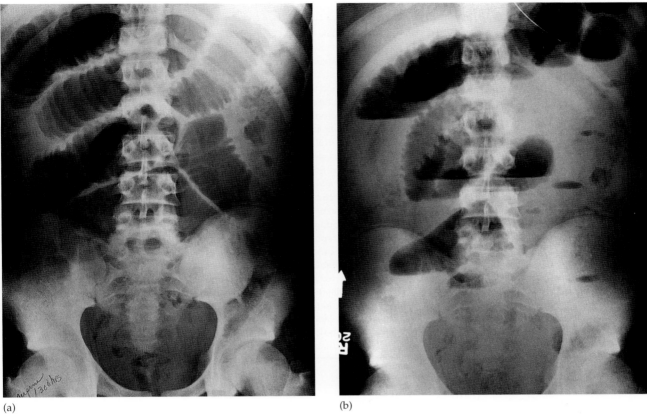

(a)　　　　　　　　　　　　　　　　　　　　　(b)

Fig. 3.2 Small bowel obstruction due to adhesions. (a) Supine. (b) Erect. The jejunal loops are markedly dilated and show air–fluid levels in the erect film. The jejunum is recognized by the presence of valvulae conniventes. The 'stack of coins' appearance is well demonstrated in the supine film. Note the large bowel contains less gas than normal.

The colon is recognized by its haustra, which usually form incomplete bands across the colonic gas shadows. Haustra are always present in the ascending and transverse colon, but may be absent distal to the splenic flexure. The presence of solid faeces is a useful and reliable indication of the position of the colon. The number of dilated loops is another valuable distinguishing feature between small and large bowel dilatation, because even with a very redundant colon the numerous layered loops that are so often seen with small bowel dilatation are not present.

If the cause or site of the obstruction is not evident from plain films, and immediate exploratory surgery is not indicated, then computed tomography (CT) or a contrast follow-through study may be helpful. Computed tomography can demonstrate the site of obstruction by showing the location of the transition from dilated to collapsed bowel, and can confirm or exclude a mass at the site of obstruction. A contrast follow-through is less informative and takes longer to perform.

Dilatation of the bowel occurs in a number of conditions in addition to mechanical bowel obstruction, notably: paralytic ileus, acute ischaemia and inflammatory bowel disease. The radiological diagnosis of these phenomena depends mainly on the pattern of distribution of the dilated loops (see Table 3.1).

Table 3.1 Patterns of bowel dilatation in gastrointestinal conditions

Diagnosis	Pattern of bowel dilatation
Mechanical obstruction of the small bowel (Fig. 3.2)	Small bowel dilatation, but colon is normal or reduced in calibre. Computed tomography may also show any responsible tumour or inflammatory mass
Mechanical obstruction of the large bowel (Fig. 3.3)	Dilatation of the colon down to the point of obstruction. May be accompanied by small bowel dilatation if the ileocaecal valve becomes incompetent
Generalized paralytic ileus (Fig. 3.4)	Both the large and the small bowel are dilated. The dilatation often extends down into the sigmoid colon and gas may be present in the rectum. It may be difficult to differentiate from low large bowel obstruction
Localized peritonitis	Often causes dilatation of the bowel loops adjacent to the inflammatory process (which may be specifically visible on computed tomography), giving rise to the so-called sentinel loops seen, for example, in appendicitis and pancreatitis
Gastroenteritis	Variable pattern. Some patients have a normal film and some show excess fluid levels without dilatation, whereas some mimic paralytic ileus and others mimic small bowel obstruction
Small bowel infarction	May mimic obstruction of the small bowel or obstruction of the large bowel depending on the distribution of the ischaemia
Closed loop obstruction (Fig. 3.5)	The diagnosis depends on whether the loop in question contains air. If it does, as for example in a caecal or sigmoid volvulus, the dilated loop is seen filled with gas in a characteristic shape. If the closed loop is filled with fluid – the common situation in most obstructed hernias – it may not be visible
Toxic dilatation of the colon (Fig. 3.6)	Usually, the dilatation is maximal in the transverse colon; indeed, the descending colon may be narrower than normal. The haustra are lost or grossly abnormal and the swollen islands of mucosa between the ulcers can be recognized as polypoid shadows. If the transverse colon is more than 6 cm in diameter in a patient with colitis, toxic dilatation should be strongly suspected

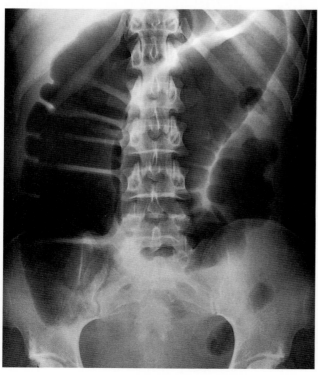

Fig. 3.3 Large bowel obstruction due to carcinoma at the splenic flexure. There is marked dilatation of the large bowel from the caecum to the splenic flexure.

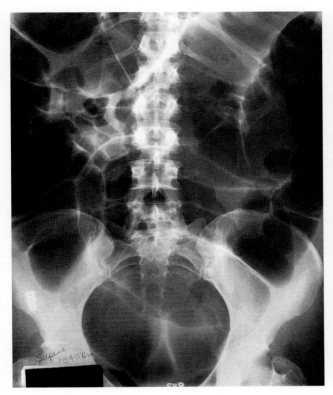

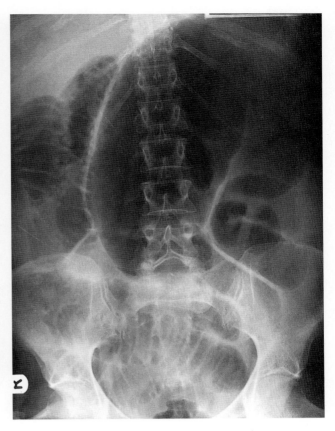

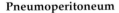

Fig. 3.4 Paralytic ileus. There is considerable dilatation of the whole of the large bowel extending well down into the pelvis. Small bowel dilatation is also seen.

Fig. 3.5 Volvulus of the caecum. The twisted obstructed caecum and ascending colon now lie on the left side of the abdomen and appear as a large gas shadow. There is also extensive small bowel dilatation from obstruction by the volvulus.

Pneumoperitoneum

The radiological diagnosis of perforation of the gastrointestinal tract is based on recognizing free gas in the peritoneal cavity (pneumoperitoneum) (Fig. 3.7). The most common cause of spontaneous pneumoperitoneum is a perforated peptic ulcer and two-thirds of such cases are recognizable radiologically. The largest quantities of free gas are seen after colonic perforation, and the smallest amounts with leakage from the small bowel. A pneumoperitoneum is very rare in acute appendicitis even if the appendix has perforated.

Free intraperitoneal air is a normal finding after a laparotomy or laparoscopy. In adults, all the air is usually absorbed within 7 days. In children, the air absorbs much faster, usually within 24 hours. An increase in the amount of air on successive films indicates continuing leakage of air.

Pneumoperitoneum under the right hemidiaphragm is usually easy to recognize on an erect abdominal film as a curvilinear collection of gas between the line of the diaphragm and the opacity of the liver. Free gas under the left hemidiaphragm is more difficult to identify because of the overlapping gas shadows of the stomach and splenic flexure of colon. Gas in these organs may mimic free intraperitoneal air when none is present.

Gas under the diaphragm is much easier to diagnose on an erect chest film than on an upright abdominal film.

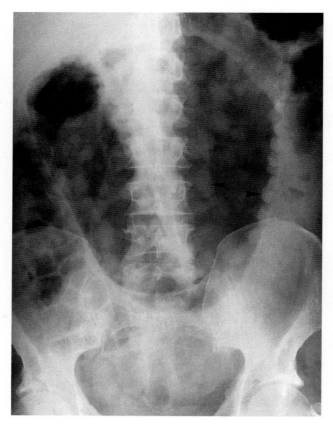

Fig. 3.6 Toxic dilatation of the large bowel from ulcerative colitis. The dilatation is maximal in the transverse colon. Note the loss of haustra and islands of hypertrophied mucosa. Two of these pseudopolyps are arrowed.

If there is doubt about the presence of a pneumoperitoneum, a lateral decubitus film will show the air collectedbeneath the flank. It is important to realize that when the patient is lying flat the free gas collects centrally beneath the abdominal wall and is very difficult to identify on supine films.

Gas in an abscess

Gas in an abdominal (Fig. 3.8) or pelvic abscess produces a very variable pattern on plain films. It may form either small bubbles or larger collections of air, both of which could be confused with gas within the bowel. Fluid levels in abscesses may be seen on a horizontal ray film. As abscesses are mass lesions, they displace the adjacent structures; for example, the diaphragm is elevated with a subphrenic abscess, and the bowel is displaced by pericolic and pancreatic abscesses. Pleural effusion or pulmonary collapse/consolidation are very common in association with subphrenic abscess. Ultrasound and CT are extensively used to evaluate abdominal abscesses (see p. 273 and 286).

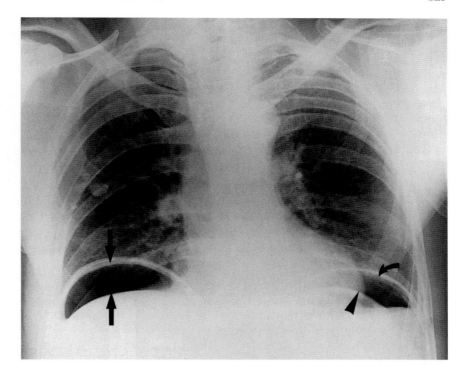

Fig. 3.7 Free gas in the peritoneal cavity. On this chest radiograph, air can be seen under the domes of both hemidiaphragms. The curved arrow points to the left hemidiaphragm and the arrow head to the wall of the stomach. The two vertical arrows on the right point to the diaphragm and upper border of the liver.

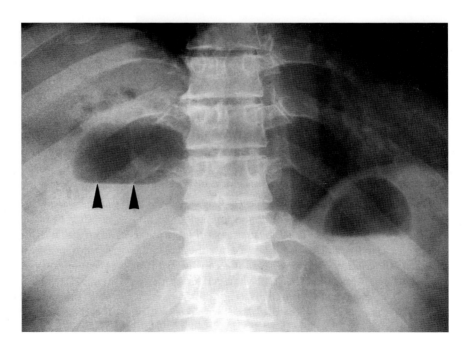

Fig. 3.8 Gas in a right subphrenic abscess. There are several collections of gas within the abscess. The largest of these contains a fluid level (arrows). The air–fluid level under the left hemidiaphragm is normal. It is in the stomach.

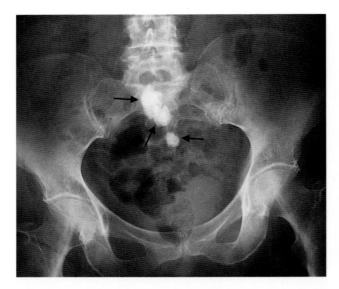

Fig. 3.13 Calcified mesenteric lymph nodes from old tuberculosis (arrows).

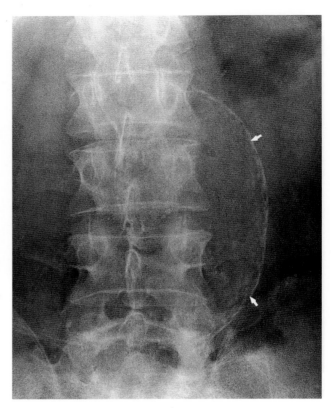

Fig. 3.14 Calcified abdominal aortic aneurysm (arrows). The aneurysm measured 8 cm in diameter on the lateral view.

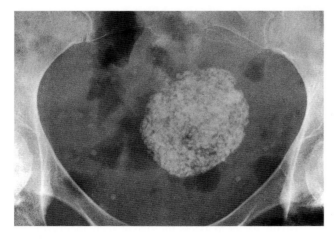

Fig. 3.15 Calcification in a large uterine fibroid.

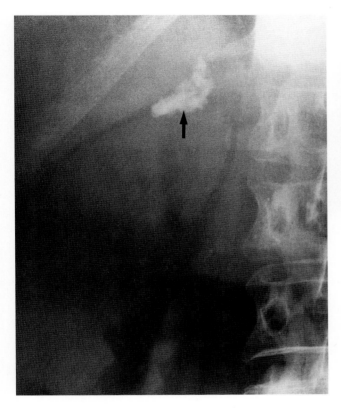

Fig. 3.16 Adrenal calcification (arrow).

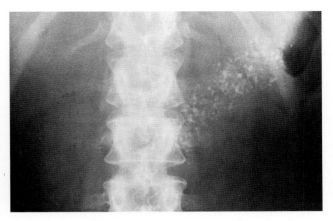

Fig. 3.17 Pancreatic calcification.

• *Malignant ovarian masses* occasionally contain visible calcium. The only benign ovarian lesion that is visibly calcified is the *dermoid cyst*, which may contain various calcified components, of which teeth are the commonest (Fig. 7.10b, p. 262).

• *Adrenal calcification* (Fig. 3.16) occurs after adrenal haemorrhage, after tuberculosis and occasionally in adrenal tumours. However, the majority of patients with adrenal calcification are asymptomatic healthy people in whom the cause of the calcification is unclear. Only a minority of patients with Addison's disease have adrenal calcification.

• *Liver calcification* occurs in hepatomas and rarely in other liver tumours. Hydatid cysts, abscesses and tuberculosis may also calcify over time.

• *Gall stones* are discussed on p. 196.

• *Splenic calcification* is rarely of clinical significance. It is seen in cysts, infarcts, old haematomas and following tuberculosis.

• *Pancreatic calcification* occurs in chronic pancreatitis. The calcifications are mainly small calculi within the pancreas. The position of the calcification usually enables the diagnosis to be made without difficulty (Fig. 3.17).

• *Faecoliths*. Calcified faecoliths may be seen in diverticula of the colon or in the appendix (Fig. 3.18). Appendiceal faecoliths are an important radiological observation, as the presence of an appendolith is a strong indication that the patient has acute appendicitis, often with gangrene and perforation. However, only a small proportion of patients with appendicitis have a radiologically visible appendolith.

• *Renal stones and other calcifications of the urinary tract* are discussed in Chapter 6.

Plain films of the liver and spleen

Substantial enlargement of the liver has to occur before it can be recognized on a plain abdominal film. As the liver enlarges it extends well below the costal margin displacing the hepatic flexure, transverse colon and right kidney downwards and displacing the stomach to the left. The diaphragm may also be elevated.

Occasionally, there is a tongue-like extension of the right lobe into the right iliac fossa. This is a normal variant known

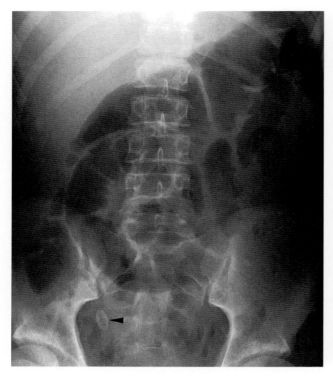

Fig. 3.18 Appendolith. The oval calcified shadow (arrow) is a faecolith in the appendix. The patient had perforated appendicitis. Note the dilated loops of small bowel in the centre of the abdomen due to peritonitis – the so-called sentinel loops.

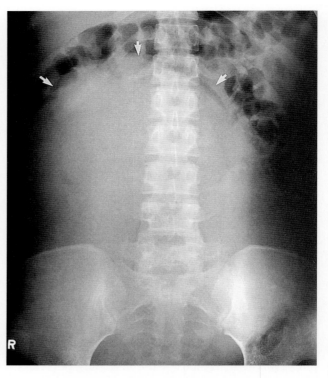

Fig. 3.19 Mass arising out of pelvis (arrows) displacing bowel to the sides of the abdomen. The mass was a large cystadeno-carcinoma of the ovary.

as a *Reidl's lobe* and should not be confused with generalized liver enlargement.

As the spleen enlarges, the tip becomes visible in the left upper quadrant below the lower ribs. Eventually, it may fill the left side of the abdomen and even extend across the midline into the right lower quadrant. The splenic flexure of the colon and the left kidney are displaced downwards and medially, and the stomach is displaced to the right.

Abdominal and pelvic masses

Attempting to diagnose the nature of an abdominal mass on a plain film is notoriously difficult, and ultrasound, CT or MRI are the appropriate imaging modalities. The site of the mass, displacement of adjacent structures and presence of calcification are important diagnostic signs but plain films are unable to distinguish between solid and cystic masses.

An enlarged bladder can be seen as a mass arising from the pelvis displacing loops of bowel. In females, uterine and ovarian enlargement also appear as masses arising from the pelvis. Ovarian cysts can become very large, almost filling the abdomen and displacing the bowel to the sides of the abdomen (Fig. 3.19).

Retroperitoneal tumours and lymph nodes, when large, become visible on plain films. Renal masses, especially cysts and hydronephrosis, can become large and appear as masses in the flank. With retroperitoneal masses the outline of the psoas muscle may become invisible.

4

Gastrointestinal Tract

The previous chapter discussed plain films in detail, but for most intestinal disorders some form of endoscopy or imaging examination is necessary.

Endoscopy is often the first investigation, because it shows mucosal lesions directly and also allows biopsy material to be obtained. Imaging is pivotal for showing processes that cannot be diagnosed or assessed endoscopically, for example to visualize the bowel beyond a stricture that cannot be traversed by an endoscope. The indications for barium examinations have dramatically reduced as endoscopy services have developed. Computed tomography (CT) techniques such as CT pneumocolon and virtual colonoscopy have now been widely taken up, magnetic resonance imaging (MRI) is now used routinely for the local staging of rectal carcinoma, and fluorodeoxyglucose positron emission tomography (FDG-PET) is used to identify sites of metastatic disease in selected patients with a primary carcinoma of the gastrointestinal (GI) tract.

Imaging techniques – general principles

Contrast examinations

Barium sulphate is the best contrast medium for demonstrating the gastrointestinal tract on conventional radiographic studies, e.g. fluoroscopy (screening). It produces excellent opacification, good coating of the mucosa and is completely inert. Its disadvantages are that the barium may solidify and impact proximal to a colonic or rectal stricture, and it may cause a severe inflammatory peritonitis if there is a barium leak from the bowel. In addition, patients must

Diagnostic Imaging, 6th Edition. By Peter Armstrong, Martin Wastie and Andrea Rockall. Published 2009 by Blackwell Publishing. ISBN: 978-1-4051-7039.

be reasonably mobile in order to undertake a complete barium study. A water-soluble contrast medium, such as Gastrografin, is predominantly used when perforations or anastomotic leaks are suspected (as it does not cause an inflammatory peritonitis), in cases where small bowel obstruction is suspected and in specific circumstances in paediatric patients. It has several disadvantages: it is hypertonic and soon becomes diluted; it is an irritant should it inadvertently enter the lungs; and it is less radio-opaque than barium.

Most barium and Gastrografin examinations are carried out under fluoroscopic control so that the passage of contrast can be observed on a television monitor and the radiologist can position the patient to demonstrate and record clearly any abnormality. One of the values of fluoroscopy is to ensure that an abnormality has a constant appearance. Peristaltic waves are transitory and so can be easily distinguished from a true narrowing, which is constant.

Barium examinations of stomach and colon (and in some cases small bowel) are usually undertaken using a double-contrast technique: the mucosa is initially coated with barium and then the lumen is distended by introducing air or some other gas, often in combination with an injection of a short-acting smooth muscle relaxant.

Computed tomography

Unlike conventional barium examinations and endoscopic procedures, CT can show the full width of the wall of the structures in question as well as surrounding fat. Modern multidetector CT scanners with 64 detectors or more, allow very rapid acquisition of high-resolution images, which may be reformatted into other imaging planes such as sagittal or coronal planes. In addition, the lumen of the gastrointestinal tract may be evaluated using either Gastrografin as the contrast agent, e.g. standard abdominal CT, or air as the contrast agent, e.g. CT pneumocolon and virtual colonoscopy (see p. 160). Computed tomography is therefore useful for diagnosing and staging GI tumours, as well as for assessing the complications of treatment such as surgery and chemotherapy. It can be used in elderly or infirm patients, because a CT examination is much less demanding for the patient than either a barium enema or colonoscopy. CT can be used to diagnose appendicitis and is useful in patients with intestinal obstruction and suspected damage to the bowel wall following trauma.

Ultrasound examinations

Ultrasound can detect intra-abdominal fluid and assess the bowel wall in certain situations, but gives limited information about the bowel mucosa. Ultrasound is used for the diagnosis of infantile pyloric stenosis, intussusception and in cases of suspected appendicitis when the diagnosis is not obvious clinically (see Fig. 4.65, p. 169). The use of endoscopic ultrasound is a specialized procedure which has a variety of uses, notably assessing the depth of invasion of tumours in the oesophagus, gastric or rectal wall and diagnosing small tumours in the pancreas and wall of the duodenum.

MRI

Magnetic resonance imaging of the gastrointestinal tract is limited, due to artefacts caused by peristalsis of the bowel. Currently, its major use is for assessing the local spread of rectal carcinoma prior to surgical resection, and for assessing perianal fistula and abscess formation (see Fig. 4.43, p. 156). The role in the assessment of oesophageal cancer is currently under development, and some progress is being made in the evaluation of the large and small bowel on MRI, using newly developed fast MR sequences and specific oral contrast media.

Nuclear medicine

Nuclear medicine studies are used for assessing bowel transit, particularly gastric emptying. Labelled white cells can detect sites of inflammatory bowel disease and sepsis and certain radiopharmaceuticals can localize neuroendocrine tumours in the GI tract. FDG-PET and FDG-PET/CT are used to demonstrate metastases in patients with a malignancy of the gastrointestinal tract.

Basic descriptive terms

A number of basic terms are used to describe the appearances on imaging studies of the gastrointestinal tract:
• *Mucosal pattern*. The normal mucosa of the stomach and small bowel is thrown into folds, which are exaggerated by peristaltic contractions, whereas the mucosa of the distended colon and rectum is smooth. Diseased mucosa may be abnormally smooth or abnormally irregular.
• *Ulceration*. An ulcer is a breach of a mucosal surface that becomes visible when the crater contains barium (Fig. 4.1).
• *Filling defect* is a term used to describe any process which prevents the normal filling of the lumen. There are three types of filling defects: intraluminal filling defects (e.g. food), which are surrounded by barium (Fig. 4.2a); intramural filling defects (e.g. a carcinoma or leiomyoma), which cause an indentation on the lumen and are not completely surrounded by barium (Fig. 4.2b); and extramural filling defects compressing the lumen from the outside (e.g. enlarged pancreas or lymph nodes), in which the mucosa is preserved but is stretched over the filling defect (Fig. 4.2c).
• *A stricture* is a circumferential narrowing. A stricture must be differentiated from the transient narrowing which occurs with normal peristalsis. A stricture may have tapering ends (Fig. 4.3a) or it may end abruptly and have overhanging edges giving an appearance known as 'shouldering' (Fig. 4.3b). Shouldering is an important radiological sign of malignancy.

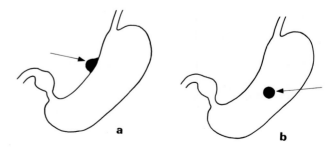

Fig. 4.1 Ulceration. (a) In profile the ulcer is seen as an outward projection (arrow). (b) *En face* the ulcer appears rounded (arrow).

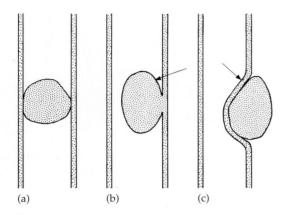

Fig. 4.2 Filling defects in the bowel. (a) Intraluminal. (b) Intramural. Note the sharp angle (arrow) made with the wall. (c) Extramural. There is a shallow angle (arrow) with the wall of the bowel.

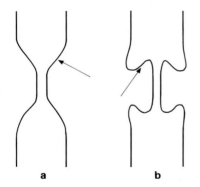

Fig. 4.3 Stricture. (a) Tapering ends (arrow). (b) Overhanging edges or shouldering (arrow).

Oesophagus

Techniques

Plain films

Plain films do not normally show the oesophagus unless it is very dilated (e.g. achalasia), but they are of use in demonstrating an opaque foreign body such as a bone lodged in the oesophagus (Fig. 4.4a). Plain films are also used to check the position of a nasogastric tube, to ensure that the tube travels down through the oesophagus and into the stomach, rather than down into one of the main bronchi or an oesophageal pouch (Fig. 4.4b and c).

The barium swallow is the standard contrast examination employed to visualize the oesophagus. The use of CT and endoscopic ultrasound is limited to the assessment of oesophageal carcinoma.

Barium examination of the oesophagus

The patient swallows a gas-producing agent to distend the oesophagus, followed by barium, and its passage down the oesophagus is observed on a television monitor. Films are taken with the oesophagus both full of barium to show the outline, and following the passage of the barium to show the mucosal pattern.

The oesophagus has a smooth outline when full of barium. When empty and contracted, barium normally lies in between the folds of mucosa, which appear as three or four long, straight parallel lines (Fig. 4.5).

Peristaltic waves can be observed during fluoroscopy. They move smoothly along the oesophagus to propel the barium rapidly into the stomach. It is important not to confuse a contraction wave with a true narrowing: a narrowing is constant whereas a contraction wave is transitory. Sometimes the contraction waves do not occur in an orderly fashion but are pronounced and prolonged giving the oesophagus an undulated appearance (Fig. 4.6). These so-called tertiary contractions usually occur in the elderly, and in most instances they do not give rise to symptoms. Occasionally, tertiary contractions cause dysphagia.

Endoscopy is the primary investigation in patients with dysphagia. In centres where expert endoscopy is readily available, the indications for barium or Gastrografin swallows are limited to the following:
• Swallowing disorders, including confirming or excluding a pharyngeal pouch.
• Determining the length of oesophageal strictures.
• Assessing possible mild gastro-oesophageal reflux.
• Assessing the integrity of an oesophageal anastomosis.
• Following obesity reduction surgery and anti-reflux surgery.

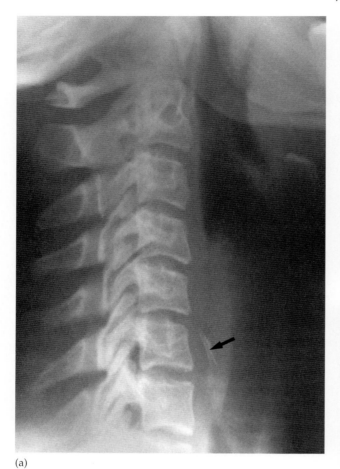

(a)

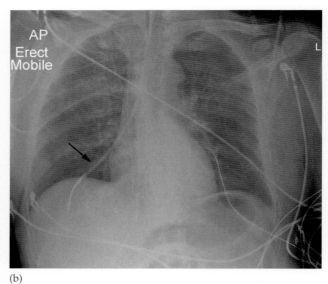

(b)

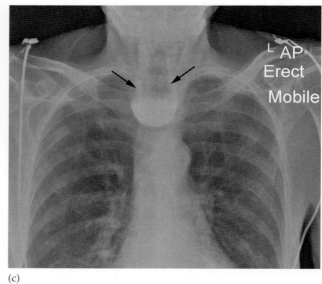

(c)

Fig. 4.4 (a) Foreign body in the oesophagus. Lateral view of the neck showing a chicken bone (arrow) lodged in the upper end of the oesophagus. (b) Nasogastric tube has been placed down the right main bronchus (arrow). (c) Nasogastric tube has coiled within an oesophageal pouch (arrows). Note that barium has been used to demonstrate the pouch.

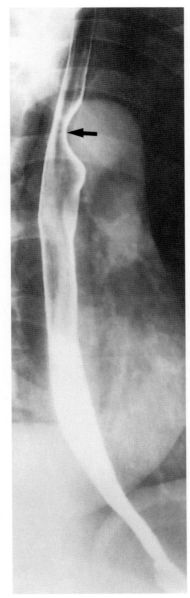

Fig. 4.5 Normal oesophagus. (a) Full of barium to show the smooth outline and indentation made by the aortic arch (arrow). (b) Film taken after the main volume of barium has passed, to show the parallel mucosal folds.

(a)   (b)

CT of the oesophagus

Computed tomography is usually performed following administration of a short-acting intravenous smooth muscle relaxant and ingestion of oral water to distend the oesophagus. Intravenous iodinated contrast medium is injected during the scan.

FDG-PET or PET/CT of oesophagus

In patients with oesophageal carcinoma, a PET study may be performed to identify any occult metastases prior to deciding whether to undertake radical surgery or to treat with radiotherapy and chemotherapy.

Oesophageal abnormalities

Oesophageal carcinoma is usually first diagnosed at upper GI endoscopy or barium swallow and the diagnosis is confirmed by biopsy at endoscopy. Carcinomas usually involve the full circumference of the oesophagus to form a stricture, which can be readily demonstrated at barium swallow examination. It may occur anywhere in the oesophagus, shows an irregular lumen with shouldered edges and is often several centimetres in length (Fig. 4.7). A soft tissue mass may be visible.

Assessing the extent of the tumour is carried out by endoscopic ultrasound and CT examination. *Endoscopic ultrasound* (EUS) is able to demonstrate the layers of the oesophageal wall and the surrounding lymph nodes. Oesophageal cancer is seen as a hypoechoic mass and the depth of invasion of the tumour into the oesophageal wall may be assessed (Fig. 4.8). Endoscopic ultrasound may also be used to assess involvement of regional lymph nodes; EUS is highly accurate in the local staging of early cancers but is limited when the endoscope does not fit into the lumen of a narrow tumour stenosis. *CT* is performed following an intravenous smooth muscle relaxant while swallowing water. The tumour is seen as a thickening of the oesophageal wall and the length of the tumour can usually be assessed (Fig. 4.9). CT may also show invasion of the mediastinum or adjacent structures, evidence of metastatic spread to lymph nodes, liver or lungs (Fig. 4.10). The role of *MRI* in staging oesophageal carcinoma is under investigation. Assessment of

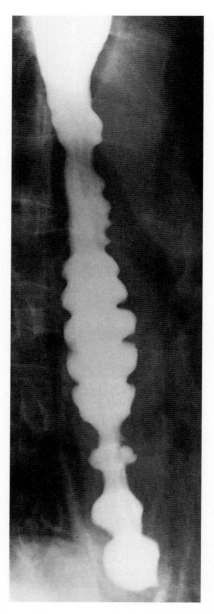

Fig. 4.6 Tertiary contractions (corkscrew oesophagus) giving the oesophagus an undulated appearance.

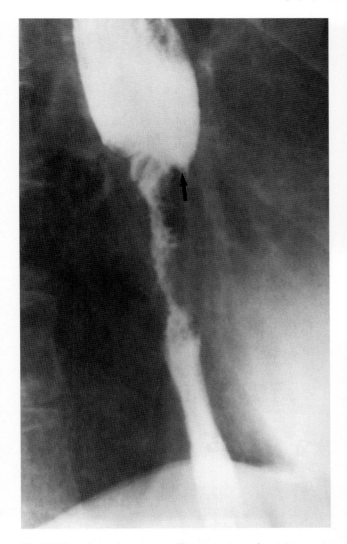

Fig. 4.7 Oesophageal carcinoma. There is an irregular stricture with shouldering (arrow) at the upper end.

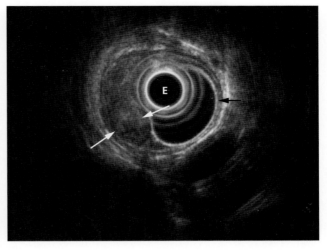

Fig. 4.8 Endoscopic ultrasound of oesophageal carcinoma. Note the thickening of the oesophageal mucosa (between white arrows). A normal part of the oesophagus is indicated by the black arrow. E, endoscope.

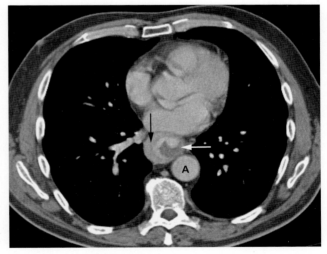

Fig. 4.9 Oesophageal cancer on CT. There is thickening and enhancement of the right lateral oesophageal wall (black arrow). In this case, the left wall of the oesophagus is relatively normal (white arrow). A, aorta.

response to treatment and follow-up of patients with carcinoma of the oesophagus is usually done with CT. *FDG-PET* or *FDG-PET/CT* is used to determine the presence of metastatic disease in selected cases and has a higher accuracy than CT in the detection of distant metastases (Fig. 4.11).

Peptic strictures can be demonstrated at barium swallow. They are found at the lower end of the oesophagus and are almost invariably associated with a hiatus hernia and gastro-oesophageal reflux and, therefore, the stricture may

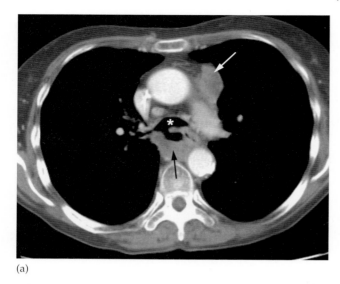

(a)

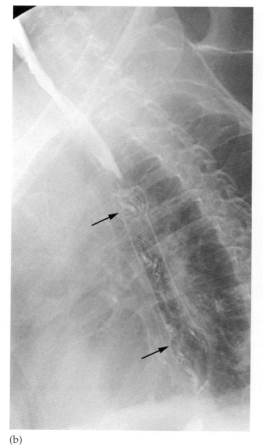

(b)

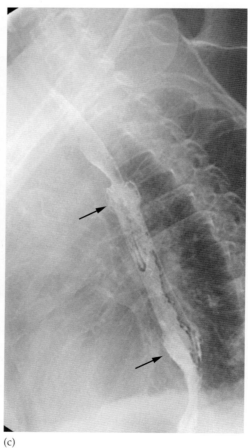

(c)

Fig. 4.10 (a) Large oesophageal cancer (black arrow) has eroded into the posterior aspect of the carina (*) forming a fistula. Enlarged lymph nodes are present in the anterior mediastinum (white arrow). (b) A stent has been placed across the fistula (arrows). (c) Barium swallow confirms occlusion of the fistula, with no leakage of barium into the bronchial tree.

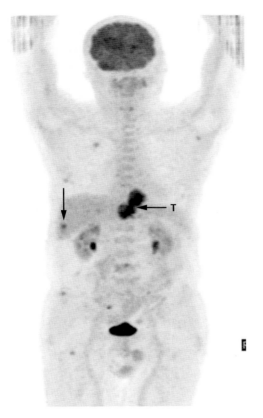

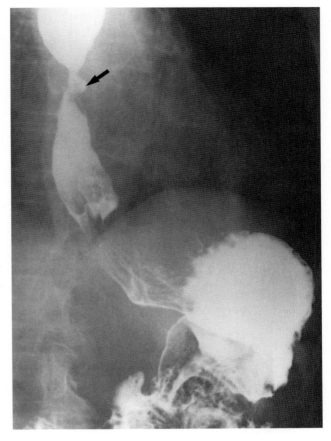

Fig. 4.11 FDG-PET/CT in a patient with oesophageal carcinoma. (a) PET component of the study demonstrates the primary tumour (T) at the lower oesophagus. In addition, there is a hot spot over the liver (long arrow).

Fig. 4.12 Peptic stricture due to gastro-oesophageal reflux in a patient with a hiatus hernia. There is a short smooth stricture at the oesophagogastric junction with an ulcer crater within the stricture (arrow).

be some distance above the diaphragm. Peptic strictures are characteristically short and have smooth outlines with tapering ends (Fig. 4.12).

Achalasia is a neuromuscular abnormality resulting in failure of relaxation at the cardiac sphincter, which presents at barium swallow examination as a smooth, tapered narrowing, always at the lower end of the oesophagus (Fig. 4.13). There is associated dilatation of the oesophagus, which often shows absent peristalsis. The dilated oesophagus usually contains food residues and may be visible on the plain chest radiograph. The lungs may show consolidation and bronchiectasis from aspiration of the oesophageal

contents. The stomach gas bubble is usually absent because the oesophageal contents act as a water seal, but this sign is not diagnostic of achalasia as it is seen in other causes of oesophageal obstruction and can occasionally be observed in healthy people.

Corrosive strictures are the result of swallowing corrosives such as acids or alkalis. They are long strictures that begin at the level of the aortic arch. As with the other benign strictures, they are usually smooth with tapered ends on barium swallow examinations, but may be irregular (Fig. 4.14).

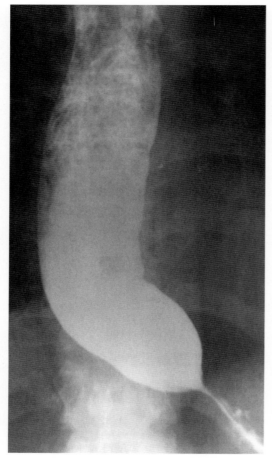

Fig. 4.13 Achalasia. The very dilated oesophagus containing food residues shows a smooth narrowing at its lower end.

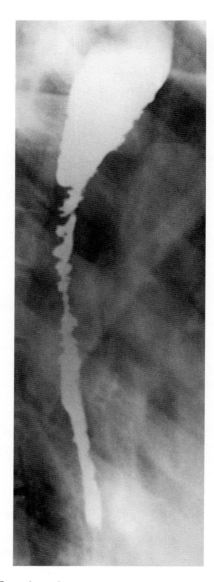

Fig. 4.14 Corrosive stricture.

Leiomyomas cause a smooth, rounded indentation into the lumen of the oesophagus. A soft tissue mass may be seen in the mediastinum indicating extraluminal extension.

An anomalous right subclavian artery, which, instead of coming from the innominate artery, arises as the last major branch from the aortic arch, gives rise to a characteristic short, smooth narrowing as it crosses behind the upper oesophagus (Fig. 4.15).

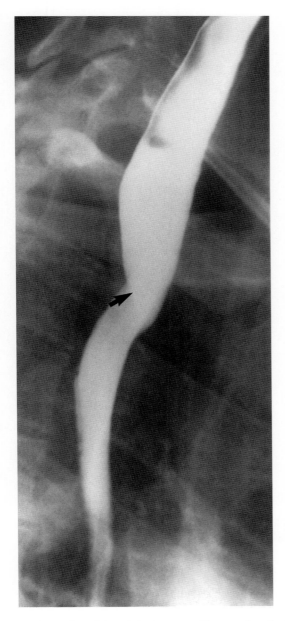

Fig. 4.15 Anomalous right subclavian artery. There is a localized indentation caused by the anomalous artery as it passes behind the oesophagus (arrow).

Dilatation of the oesophagus

There are two main types of oesophageal dilatation – obstructive and non-obstructive:

• Dilatation due to obstruction is associated with a visible stricture. The patient with a carcinoma usually presents with dysphagia before the oesophagus becomes very dilated. On the other hand, a markedly dilated oesophagus indicates a very long-standing condition, usually achalasia or occasionally a benign stricture.

• Dilatation without obstruction occurs in scleroderma. The disease involves the oesophageal muscle resulting in dilatation of the oesophagus, which resembles an inert tube with no peristaltic movement so that barium does not flow from the oesophagus into the stomach unless the patient stands upright.

An oesophageal web is a thin, shelf-like projection arising from the anterior wall of the cervical portion of the oesophagus. To demonstrate it, that part of the oesophagus must be full of barium (Fig. 4.16). A web may be an isolated finding, but the combination of a web, dysphagia and iron deficiency anaemia is known as Plummer–Vinson syndrome.

Oesophageal diverticula are saccular outpouchings, which are often seen as chance findings, in the intrathoracic portion of the oesophagus. One type of diverticulum, the pharyngeal pouch or Zenker's diverticulum (Fig. 4.17) is important as it may give rise to symptoms caused by retention of food and pressure upon the oesophagus. A pharyngeal pouch arises through a congenital weakness in the inferior constrictor muscle of the pharynx and comes to lie behind the oesophagus near the midline. It may reach a very large size and can cause displacement and compression of the oesophagus.

In *oesophageal atresia*, the oesophagus ends as a blind pouch in the upper mediastinum. Several different types exist (Fig. 4.18), but the most frequent is for the upper part of the oesophagus to be a blind sac with a fistula between the lower segment of the oesophagus and the tracheobronchial tree. A plain abdominal film will show air in the bowel if a fistula is present between the tracheobronchial tree and the oesophagus distal to the atretic segment.

The diagnosis of oesophageal atresia is made by passing a soft tube into the oesophagus and showing that the tube holds up or coils in the blind-ending pouch. The use

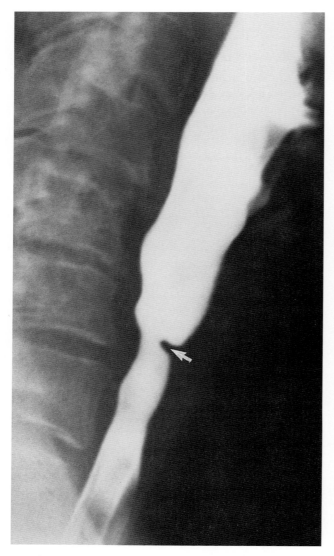

Fig. 4.16 Oesophageal web. There is a shelf-like indentation (arrow) from the anterior wall of the upper oesophagus.

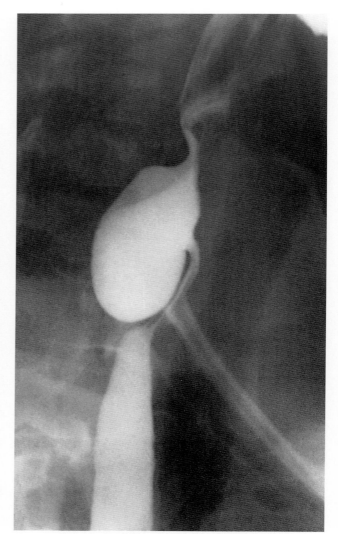

Fig. 4.17 Pharyngeal pouch (Zenker's diverticulum). The pouch is lying behind the oesophagus, which is displaced forward.

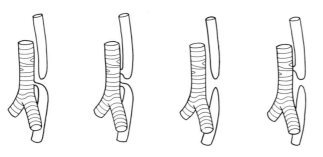

Fig. 4.18 Oesophageal atresia. Diagram of the various types. The first two types also have an oesophagotracheal fistula distal to the atretic segment and will show air in the stomach.

of contrast agents is potentially dangerous because the contrast may cause respiratory problems if it spills over into the trachea.

Stomach and duodenum

Techniques

Barium meal examination

Barium meal examination is now rarely performed. The usual technique involves instructing the patient to fast for at least 6 hours prior to the examination. The stomach is distended with a gas-producing agent, and an intravenous injection of a short-acting smooth muscle relaxant is often given. The patient drinks about 200 ml of barium. Films are taken in various positions with the patient both erect and lying flat, so that each part of the stomach and duodenum is shown distended by barium and also distended with air but coated with barium to show the mucosal pattern (Fig. 4.19). The duodenal cap or bulb arises just beyond the short pyloric canal, and the duodenum forms a loop around the head of the pancreas to reach the duodeno-jejunal flexure. Diverticula arising beyond the first part of duodenum are a common finding and are usually without clinical significance (Fig. 4.20).

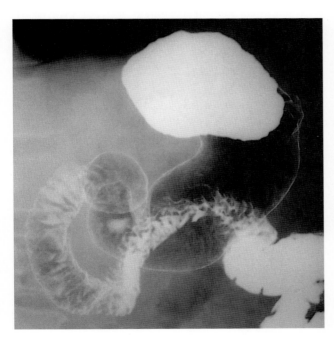

Fig. 4.19 Normal stomach and duodenum: double-contrast barium meal. On this supine view, barium collects in the fundus of the stomach. The body and the antrum of the stomach together with the duodenal cap and loop are coated with barium and distended with gas. Note how the fourth part of the duodenum and duodenojejunal flexure are superimposed on the body of the stomach.

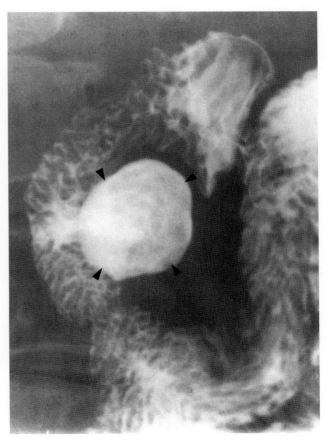

Fig. 4.20 Duodenal diverticulum arising from the second part of the duodenum (arrows).

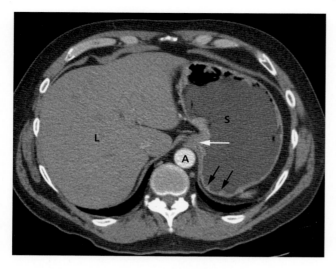

Fig. 4.21 CT of normal stomach. The stomach has been distended by oral water contrast and the use of an intravenous smooth muscle relaxant. Some normal rugal folds are still visible (black arrows). Note the gastro-oesophageal junction (white arrow). S, stomach; L, liver; A, aorta.

CT of the stomach and duodenum

Accurate assessment of the stomach on CT requires good patient preparation and fastidious technique. Firstly, the patient must not eat for 6 hours prior to the CT to ensure that no food residues remain in the stomach, which could obscure or mimic disease. The patient is usually given about 100 ml of tap water to drink as well as a smooth muscle relaxant, in order to distend the stomach and duodenum (Fig. 4.21). If the stomach is not distended during the scan, any thickening of the gastric wall could be misinterpreted as being a mass. During the scan, intravenous iodinated contrast medium is infused to demonstrate enhancement of both the normal structures as well as to distinguish the enhancement characteristics of any abnormality.

Upper GI endoscopy is widely used as the initial investigation in patients with possible disease of the stomach and duodenum. It enables the mucosa of the stomach and duodenum to be directly inspected and biopsied. The main indications for its use can be summarized as:
• Demonstrating mucosal lesions such as gastritis, ulceration or carcinoma.

• Investigating persistent dyspepsia.
• Detecting *Helicobacter pylori* infection.
• Assessing healing of an ulcer.
• Examining patients after gastric surgery.
• Diagnosing the cause of acute bleeding from the upper gastrointestinal tract.
• Making a histological diagnosis of an abnormality shown on a barium meal.

Therefore, in centres where expert endoscopy is readily available, the indications for imaging are highly specific. Contrast radiography (barium or Gastrografin meal) is used for:
• Failed gastroscopy.
• Assessment of duodenal strictures which cannot be characterized or navigated on endoscopy.
• Assessment of functional patency/gastric emptying following gastroenterostomy or anti-obesity surgery.
• To confirm or rule out anastomotic leak following gastric surgery (a water-soluble contrast agent is used rather than barium).
CT can be used to:
• Stage the extraluminal extent of any disease, notably carcinoma, discovered at endoscopy.
• Further evaluate the stomach if there is a suspicion of an external mass compressing the stomach.

Specific diseases of the stomach and duodenum

Peptic ulcer (Fig. 4.22)

Gastric ulcers may be benign or malignant so confirmation at gastroscopy is routinely undertaken, whereas duodenal ulcers are almost invariably benign. Ulcers are identified as projections of barium beyond the mucosal profile. With duodenal ulceration, the duodenal cap (bulb) may be very deformed by scarring.

Gastric carcinoma

Because of the much better prognosis, emphasis is placed on the diagnosis of early gastric cancer which is confined to the mucosa. In the past, high-quality barium meal examination has been used as a screening tool in some countries to detect early gastric carcinoma. However, gastroscopy has now almost completely taken over this role.

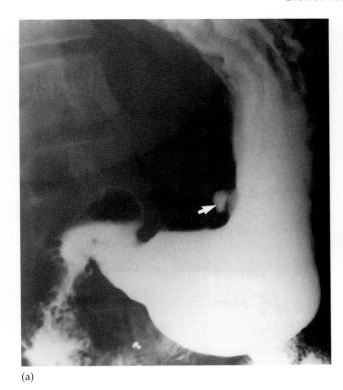

(a)

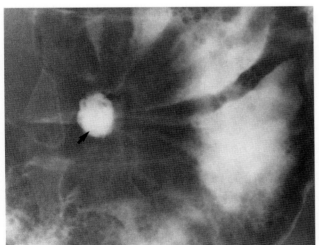

(b)

Fig. 4.22 Benign ulcer. (a) In profile, the ulcer (arrow) projects from the lesser curve of the stomach. (b) *En face* the ulcer (arrow) is seen as a rounded collection of barium.

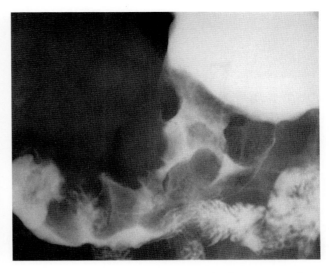

Fig. 4.23 Gastric carcinoma on barium study. There are a number of large filling defects in the antrum and body of stomach.

At barium examination, gastric carcinoma typically produces an irregular filling defect with alteration of the normal mucosal pattern (Fig. 4.23).

CT is the main imaging modality for the pre-operative staging of patients with gastric cancer as it can show the extent of the primary tumour (Fig. 4.24). Endoscopic ultrasound may be used in some cases for local staging of early gastric cancer, but CT is required for full evaluation. Direct infiltration of surrounding structures may be assessed and the presence of enlarged lymph nodes and liver metastases can be recorded for the purposes of tumour staging and determining the best treatment for the patient (Fig. 4.24b). FDG-PET and FDG-PET/CT do not have a clear role in the primary staging of gastric cancer due to the normal uptake of FDG by the gastric mucosa.

Other gastric tumours

Gastrointestinal stromal cell tumours (GIST) arise from the wall of the stomach resulting in a smooth, round submucosal filling defect, which may ulcerate as the tumour enlarges. Gastrointestinal stromal cell tumours are a group of tumours which are usually benign and well differentiated,

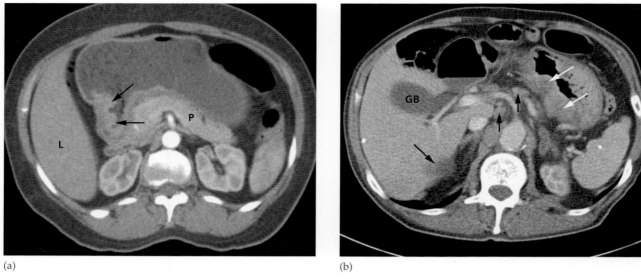

Fig. 4.24 Gastric carcinoma on CT. (a) A focal ulcer is seen arising in the antrum (arrows). (b) In a different patient, there is diffuse thickening of the wall of the stomach (white arrows). Several lymph nodes (short black arrows) and a liver metastasis (long black arrow) are also seen. L, liver; P, pancreas; GB, gallbladder.

with several different subtypes, such as a leiomyoma-type (Fig. 4.25), neural-type or non-differentiated type. Gastrointestinal stromal cell tumours may occur anywhere in the GI tract but 60–70% occur in the stomach. A leiomyoma is a submucosal tumour which, as well as projecting into the lumen of the stomach, may have a large extraluminal extension that can be easily recognized at CT.

Neuroendocrine tumours of the stomach and duodenum include gastric carcinoid tumours and gastrinomas. These tumours are often small but cause symptoms due to the secretion of hormones. Gastrinomas usually secrete gastrin, resulting in increased gastric acidity and peptic ulceration. Gastrinomas are often very small and typically enhance brightly in the arterial phase (Fig. 4.26).

Gastric polyps

Gastric polyps may be single or multiple. They may be sessile or have a stalk. Even with high-quality radiographs it is often impossible to distinguish benign from malignant polyps. For this reason, gastroscopy with biopsy or operative removal is invariably carried out on all suspected polyps.

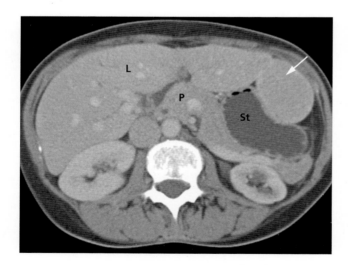

Fig. 4.25 Gastrointestinal stromal tumour (GIST). There is a smooth ovoid mass arising from the anterior wall of the stomach (arrow). This causes an indentation of the stomach. St, stomach; L, liver; P, pancreas.

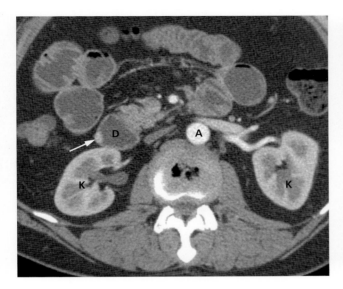

Fig. 4.26 Duodenal gastrinoma. The duodenum has been distended using a smooth muscle relaxant and oral water. The tiny gastrinoma is seen as a brightly enhancing lesion in the wall of the duodenum (arrow), on the arterial phase of enhancement. D, duodenal lumen; A, aorta; K, kidney.

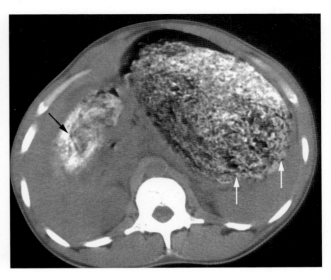

Fig. 4.28 CT of a bezoar. The stomach is distended by a large mass of hair mixed with oral contrast (white arrows). The antrum is also distended by the ingested material (black arrow).

Lymphoma

The stomach is the most frequent site of lymphoma involving the gastrointestinal tract, either as primary disease or by infiltration from adjacent nodes. The appearance of primary gastric lymphoma is typically of an extensive area of diffuse thickening of the gastric wall (Fig. 4.27). There may be extensive, bulky lymphadenopathy adjacent to the tumour. The appearance may mimic gastric carcinoma.

Intraluminal defects within the stomach include food or blood following a haematemesis. Sometimes ingested fibrous material, such as hair, may intertwine forming a ball or bezoar (Fig. 4.28).

Gastric outlet obstruction

In most patients, barium leaves the stomach within a few minutes of the smooth muscle relaxant wearing off, but in others this only occurs after the patient has been lying on the right side for some time. Prolonged delay in a patient with a dilated stomach containing food residues needs to be explained. In adults the causes of gastric outlet obstruction are listed in Box 4.1.

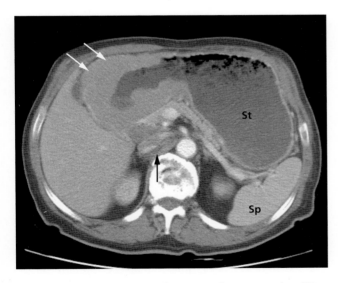

Fig. 4.27 Gastric lymphoma in the antrum, demonstrated on CT (white arrows). Lymphadenopathy surrounds the inferior vena cava (black arrow). St, stomach; Sp, spleen.

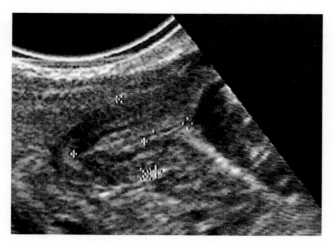

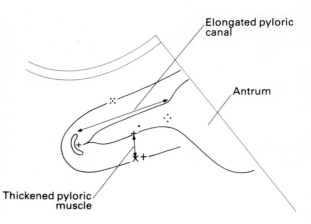

Fig. 4.29 Pyloric stenosis. Ultrasound scan in a neonate showing a thickened elongated pyloric canal.

Box 4.1 Causes of gastric outlet obstruction

- Chronic duodenal ulceration. The diagnosis depends on demonstrating a very deformed, stenosed duodenal cap. It may or may not be possible to identify an actual ulcer crater
- Carcinoma of the antrum
- Duodenal, ampullary and pancreatic carcinoma
- Acute or chronic pancreatitis, including pseudocyst formation
- Poor functional patency of a gastroenterostomy
- Pyloric stenosis in infants

In infants, pyloric stenosis is by far the commonest cause of gastric outlet obstruction. Often, the diagnosis is made clinically and can be confirmed with ultrasound, which has superseded the barium meal. Ultrasound shows a thickened, elongated pyloric canal (Fig. 4.29).

Hiatus hernia

A hiatus hernia is a herniation of the stomach into the mediastinum through the oesophageal hiatus in the diaphragm. It is a common finding. Two main types of hiatus hernia exist: sliding and rolling. An alternative name for a rolling hernia is 'para-oesophageal' (Fig. 4.30).

Fig. 4.30 Hiatus hernia. (a) Sliding: a portion of the stomach and the gastro-oesophageal junction are situated above the diaphragm. (b) Rolling or para-oesophageal: the gastro-oesophageal junction is below the diaphragm.

The commoner type is the sliding hiatus hernia, where the gastro-oesophageal junction and a portion of the stomach are situated above the diaphragm (Fig. 4.31). The cardiac sphincter is usually incompetent, so reflux from the stomach to the oesophagus occurs readily and

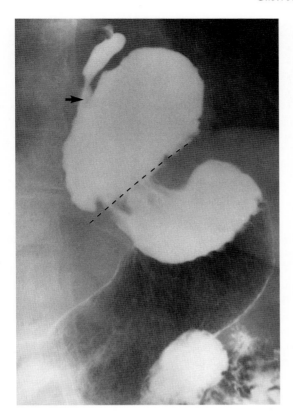

Fig. 4.31 Sliding hiatus hernia. The fundus of the stomach and the gastro-oesophageal junction (arrow) have herniated through the oesophageal hiatus and lie above the diaphragm (dotted line).

this may cause oesophagitis, ulceration or peptic stricture. A small sliding hernia may be demonstrated in most people during a barium meal examination, provided that enough manoeuvres have been undertaken to increase intra-abdominal pressure. It is, therefore, difficult to assess the significance of a small hernia with little or no reflux.

In a rolling or para-oesophageal hernia the fundus of the stomach herniates through the diaphragm, but the oesophagogastric junction often remains competent below the diaphragm.

A large hernia, particularly one of the para-oesophageal type, may not be reduced when the patient is in the erect position. In these instances the hiatus hernia will be seen on chest films and on CT (Fig. 4.32).

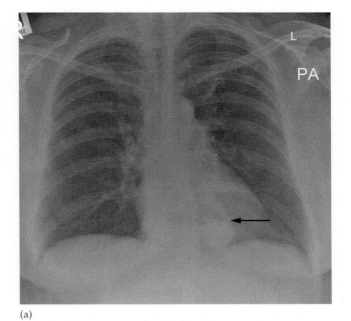

(a)

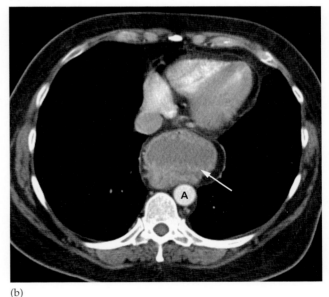

(b)

Fig. 4.32 Hiatus hernia. (a) Chest x-ray demonstrates a rounded mass with an air fluid level projected behind the heart shadow. (b) CT in the same patient demonstrates the fundus of the stomach extending up into the posterior mediastinum (arrow). A, aorta.

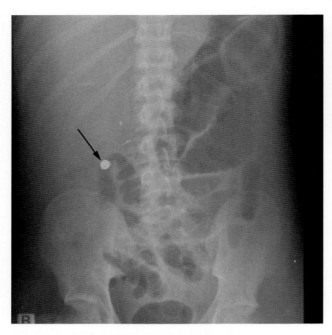

Fig. 4.33 A capsule endoscope is demonstrated within a loop of small bowel. A nasogastric tube is also present, projected over the left upper quadrant.

Small intestine

The small bowel remains one of the most difficult organs to evaluate. Fibre-optic endoscopy cannot be performed due to the long and tortuous nature of the small intestine. Capsule endoscopy, which requires the patient to ingest a tiny capsule containing a camera, may be helpful in some cases (Fig. 4.33). The capsule is ultimately passed with the faeces and may provide information concerning luminal or mural abnormalities of the small bowel.

Techniques

The standard imaging techniques and their indications are:
- *Small bowel follow-through (small bowel meal)* (Fig. 4.34). The patient drinks about 200–300 ml of barium and its passage through the small intestine is observed by taking films at regular intervals until the barium reaches the colon. This can be a time-consuming procedure and usually takes 2–3 hours, but the transit time is very variable. The indications for a barium examination of the small bowel are listed in Box 4.2.
- Enteroclysis (small bowel enema) (Fig. 4.35) distends the bowel and gives excellent mucosal detail, and is an alternative to a small bowel follow-through. The disadvantage is that it requires intubation with a nasoduodenal tube, which is passed to the duodenojejunal flexure, usually resulting in an increased radiation dose. Barium is injected through the tube followed by water or methyl cellulose to propel the barium through the small bowel allowing distension of bowel and a double contrast effect.
- CT of the small bowel has a role in small bowel disease as it can show thickening of the bowel wall, an important sign of inflammatory bowel disease and lymphoma and occasionally mucosal irregularity and small bowel neoplasms. The patient is fasted for 4–6 hours prior and then may be given oral Gastrografin or water to delineate the small bowel. In some cases, an intravenous bowel relaxant is injected. CT enteroclysis may also be performed with contrast being infused into the small bowel via a nasoduodenal tube, followed by CT. Intravenous iodinated contrast medium is injected to demonstrate vessels and enhancing structures.
- Ultrasound has a limited role in the investigation of small bowel pathology. In some cases, it can demonstrate small bowel thickening and free fluid associated with inflammatory conditions or, rarely, the presence of an intussusception.

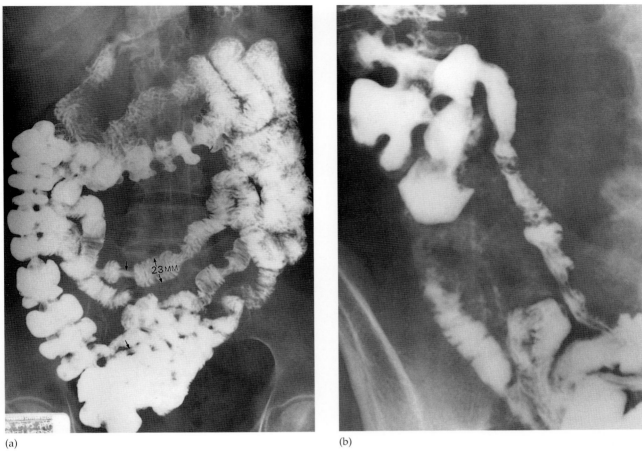

(a)   (b)

Fig. 4.34 (a) Normal barium follow-through. The small intestine, ascending and transverse colon are filled with barium. The jejunum in the left side of the abdomen has a much more marked mucosal fold pattern than the ileum, which is lying in the pelvis. When a peristaltic wave contracts the bowel, the mucosal folds lie longitudinally (arrows). Note the way of measuring the diameter of the bowel. In the pelvis the loops overlap and details of the bowel become hidden. (b) Normal terminal ileum.

• The use of MRI for assessment of the small bowel is under development in several centres, including research into the best MR sequences, oral contrast media and MR enteroclysis. Fast breath-hold sequences and smooth muscle relaxants are used to reduce movement artefacts and improve the clarity of the image.

• Nuclear medicine techniques, using meta-iodo-benzyl guanadine (MIBG) or octreotide, may be used in cases of suspected neuroendocrine or carcinoid tumours. 99m-Technetium may be used to detect Meckel's diverticulum.

Normal appearances of the small bowel

The normal small intestine (Fig. 4.34) occupies the central and lower abdomen, usually framed by the colon. The terminal portion of the ileum enters the medial aspect of the caecum through the ileocaecal valve. As the terminal ileum may be the first site of disease, this region is often fluoroscoped and observed on a television monitor so that peristalsis can be seen and films can be taken with the terminal ileum unobscured by other loops of small intestine.

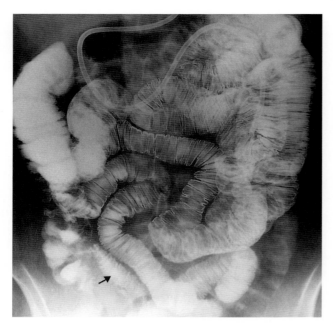

Fig. 4.35 Normal enteroclysis (small bowel enema). This technique gives good mucosal detail. The arrow points to the terminal ileum. Note that a tube has been passed through the stomach into the jejunum.

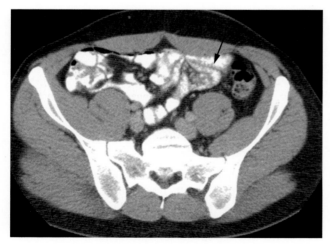

Fig. 4.36 Normal CT of the small bowel. The small bowel contains Gastrografin contrast medium. Note the feathery appearance of the jejunal loops (arrow).

The barium forms a continuous column defining the diameter of the small bowel, which is normally not more than 25 mm unless enteroclysis has been performed. Transverse folds of mucous membrane project into the lumen of the bowel and barium lies between these folds, which appear as lucent filling defects of about 2–3 mm in width. The appearance of the mucosal folds depends upon the diameter of the bowel. When distended, the folds are seen as lines traversing the barium column known as valvulae conniventes. When the small bowel is contracted the folds lie longitudinally, and when it is relaxed the folds assume an appearance described as feathery. The mucosal folds are largest and most numerous in the jejunum and tend to disappear in the lower part of the ileum.

On CT, the small bowel is seen as multiple loops usually containing oral water or Gastrografin contrast medium. The lumen of each loop should not exceed 25 mm unless enteroclysis has been performed (Fig. 4.36). The wall of the small bowel may not be properly assessed unless the small bowel is distended. Images may be reformatted to review the appearances of the bowel wall in coronal or sagittal planes.

Signs of disease on imaging examinations of the small intestine

Dilatation

Dilatation usually indicates malabsorption, paralytic ileus or small bowel obstruction (Fig. 4.37). A diameter over 30 mm is definitely abnormal, but it is important to make sure that two overlapping loops are not being measured.

Mucosal abnormality

The mucosal folds become thickened in many conditions, e.g. malabsorption states, oedema or haemorrhage in the bowel wall, and when inflamed or infiltrated (Fig. 4.38). As mucosal fold thickening occurs in many diseases, it is not possible to make a particular diagnosis unless other more specific features are present.

Narrowing

The only normal narrowings are those caused by peristaltic waves. They are smooth, concentric and transient, with

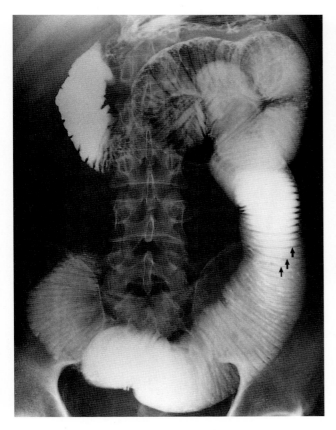

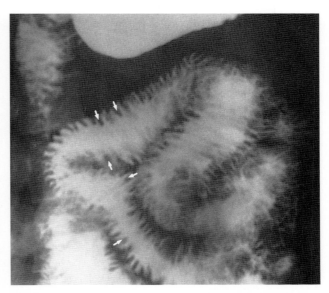

Fig. 4.38 Mucosal abnormality with infiltration of the bowel, in this case from oedema. The mucosal folds become thickened. Some of the thickened folds are arrowed.

Fig. 4.37 Dilatation from small bowel obstruction. The diameter of the bowel is greatly increased. The feathery mucosal pattern is lost and the folds appear as thin lines traversing the bowel, known as valvulae conniventes (arrows).

normal mucosal folds traversing them and normal bowel proximally. The common causes of strictures are Crohn's disease (Fig. 4.39), tuberculosis and lymphoma. Strictures do not contain normal mucosal folds and usually result in dilatation of the bowel proximally.

Ulceration

The outline of the small bowel should be smooth apart from the indentation caused by normal mucosal folds. Ulcers appear as spikes projecting outwards, which may be shallow or deep (Fig. 4.40). Ulceration is seen in Crohn's disease, tuberculosis and lymphoma. When there is a com-

bination of fine ulceration and mucosal oedema, a 'cobble-stone' appearance may be seen.

Specific diseases of the small intestine

Crohn's disease

Crohn's disease is a disease of unknown aetiology characterized by localized areas of non-specific chronic granulomatous inflammation, which nearly always affects the terminal ileum. In addition, it may cause disease in several different parts of the small and large intestine, often leaving normal intervening bowel, the affected parts being known as skip lesions.

The major signs on barium examinations (Fig. 4.41) that may be seen in isolation or combination include:
• Strictures, which are extremely variable in length. Sometimes a loop of bowel is so narrow, either from spasm or oedema and fibrosis in the bowel wall, that its appearance has been called 'the string sign'.
• Contraction of the caecum may be seen, particularly when there is visible disease in the terminal ileum.

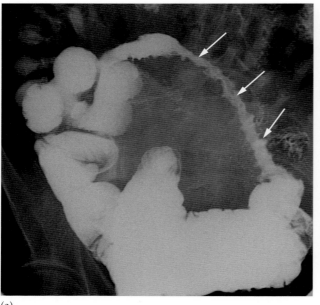

(a)

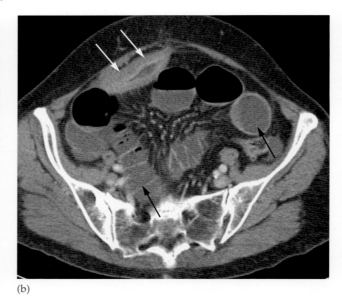

(b)

Fig. 4.39 Narrowing. (a) There is a long stricture (arrows) in the ileum due to Crohn's disease. There is an abnormal mucosal pattern. There is also separation of the abnormal segment from the other loops of bowel. (b) CT in the same patient demonstrates marked thickening of the abnormal loop of small bowel, with a narrowed lumen (white arrows). Several dilated loops of small bowel are also seen (black arrows), due to some obstruction at the level of the stricture.

• Dilatation of the bowel may be seen proximal to narrowed areas.

• Ulcers are seen which are sometimes quite deep. Fine ulceration combined with mucosal oedema gives rise to the so-called 'cobblestone' appearance.

• Thickening, distortion or effacement of mucosal folds.

• Separation of loops of bowel, due to bowel wall thickening or an inflammatory mass.

• Fistulae to other small bowel loops, colon, bladder or vagina (Fig. 4.42). When the fistula is between adjacent loops of small intestine it can be difficult to detect.

• Signs of malabsorption (see below).

Ultrasound may be helpful in identifying thickened loops of bowel, as well as abscess collections in the lower abdomen. On CT, involved loops of bowel have a thick-walled appearance with streaky high density of the surrounding mesenteric fat, due to surrounding oedema and inflammatory change. CT may be used to delineate the extent of an abscess collection and may be used to undertake percutaneous

drainage of the abscess. When Crohn's disease affects the anal canal, peri-anal fistula often results. MRI is often used to demonstrate the position and extent of the fistula. In particular, MRI is used in suspected complex fistulae, where there may be extension into the pelvis above the levator plate or extension through the sphincter into the ischio-rectal fossae (Fig. 4.43).

Small bowel ischaemia

Intestinal infarction, a serious life-threatening condition, is caused by occlusion of the superior mesenteric artery, either due to a thrombosis or an embolus (Fig. 4.44). There may be thickening and oedema of the wall of the small bowel, and gas may be seen within the bowel wall. Perforation may occur, with free gas seen within the peritoneal cavity. There may be air within the superior mesenteric vein or portal vein system in severe cases. The features are best demonstrated on CT.

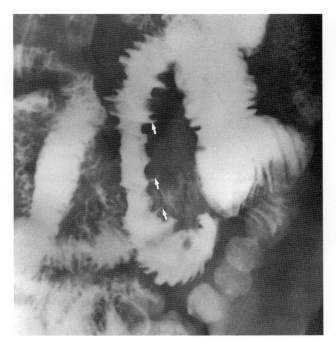

Fig. 4.40 Ulceration. Abnormal loops of bowel in Crohn's disease showing the ulcers as outward projections (arrows).

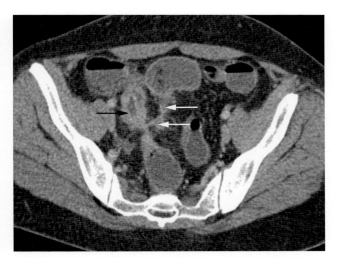

Fig. 4.42 CT of a fistula (white arrows) between the ileum and the sigmoid colon in a patient with Crohn's disease. Note the thickened and inflamed loop of ileum (black arrow).

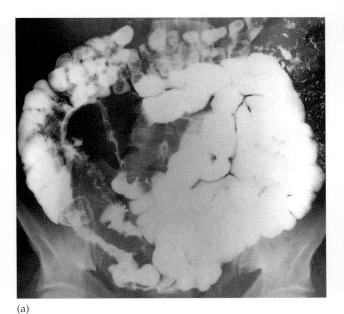

(a)

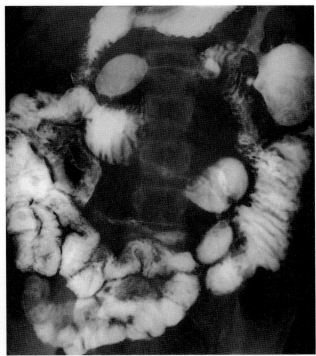

(b)

Fig. 4.41 Crohn's disease. (a) Many of the features are illustrated in this film. There are long strictures affecting different loops of ileum. The outlines of the strictures are irregular due to ulceration. Note how the affected loops lie separately, displaced from other loops because of the presence of inflammatory masses. (b) In this patient there are several strictures with dilatation of the bowel proximal to the strictures.

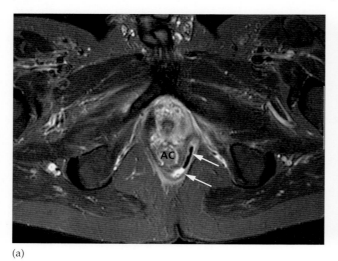
(a)

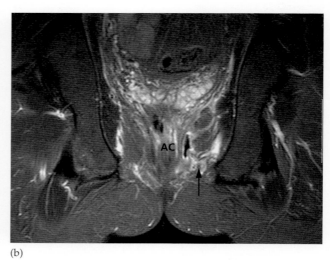
(b)

Fig. 4.43 Perianal fistula in Crohn's disease on MRI. (a) Axial MRI using a specialized sequence which is T2-weighted with fat saturation (STIR sequence) demonstrates air and fluid within a cavity which runs in the left intersphincteric space, involving the external sphincter (arrows). (b) Coronal STIR demonstrates the air within the fistula as well as bright inflammatory change in the ischio-rectal fat (arrow). AC, anal canal.

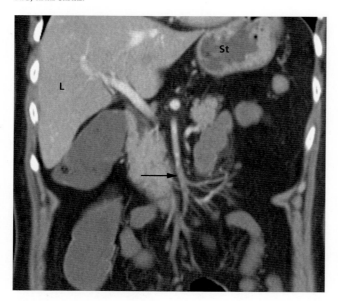

Fig. 4.44 Occlusion of the superior mesenteric artery (SMA). CT coronal reformat demonstrates non-enhancement of the SMA in a patient with severe abdominal pain (arrow). L, liver; St, stomach.

Tuberculosis

Tuberculosis of the small bowel is indistinguishable from Crohn's disease on barium examination. It commonly affects the ileocaecal region and also causes contraction of the caecum. On CT, there may be signs of diffuse peritoneal involvement, with ascites, thickening of the omentum, peritoneal and serosal nodules, and lymph node enlargement. These appearances may be indistinguishable from a disseminated intraperitoneal malignancy and ultrasound or CT-guided biopsy is usually required to establish the diagnosis.

Lymphoma

The infiltration in the wall of the bowel with lymphoma gives an appearance that is often extremely difficult to distinguish from Crohn's disease. Features that may help differentiate the two conditions on barium examinations are small mucosal filling defects due to tumour nodules (Fig. 4.45), and displacement of loops caused by enlarged mesenteric lymph nodes. Enlargement of the liver and spleen may also be present. CT and ultrasound can show very marked thickening of the bowel wall (Fig. 4.46), which can help differentiate between Crohn's disease and lymphoma. CT can also demonstrate mesenteric and para-aortic

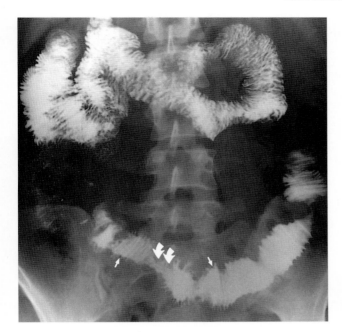

Fig. 4.45 Lymphoma. Lymphomatous infiltration has occurred in the lower loops of bowel causing thickening of the mucosal folds (small arrows) and discrete filling defects due to tumour nodules (curved arrows).

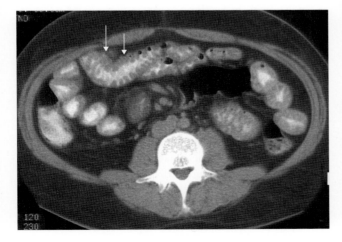

Fig. 4.46 Lymphoma. CT with the bowel opacified by contrast agent. The wall of all the bowel loops is considerably thickened. The arrows point to a portion of bowel which is particularly involved by lymphoma.

lymphadenopathy and lymphomatous deposits in the liver and spleen.

Malabsorption

A number of disorders result in defective absorption of foodstuffs, minerals or vitamins. The definitive test for malabsorption is jejunal biopsy.

The imaging signs that may occur with any of the causes of malabsorption are (Fig. 4.47):
• Small bowel dilatation, the jejunum being affected more than the ileum.
• Thickening of mucosal folds.
• The barium may be diluted by the excessive fluid in the small bowel and so appears less dense.

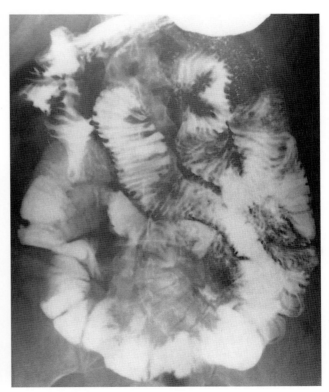

Fig. 4.47 Malabsorption. The bowel is dilated and the mucosal folds thickened. In the lower loops the barium appears less dense due to it becoming diluted. No specific cause for the malabsorption can be detected, which in this case was due to gluten enteropathy.

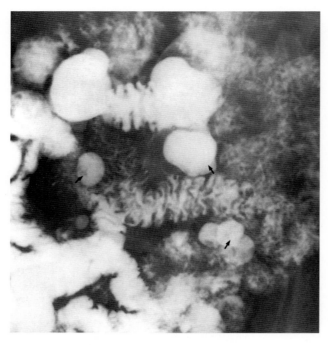

Fig. 4.48 Diverticulosis. A number of diverticula of varying size are arising from the small bowel. Some of these are arrowed.

The use of the barium follow-through in malabsorption is mainly confined to demonstrating a structural abnormality causing the malabsorption, notably:
• Crohn's disease (see p. 153).
• Lymphoma (see p. 156).
• Anatomical abnormalities, e.g. decreased length of small bowel available for absorption, such as surgical resection or a fistula short-circuiting a length of small bowel.
• Stagnation of bowel contents, allowing bacterial overgrowth, which utilizes nutrients from the bowel lumen, caused by:
  (a) Multiple small bowel diverticula (Fig. 4.48).
  (b) A dilated loop cut off from the main stream of the bowel in which there is delayed filling and emptying (blind loop).
  (c) A dilated loop proximal to a stricture (stagnant loop).

Acute small bowel obstruction

Acute small bowel obstruction can be due to a variety of causes, notably peritoneal adhesions, usually postoperatively or following previous peritoneal inflammation, obstruction in hernial orifices, Crohn's disease, at the site of twisting in volvulus, or occasionally due to metastatic carcinoma, lymphoma or even primary small bowel tumours. A barium examination is not carried out in most cases of obstruction as the diagnosis is usually made on clinical history and examination with the help of plain abdominal films (p. 121). If the cause of small bowel obstruction is evident clinically, e.g. in a patient with a strangulated hernia or known widespread malignancy, further imaging is rarely required. However, if the cause of the obstruction is not evident, then a contrast follow-through study may be helpful. Water-soluble contrast is used in preference to barium. If the contrast is seen within the large bowel at 24 hours, conservative management is likely to be successful, because the degree of obstruction is likely to be minor. If there is mechanical obstruction in the proximal small bowel, then the contrast will remain in the dilated stomach and proximal small bowel at 24 hours.

Computed tomography can be a useful technique in selected cases to demonstrate the site of obstruction by showing the location of the transition from dilated to collapsed small bowel and also to confirm or exclude a mass at the site of obstruction (Fig. 4.49). No imaging technique can directly demonstrate adhesions, the commonest cause of small bowel obstruction.

Malrotation

During intrauterine life, the bowel undergoes a series of rotations. Failure of the normal rotation may result in the small bowel being situated in the right side of the abdomen and the colon on the left side. However, in children it is important to recognize even minor degrees of malrotation, as the condition predisposes to intestinal volvulus, which is often a surgical emergency. Malrotation is diagnosed when the duodenojejunal flexure is displaced downwards and to the right of its normal position, which should be level with the duodenal cap and to the left of the spine.

Worm infestation

Roundworms (*Ascaris*) are commonly encountered worms, large enough to be seen as filling defects in the lumen of the bowel (they may grow up to 35 cm long) (Fig. 4.50).

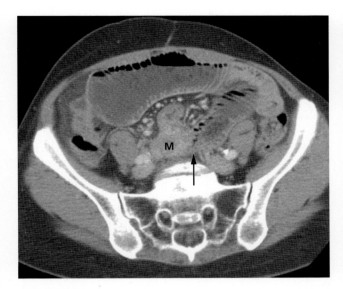

Fig. 4.49 CT of small bowel obstruction in a patient with recurrent ovarian cancer. There is an abrupt change in caliber of the dilated small bowel lumen (arrow) where a mass is infiltrating the bowel wall (M).

The worms themselves may ingest the barium to have their own barium meal and barium may be seen in their digestive tracts.

Large intestine

Techniques

Colonoscopy is now the gold standard for examining the colonic mucosa. The technique allows direct inspection of the mucosal surface of the bowel and may be used for diagnostic or therapeutic biopsy or resection of mucosal lesions. Colonoscopy may fail for several reasons:

- Incomplete colonic evaluation.
- Impassable stricture.
- Patient intolerance.
- Increased risk of perforation, e.g. in extensive or severe acute colitis.

If the colonoscopist fails to reach the caecum, the large bowel may be investigated by performing either a barium enema or a CT pneumocolon.

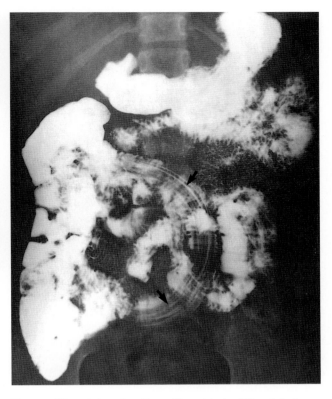

Fig. 4.50 Worm infestation. Several long tubular filling defects (arrows) due to roundworms (*Ascaris*) in the small bowel.

Barium enema

Firstly, the bowel is prepared by means of aperients or washout to rid the colon of faecal material, which might otherwise mask small lesions and cause confusion by simulating polyps. Barium is run into the colon under gravity through a tube inserted into the rectum. Air is then blown in to push the barium around the colon with the result that the colon is distended with air and the mucosa coated with barium, giving the 'double contrast' effect. Films are taken in various projections so that all the loops of colon are unravelled.

Barium enema examination is particularly helpful in patients with extensive diverticular disease being prepared for resection: the length of involved bowel can be clearly delineated for the surgeon. Colonic carcinoma is also well demonstrated, but CT pneumocolon (see below) has the advantage of allowing not only diagnosis of the tumour but also the demonstration of metastatic disease.

CT pneumocolon

Computed tomography pneumocolon has superseded barium enema as the method of choice for identifying malignant tumours of the colon when colonoscopy has failed. The technique is also used in patients who are frail and with poor mobility, in which case colonoscopy (and barium enema) would be difficult to undertake. The patient is given a purgative to clean the colon prior to the CT examination and a smooth muscle relaxant is given by injection. A rectal tube is inserted and the colon is distended with gas (CO_2 or air). The only contrast medium that is administered, other than the gas, is an intravenous contrast agent to enhance any tumours that may be present. Neither barium nor Gastrografin is used. One scan is obtained with the patient supine, followed by a second scan with the patient prone. In some centres, an alternative for frail and immobile patients, which avoids the use of aperients, is to fill the colon with contrast by giving oral contrast some time before the examination and a CT of the abdomen is then performed.

With multidetector CT and the appropriate software, the CT pneumocolon images can be viewed as sectional images in any desired plane. They can also be reconstructed to a three-dimensional display and viewed as *virtual colonoscopy* (see Fig. 4.75, p. 175). Virtual colonoscopy requires a substantial amount of time and training to interpret.

Sigmoidoscopy is performed in almost every patient in whom a barium enema or CT pneumocolon is requested, because lesions in the rectum, especially mucosal abnormalities, may be missed.

MRI

Magnetic resonance imaging of the colon is challenging, due to movement artefacts from bowel peristalsis. This can be overcome to some extent using a smooth muscle relaxant and rapid sequences. MRI is mainly used to evaluate the rectum and anal canal, where movement artefacts are minimal. No specific patient preparation is required.

Nuclear medicine studies

Intestinal transit time may be evaluated using an oral radiopharmaceutical in patients with chronic constipation. The presence of inflammation may be assessed using indium-111 or technetium HMPAO-labelled white cells in patients with ulcerative colitis.

Normal colon

The radiological anatomy of the normal colon is shown in Fig. 4.51. Certain features are worth emphasizing.

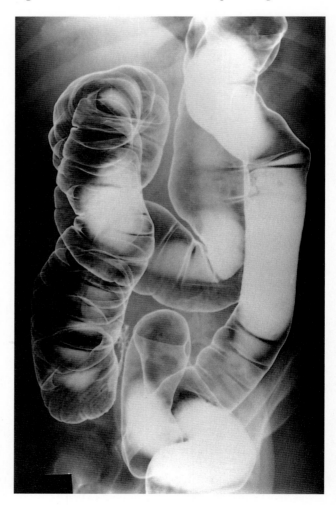

Fig. 4.51 Normal double-contrast barium enema.

The length of the colon is very variable and sometimes there are redundant loops, particularly in the sigmoid and transverse colon. The caliber decreases from the caecum to the sigmoid colon.

The caecum is usually situated in the right iliac fossa, but it may be seen under the right lobe of the liver or even in the centre of the abdomen if it possesses a long mesentery. The lips of the ileocaecal valve may project into the caecum and cause a filling defect, which must not be mistaken for a tumour. Filling of the terminal ileum and appendix with rectal contrast may occur, but if they do not fill no significance can be attached to this.

Haustra can usually be recognized in the whole of the colon, although they may be absent in the descending and sigmoid regions. The outline of the descending colon, apart from the haustra, is smooth.

Imaging signs of disease of the large intestine

Narrowing of the lumen

Narrowing of the colon may be due to spasm, stricture formation or compression by an extrinsic mass. *Spasm* is often seen in normal patients and, providing it is an isolated finding, it can be ignored. Spasm is also seen in conjunction with diverticular disease and various inflammatory disorders. The main causes of *stricture* formation are listed in Box 4.3.

When attempting to diagnose the nature of a stricture in the colon the following points should be borne in mind:
• *Neoplastic strictures* have shouldered edges, an irregular

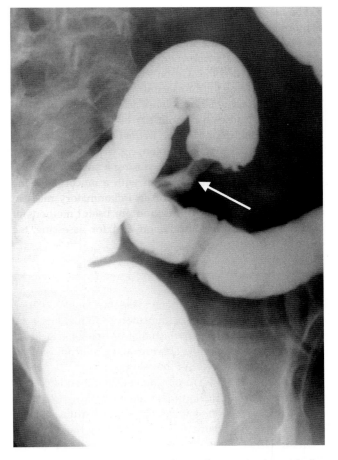

Fig. 4.52 Stricture. A short circumferential narrowing is seen in the sigmoid colon (arrow) from a carcinoma.

Box 4.3 Causes of narrowing of the colonic lumen

• Carcinoma
• Diverticular disease
• Crohn's disease
• Ischaemic colitis

Rarer causes:
• Tuberculosis
• Lymphogranuloma venereum
• Amoebiasis
• Radiation fibrosis

lumen and are rarely more than 6 cm in length (Fig. 4.52), whereas benign strictures classically have tapered ends, a relatively smooth outline and may be of any length.
• *Ulceration* may be seen in strictures due to Crohn's disease, and sacculation of the colon is a feature of ischaemic strictures.
• *Narrowing due to diverticular disease* is usually accompanied by other signs of diverticular disease. It is sometimes impossible to distinguish a stricture due to a carcinoma in an area of diverticular disease from a stricture due to diverticular disease.

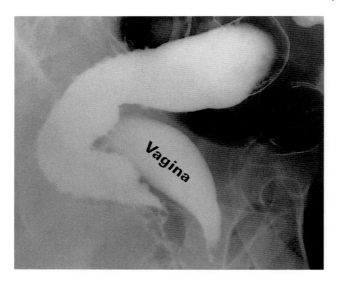

Fig. 4.62 Crohn's disease – rectovaginal fistula. During the barium enema, filling of the vagina with barium occurred. Note the ulceration in the rectum.

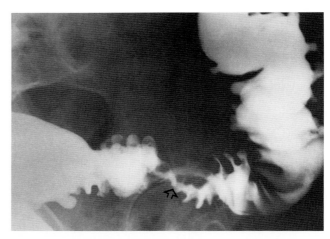

Fig. 4.64 Diverticular disease. A stricture is present (arrow). Although there is recognizable diverticular disease at both ends of the stricture, it is impossible to exclude definitely a carcinoma.

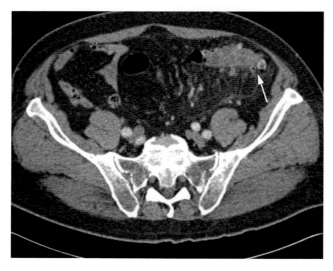

Fig. 4.63 Diverticular disease. Numerous diverticula are seen as out-pouchings from the sigmoid colon (arrow). There is marked stranding of the surrounding fat planes. In this case, there is no associated abscess.

in the pericolic region or within the structure to which the fistula has occurred. An abscess is most readily diagnosed with CT. Occasionally, diverticula perforate directly into

the peritoneal cavity causing peritonitis, and free intraperitoneal air should be looked for on a plain abdominal film if necessary. A stricture with or without local abscess formation (Fig. 4.64) may occur. Usually, this is clearly within an area of recognizable diverticular disease. It is, however, often impossible to differentiate such a stricture from a carcinoma occurring coincidentally in a patient with diverticular disease.

Appendicitis

In most cases, the diagnosis of appendicitis is obvious clinically and imaging is unnecessary. In cases of doubt the diagnosis can be made with ultrasound, which shows a distended non-compressible appendix with a thickened oedematous wall, often accompanied by free fluid within the pelvis (Fig. 4.65a). An appendicolith may be visible within the appendix as a hyperechoic area casting an acoustic shadow (Fig. 4.65b). Similar changes can be demonstrated with CT. An appendix abscess can be diagnosed with CT (Fig. 4.66) or ultrasound as a mass in the right iliac fossa.

Ischaemic colitis

Acute infarction of the large bowel is very rare. Ischaemia is usually a more chronic process giving rise, initially, to

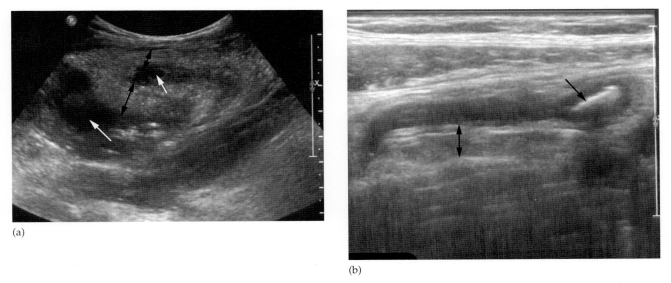

(a)

(b)

Fig. 4.65 Appendicitis. (a) Longitudinal ultrasound scan demonstrates marked thickening of the wall of the appendix (double head arrows). Fluid is seen within the lumen and surrounding the appendix (white arrows). (b) An appendicolith is seen in the tip of the appendix in a different patient (black arrow).

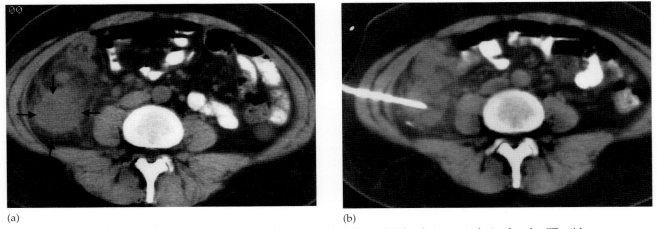

(a)   (b)

Fig. 4.66 Appendix abscess. (a) CT shows a mass (arrows) in the right iliac fossa. (b) The abscess was drained under CT guidance.

mucosal oedema and haemorrhage, which may resolve. In the later stages, a stricture may form. The findings on barium enema depend on the stage at which the examination is performed.

Mucosal haemorrhage and oedema may be recognized by observing multiple smooth indentations into the lumen of the bowel, resembling thumb prints (Fig. 4.67a). If stricture formation occurs, the stricture will be smooth and have tapered ends. The site is usually centred between the splenic flexure and the sigmoid colon because these are the regions of the colon with the most vulnerable blood supply (Fig. 4.67b). Sacculations may be seen arising from one side of the strictured area.

Pneumatosis coli

In this unusual condition, gas-filled spaces are present in the wall of the bowel. These cyst-like spaces do not communicate with the lumen. They can be identified on a plain film of the abdomen, but the diagnosis is much easier with a barium enema where the cysts cause smooth translucent filling defects projecting from the wall of the bowel (Fig. 4.68). The appearance could be confused with intramural haemorrhage and oedema, or with colitis if the presence of air within the cysts is not appreciated.

Volvulus

In a volvulus a loop of bowel twists on its mesentery. This happens most frequently in the sigmoid colon, particularly when it is redundant, and less often in the caecum. The twisted loop becomes greatly distended and the bowel proximal to the volvulus is obstructed by the twist and may, therefore, also be dilated.

The diagnosis is usually made on the plain abdominal films (see p. 123), but a barium enema or CT may be helpful in doubtful cases so that, if confirmed, non-operative reduction of the volvulus may be attempted. This will show a smooth, tapered narrowing (Fig. 4.69) from twisting of the colon, with marked dilatation of the bowel proximal to the twist.

Intussusception

An intussusception is the invagination of one segment of the

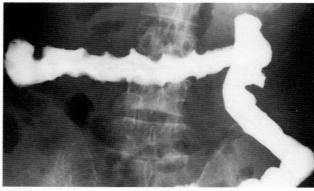

(a)

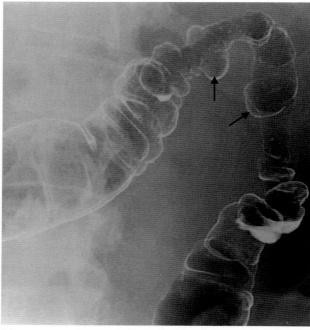

(b)

Fig. 4.67 Ischaemic colitis. (a) Mucosal haemorrhage and oedema have caused indentations resembling thumb prints in the transverse colon. (b) A long smooth stricture involving the splenic flexure with sacculations arising from the colon (arrows) in another patient.

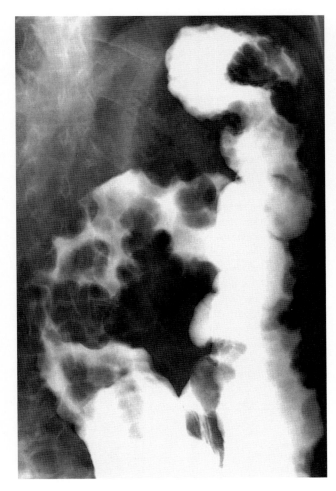

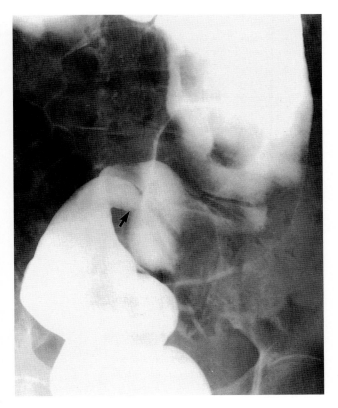

Fig. 4.69 Volvulus. A smooth narrowing is seen in the sigmoid colon where the colon has twisted (arrow). Note the dilated colon proximal to this.

Fig. 4.68 Pneumatosis coli. Part of the colon showing numerous translucencies in the wall of the colon owing to many gas-filled cysts.

bowel into another. Infants and young children are much more liable to intussusception than adults.

By far the commonest type is an *ileocolic intussusception*, namely ileum invaginating into the colon. Other types are *colocolic*, when the colon invaginates into another part of the colon, and *ileo-ileal* when the ileum invaginates into a more distal segment of ileum.

The diagnosis of intussusception in children is often made using ultrasound, by diagnosing an abdominal mass often with a hyperechoic centre (Fig. 4.70). In infants and young

children, in particular, the diagnosis is often confirmed by an enema with air or carbon dioxide as the contrast agent, and an attempt at reduction of the intussusception is made using the increased pressure of the introduced air or carbon dioxide. When gas is insufflated *per rectum* under fluoroscopic or ultrasound control, the flow of gas will be obstructed by the leading edge of the intussusception and an attempt at pneumatic reduction can be made in order to avoid a laparotomy (Fig. 4.71). If such a reduction is to be safely carried out, the child should have no clinical signs of peritonitis. The longer the symptoms have been present, the greater the risk of perforating gangrenous bowel.

In adults, intussusception is almost always due to the presence of a neoplasm, typically in the submucosa, such as

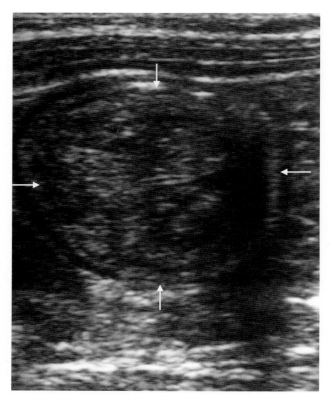

Fig. 4.70 Intussusception. Ultrasound of upper abdomen showing the intussusception as a mass (arrows).

lymphomatous deposits or melanoma metastases. The diagnosis is usually made on CT. A sausage-shaped mass is demonstrated, which has mesenteric fat within the lumen of the intussuscipiens (Fig. 4.72). Surgical treatment is invariable.

Colorectal tumours

Polyps

The word 'polyp' means a small mass of tissue arising from the wall of the bowel projecting into the lumen. They are best investigated by endoscopy, but may be found at barium enema or CT pneumocolon. It is often impossible on radiological grounds to exclude frank malignancy in a polyp in an adult. However, only a tiny minority of polyps less than 1 cm in size, and very few less than 2 cm, are cancers. The

features that suggest malignancy are a diameter of more than 2 cm, a short thick stalk or an irregular surface.

Polyps may be sessile or on a stalk, single or multiple. The common polyps are:
• *Adenomatous polyps* (Fig. 4.73). These are benign neoplasms but have a predisposition to malignant change. They are, therefore, removed endoscopically when discovered, regardless of whether or not an individual polyp is believed to be responsible for symptoms. Polyps may first be discovered because of a positive faecal occult blood test or may present with overt bleeding. They may be single or multiple and are found most frequently in the rectosigmoid region. In *familial polyposis* they are numerous and one or more will, in time, undergo malignant change.
• *Villous adenomas* are benign sessile tumours showing a sponge-like appearance owing to barium trapped between the villous strands. They are usually large when first discovered and are frequently mistaken for faeces. The common sites are the rectum and the caecum. There is a high incidence of malignant change.
• *Polypoid adenocarcinomas*.
• *Juvenile polyps*. Almost all isolated polyps in children are benign. They are probably developmental in origin.
• *Inflammatory polyps (pseudopolyps)* are seen in ulcerative colitis.
• *Hyperplastic or metaplastic polyps*.

Carcinoma

Carcinomas may arise anywhere in the colon and rectum but they are commonest in the rectosigmoid region and caecum. The appearance and behaviour of a carcinoma in these two sites are usually quite different. The patient with a rectosigmoid carcinoma often has an annular stricture and presents with alteration in bowel habit and obstruction, whereas with a caecal carcinoma the tumour can become very large without obstructing the bowel, so anaemia and weight loss are the common presenting features.

A barium enema shows annular carcinomas as an irregular stricture with shouldered edges (see Fig. 4.52, p. 161). Such strictures are rarely more than 6 cm in length. The polypoid or fungating carcinoma causes an irregular filling defect projecting into the lumen of the bowel.

Multiple primary tumours must be excluded, as a patient with one carcinoma of the colon has a higher than normal

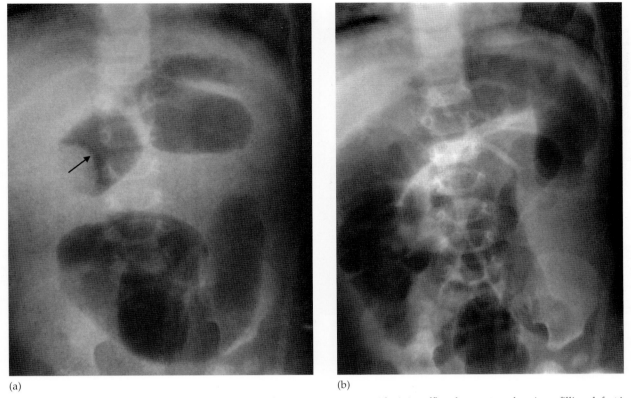

(a)

(b)

Fig. 4.71 Intussusception. (a) Film taken during reduction of the intussusception with air insufflated *per rectum* showing a filling defect in the transverse colon (arrow) owing to ileum invaginated into the colon. (b) Later film showing that the intussusception has been reduced with air filling the caecum and entering the small bowel.

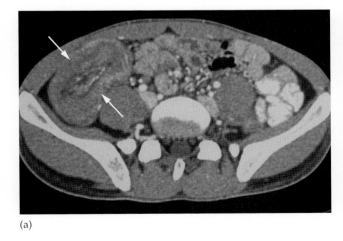

(a)

Fig. 4.72 Intussusception due to a tumour on CT. (a) Axial and (b) coronal reformat demonstrates a sausage-shaped mass in the right iliac fossa (arrows). Mesenteric fat and vessels are seen in the centre of the mass.

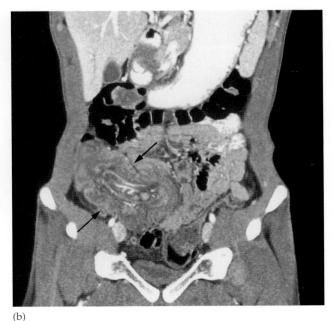

(b)

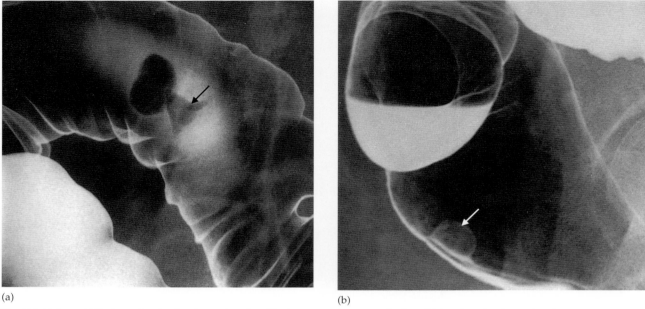

(a)

(b)

Fig. 4.73 Polyps. (a) Pedunculated polyp (arrow) outlined by barium in the sigmoid colon. (b) Sessile polyp (arrow) in the rectum.

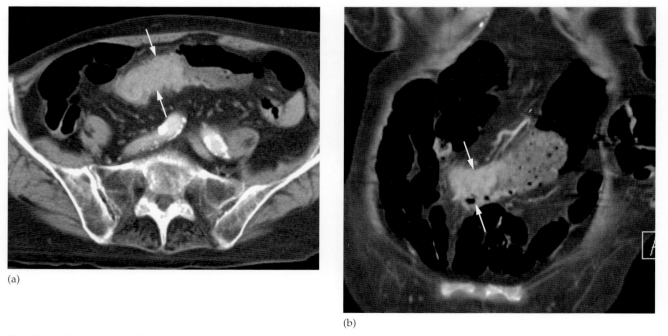

(a)

(b)

Fig. 4.74 Colon carcinoma. (a) Standard axial CT acquired on thin sections showing a tumour (arrows) in the transverse colon. (b) Coronal reformat of the same tumour.

risk of developing a second colonic cancer, which may be present simultaneously or after the first tumour has been removed.

CT (Fig. 4.74), particularly CT pneumocolon (Fig. 4.75), is an alternative examination to a barium enema for the diagnosis of a colonic carcinoma. A carcinoma can be recognized as thickening of the bowel wall and an irregular narrowing of the lumen of the colon.

MRI is the method of choice for accurate pre-operative assessment of the local extent of *rectal carcinoma*. High resolution T2-weighted images through the tumour can accurately delineate the rectum, as well as the mesorectal fat and mesorectal fascia which surround the rectum (Fig. 4.76). The mesorectal fascia is an important anatomical landmark, as it represents the surgical plane of dissection during rectal cancer surgery. The distance between tumour invading the mesorectal fat and the mesorectal fascia can be measured and the surgical resection margin can be safely predicted. The possibility of an involved surgical margin can be accurately predicted (Fig. 4.77) and may significantly influence the treatment planning. The role of endoscopic ultrasound in rectal cancer is limited to very early stage disease as some tumours cannot be adequately evaluated.

Staging colorectal carcinoma. CT can be used to demonstrate metastases to the liver or lungs and to identify para-aortic nodal disease. If the initial investigation is CT, then staging and initial diagnosis are accomplished with a single examination. In most cases, the local extent of tumours that are to be operated upon is assessed at surgery, although in locally advanced disease (Fig. 4.78), infiltration of the abdominal or pelvic organs, or abdominal or pelvic walls can be demonstrated on CT. FDG-PET or FDG-PET/CT are not currently used routinely for initial staging of colorectal cancer due to limited availability; however, this has been shown to be more sensitive than CT in the detection of metastatic sites of disease and in suspected

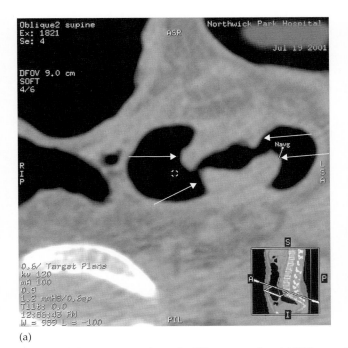

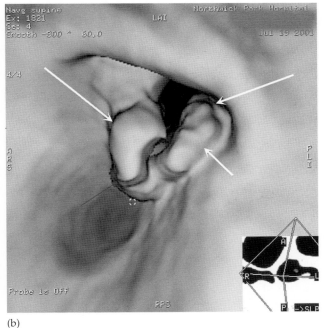

(a) (b)

Fig. 4.75 Colon carcinoma shown by CT pneumocolon. (a) Oblique axial section showing a stricture with classic shouldered edges (arrows). (b) Virtual colonoscopy demonstrating the irregularly shaped tumour (arrows).

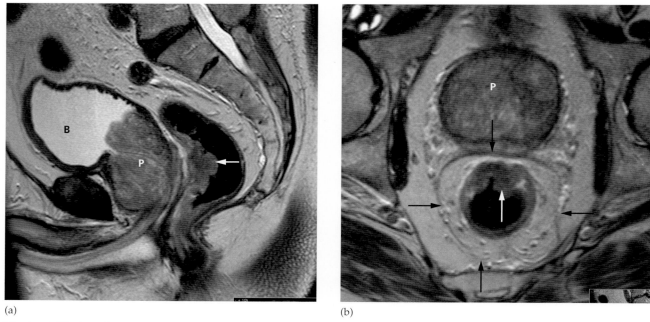

(a)

(b)

Fig. 4.76 MRI of rectal carcinoma. (a) Sagittal T2-weighted image demonstrates a polypoid growth arising from the anterior wall of the rectum (white arrow). Note benign hyperplasia of the prostate (P). (b) Axial image of the same tumour. Note the mesorectal fascia (black arrows) which encases the mesorectal fat and the rectum.

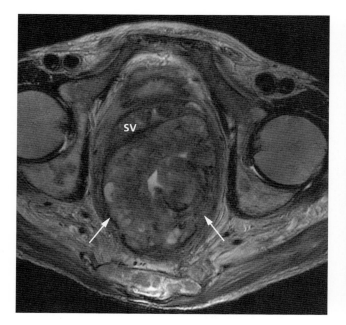

Fig. 4.77 MRI of advanced rectal carcinoma. The tumour (arrows) has completely invaded the perirectal fat and fascia and there is infiltration of the seminal vesicles (SV).

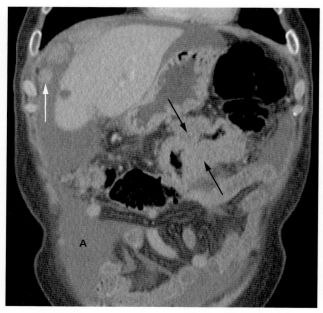

Fig. 4.78 Locally advanced cancer of the transverse colon (black arrows), on a CT coronal reformat. Multiple peritoneal metastases (white arrow) are seen beneath the diaphragm and there is ascites (A) consistent with metastatic disease.

recurrent disease, and is used in selected patients to help plan the best treatment.

Hirschsprung's disease (congenital aganglionosis)

Hirschsprung's disease is due to absence of ganglion cells beyond a certain level in the colon, usually in the sigmoid or rectosigmoid region. In time, the colon proximal to the aganglionic segment becomes grossly distended, but in those patients who present soon after birth the dilatation may not be obvious.

The aganglionic segment, usually the rectum, is either normal or small at barium enema and the diagnosis depends on recognizing the transition from the normal or reduced caliber colon to the dilated colon (Fig. 4.79). To prevent the danger of water intoxication from the dilated colon, the colon is not washed out before the barium enema.

The barium introduced is usually limited to the amount required to show the zone of transition from aganglionic to dilated bowel.

Idiopathic megacolon (functional megacolon)

The cause of idiopathic megacolon is believed to be chronic constipation. Both the rectum and colon are dilated and contain a large amount of faeces. The large-sized rectum serves as a differentiating feature from Hirschsprung's disease.

Anal fistula and perianal abscess

Most anal fistulae are simple low tracks that can be assessed by clinical examination and do not require imaging. MRI is the best method of demonstrating the course of

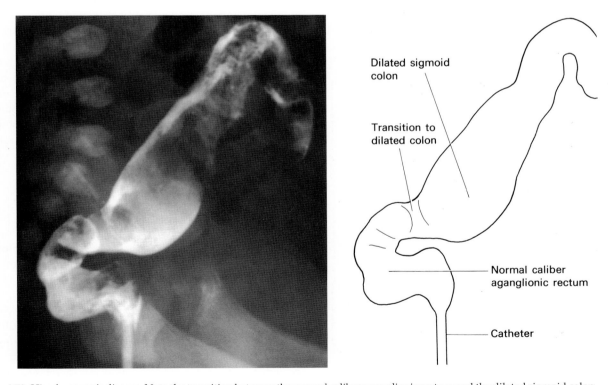

Fig. 4.79 Hirschsprung's disease. Note the transition between the normal caliber aganglionic rectum and the dilated sigmoid colon.

an anal fistula and in complex or recurrent cases is used to help plan the surgical approach (see Fig. 4.43, p. 156).

Imaging in the investigation of the acute abdomen

The term 'acute abdomen' refers to the rapid onset of symptoms, such as pain, nausea and vomiting, which may indicate serious intra-abdominal pathology. The differential diagnosis is wide (see Box 4.4).

A careful history and physical examination are always needed when evaluating a patient with suspected acute abdomen. The diagnostic imaging aspects of the specific conditions are discussed in the relevant sections of this and other chapters. The following discussion concentrates on the *role* of various imaging investigations in patients with an acute abdomen.

Plain films

The diagnosis of *perforation of the gastrointestinal tract* is aided by demonstrating a spontaneous pneumoperitoneum

Box 4.4 Common causes of 'acute abdomen'

- Small bowel obstruction
- Large bowel obstruction
- Paralytic ileus
- Acute appendicitis/Meckel's diverticulum
- Peptic ulcer disease
- Diverticulitis
- Severe colitis
- Intra-abdominal abscess
- Gastroenteritis
- Acute intestinal ischaemia/infarction
- Acute cholecystitis
- Acute pancreatitis
- Ectopic pregnancy
- Pelvic inflammatory disease
- Leaking/ruptured abdominal aortic aneurysm
- Acute thoracic disease, e.g. myocardial infarction or pneumonia
- Renal tract pathology

on plain abdominal or chest films (see Chapter 3, p. 125). Erect chest x-rays are usually requested at the same time as an abdominal film to exclude acute pulmonary conditions that can cause acute abdominal pain, notably pneumonia close to the diaphragm, and because an upright chest x-ray is a more sensitive method for detecting a pneumoperitoneum than an abdominal x-ray film, even when the abdominal film is taken in the upright position.

Dilatation of the bowel is the cardinal sign of *intestinal obstruction* on plain abdominal films, and the pattern of dilatation is the key to the radiological distinction between small and large bowel obstruction (see p. 119, Chapter 3 for description of plain film findings).

Barium or Gastrografin follow-through

If the cause or site of intestinal obstruction is not evident from clinical examination (e.g. strangulated hernia, previous surgery, widespread malignancy) and plain films, and providing immediate exploratory surgery is not indicated, a contrast follow-through study may be helpful. *Gastrografin* is used in preference to barium. If the contrast agent is seen within the large bowel at 24 hours, conservative management is likely to be successful. If there is mechanical obstruction in the proximal small bowel, then the contrast will remain in the dilated stomach and proximal small bowel at 24 hours. Unfortunately, in distal small bowel obstruction, the contrast becomes too diluted to determine the nature of any obstruction, but the absence of contrast in the large bowel does indicate that the obstruction is in the small bowel.

Ultrasound

Transabdominal ultrasound is an easily performed procedure in acutely ill patients, which can be a bedside procedure if necessary. It is, therefore, a useful test for a variety of acute abdominal conditions, particularly for imaging acute disease of the biliary, urinary and gynaecological tracts, and for imaging the acute abdomen in children, notably when looking for pyloric stenosis and intussusception. But ultrasound has the disadvantage that gas in the gastrointestinal tract, which is often a particular feature in many acute abdominal conditions, absorbs sound and, therefore, creates substantial blind spots.

Computed tomography

Computed tomography provides similar information to ultrasound, but without blind spots, and is being increasingly used, often as the initial imaging examination. CT provides much more information than plain films because it shows not only the gas inside and outside the bowel more sensitively and in more detail than on plain film, but it also demonstrates the abdominal wall, the peritoneal cavity and the state of all the solid organs within the abdomen. CT is, therefore, the best overview technique to demonstrate ascites, bowel perforation or inflammation (Fig. 4.80), and many acute disorders of the liver, spleen, pancreas and kidneys. It can be a useful technique in selected cases of intestinal obstruction to demonstrate the site of obstruction by showing the location of the transition from dilated to collapsed bowel, and also to confirm or exclude a mass at the site of obstruction, although the commonest cause of small bowel obstruction, adhesions, are not usually visible. CT is also valuable for triaging patients with non-specific acute abdominal pain, particularly in patients with marked obesity, unclear ultrasound findings, possible bowel obstruction, and multiple lesions, and is the examination of choice in patients with palpable abdominal masses, suspected abdominal aortic aneurysm or retroperitoneal disease.

Imaging investigation of acute bleeding from the gastrointestinal tract

The gold standard investigation for acute GI haemorrhage is endoscopy. The source of haemorrhage in the upper GI tract (i.e. within the oesophagus, stomach or duodenum) can usually be diagnosed at endoscopy. In lower GI haemorrhage (including the small and large bowel), the source of bleeding is within the colon and rectum in over 95% of cases. In most cases, the acute bleed resolves spontaneously, and then the bowel may be prepared with purgatives for diagnostic colonoscopy. If, however, there is uncontrolled lower GI haemorrhage, then mesenteric arteriography is indicated to identify the source of bleeding, by showing contrast medium in the lumen of the bowel. Identifying the location of the bleed is extremely helpful in planning optimal surgery. Sometimes arteriography also permits a diagnosis to be made, e.g. angiodysplasia or small bowel tumour. Where appropriate, it may be possible to proceed to therapeutic embolization of the feeding vessel.

If the patient is actively bleeding at a rate of more than 0.5 mL/min then nuclear medicine techniques may be employed to localize the bleeding. The patient's red blood cells are labelled with ^{99m}Tc and the patient is then imaged under a gamma camera, so that any blood collecting in the bowel will be visualized. Radionuclide imaging is very sensitive for identifying active bleeding, although localizing the exact source of bleeding can be difficult. Barium studies are never used in investigating acute GI haemorrhage, because the presence of barium may preclude other investigations.

Colonic bleeding in adults is most commonly due to diverticular disease, angiodysplasia, malignancy or inflammatory bowel disease (Crohn's and ulcerative colitis). Colonic diverticular disease is most common in the sigmoid colon. Angiodysplasia is a submucosal vascular lesion, usually found in the caecum or ascending colon, and is a fairly common cause of bleeding in elderly patients. Colonoscopy is usually performed but may be unrewarding as it

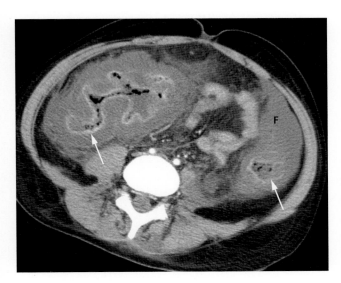

Fig. 4.80 Pseudomembranous colitis, secondary to *Clostridium difficile* infection. There is gross thickening of the colonic wall, thickened enhancing mucosa (arrows) and inflammatory changes and free fluid (F) in the surrounding tissues.

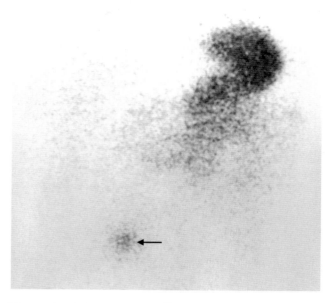

Fig. 4.81 Meckel's diverticulum. ^{99m}Tc-pertechnetate scan showing an isolated area of uptake in ectopic gastric mucosa in a Meckel's diverticulum (arrow). Normal uptake of radionuclide is seen in the stomach.

is sometimes not possible to reach the right side of the colon. Even when the caecum is reached, angiodysplasia may not be visible through the colonoscope.

The causes of bleeding in the small bowel are all rare but include benign and malignant tumours, vascular malformations, jejunal diverticula, Meckel's diverticulum and inflammatory bowel disease. Meckel's diverticulum, if it contains ectopic gastric mucosa, may be responsible for unexplained bleeding, particularly in children. Meckel's diverticulum is very difficult to demonstrate on a barium follow-through, but may be visualized with radionuclide techniques. An intravenous injection of technetium-99m (^{99m}Tc-pertechnetate) is given, which localizes in gastric mucosa. High uptake is seen in the stomach and in any gastric mucosa within a Meckel's diverticulum (Fig. 4.81).

Imaging in abdominal trauma

Initial imaging in cases of abdominal trauma is usually with plain x-ray, in order to identify free gas, in addition to bony injuries. A very rapid assessment for intra-abdominal free fluid (which is usually blood in the trauma setting) can be undertaken with FAST ultrasound (see Chapter 5, p. 192) and CT. Although ultrasound may be helpful in the detection of haemoperitoneum in the unstable patient, CT is used to detect injuries of the solid organs and the gastrointestinal tract (see Figs 5.21 and 5.46, pp. 192 and 206). Vascular injuries may also be detected. Computed tomography is performed using intravenous contrast media in order to assess the integrity of the major vessels and the vascular supply to the solid organs. Fracture of solid organs is associated with areas of low attenuation and disruption of the organ. In addition, there is adjacent haemorrhage. Perforation of the GI tract will be accompanied by free intraperitoneal air. Diaphragmatic rupture is well demonstrated by performing coronal reformats. Bone window settings must be reviewed to detect pelvic and vertebral fractures. Fractures may be displayed using reformatted coronal, sagittal and three-dimensional views, which may be helpful in surgical planning.

5

Hepatobiliary System, Spleen and Pancreas

Many different methods of imaging the hepatobiliary system and pancreas are available, notably ultrasound, computed tomography (CT), radionuclide imaging and magnetic resonance imaging (MRI). Invasive studies such as percutaneous or operative cholangiography and endoscopic retrograde cholangiopancreatography (ERCP) may be indicated. Every test has its own advantages and disadvantages. Ultrasound, for example, is particularly useful for diagnosing gall bladder disease, recognizing dilated bile ducts, diagnosing cysts and abscesses, and defining perihepatic fluid collections, whereas CT and MRI are particularly sensitive for detecting and characterizing mass lesions such as metastases and abscesses. Often the various methods complement each other, and, in practice, the imaging techniques used will depend on local expertise and may vary from centre to centre.

Although in clinical practice the liver and biliary tree are usually considered together, for the sake of clarity, we will discuss them independently. Interventional techniques designed to treat or remove gall stones and to drain the biliary system are described on p. 454.

LIVER

Imaging techniques

Ultrasound of the liver

The *normal hepatic parenchyma* (Fig. 5.1) is of uniform echogenicity, composed of medium and low level echoes, interspersed with the bright echoes of the portal triads and echo-free areas corresponding to large hepatic veins.

The normal liver displays considerable variation in size and shape. The right hepatic lobe is much larger than the left, which may be small. The falciform ligament, which contains the ligamentum teres, lies between the medial and lateral segments of the left lobe. The ligamentum teres is often surrounded by fat; the resulting echo pattern should not be confused with a mass (Fig. 5.2).

The portal vein within the liver divides into right and left branches. Running alongside the portal veins are the hepatic arteries and bile ducts, both of which are usually too small to be visualized within the liver. Surrounding these portal triads is an echo-reflective sheath of fibrous and fatty tissue. The hepatic veins run separately, increasing in diameter as they drain towards the inferior vena cava at the level of the diaphragm (Fig. 5.3).

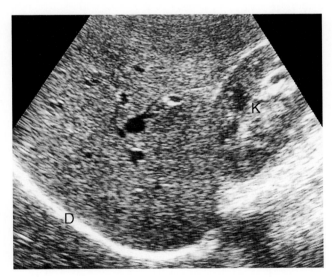

Fig. 5.1 Ultrasound of normal liver. Longitudinal scan showing uniform echo-pattern interspersed with bright echoes of portal triads and echo-free areas of hepatic and portal veins. D, diaphragm; K, right kidney.

Diagnostic Imaging, 6th Edition. By Peter Armstrong, Martin Wastie and Andrea Rockall. Published 2009 by Blackwell Publishing. ISBN: 978-1-4051-7039.

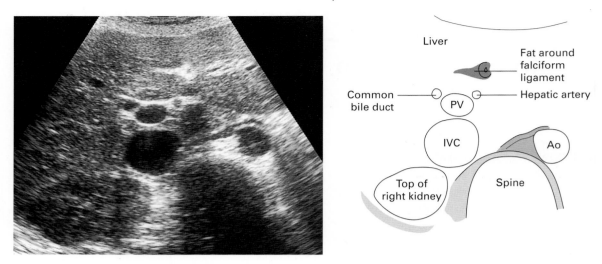

Fig. 5.2 Ultrasound of normal liver. Transverse scan across the porta hepatis. Ao, aorta; IVC, inferior vena cava; PV, portal vein.

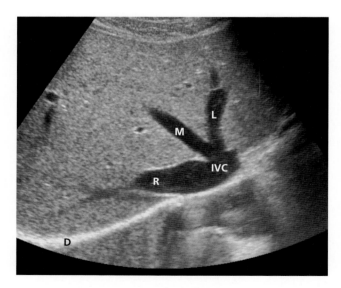

Fig. 5.3 Ultrasound of normal liver. Transverse scan through the superior portion of the liver showing the right (R), middle (M) and left (L) hepatic veins draining into the inferior vena cava (IVC) as it penetrates the diaphragm (D).

Focal masses are recognized as alterations of the normal echo pattern. They can be divided into cysts, solid masses, or complex combinations of the two. Cysts which are echo-free and have thin or invisible walls can be assumed to be benign (Fig. 5.4). Solid and complex masses (Figs 5.5 and 5.6) within the liver may be either benign or malignant in nature. Theoretically, most benign solid masses are well defined and should demonstrate a relatively sharp margin with the adjacent hepatic parenchyma, whereas malignant lesions may demonstrate a more irregular border. However, in practice it is often difficult to distinguish benign from malignant lesions unless the mass is clearly a simple cyst.

When multiple solid or complex masses are seen within the liver, metastatic disease is the likely diagnosis, especially in patients with a known primary tumour. The differential diagnoses of multiple masses are multiple abscesses, regenerating nodules in cirrhosis of the liver and multiple haemangiomas.

Diffuse parenchymal diseases such as diffuse chronic inflammation and diffuse neoplastic infiltration can cause a generalized increase in the intensity of echoes from the liver parenchyma, and are difficult to distinguish from one another.

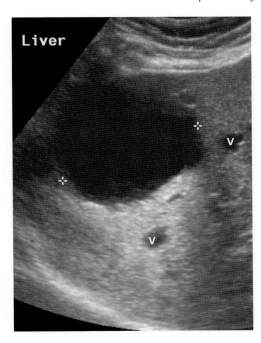

Fig. 5.4 Ultrasound of benign cyst. Note the imperceptible wall and absence echoes within the cyst. There is also posterior acoustic enhancement (increased echogenicity of structures deep to the cyst) secondary to enhanced transmission of the ultrasound waves through the water density of the cyst. V, hepatic veins.

CT of the liver

Intravenous contrast medium is usually given in order to increase the density of normal liver parenchyma and to emphasize the density difference between the normal parenchyma and lesions that enhance poorly, such as tumours or abscesses (Fig. 5.7). It is possible to visualize the different phases of liver opacification by taking scans at varying times after the injection of contrast. The liver has a dual blood supply from the hepatic artery and portal vein. Most metastases are best demonstrated as low attenuation areas during the portal venous phase on a scan taken 60–70 seconds after injection of contrast. Scanning during the arterial phase, about 30 seconds after the injection of contrast, will show lesions such as haemangiomas and some neoplasms, particularly hepatomas and highly vascular metastases (e.g. carcinoid), as areas of greater enhancement than the surrounding parenchyma.

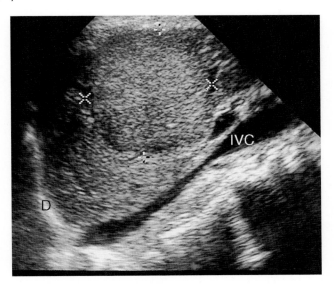

Fig. 5.5 Ultrasound of solid mass. Longitudinal scan. The cursors indicate an echogenic mass, which proved to be a metastasis. D, diaphragm; IVC, inferior vena cava.

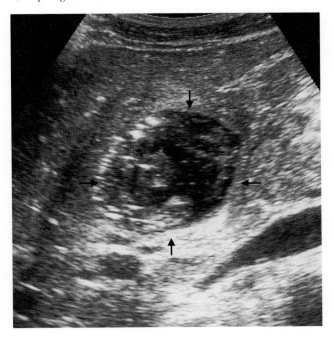

Fig. 5.6 Ultrasound of complex mass. Longitudinal scan of an abscess showing spherical mass (arrows) with areas of echogenicity both greater and less than normal liver.

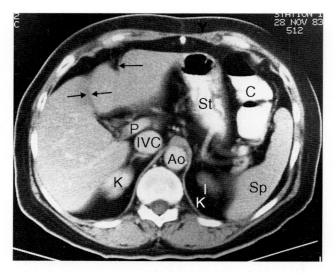

Fig. 5.7 CT scan of the normal liver through the porta hepatis (enhanced scan). A, aorta; C, colon; IVC, inferior vena cava; K, kidney; P, portal vein; Sp, spleen; St, stomach; single arrow fissure for falciform ligament, double arrow fissure for gall bladder which divides liver into right and left lobes.

Anatomically, the liver is divided into eight functionally independent segments (Fig. 5.8). Each segment has its own hepatic artery and portal venous inflow, hepatic venous drainage and biliary drainage. This classification is important in hepatic surgery as each segment can be resected without damaging those remaining. For the liver to remain viable, resections must proceed along the vessels that define the peripheries of these segments. This means that resection lines run parallel to the hepatic veins. The fissure for the gall bladder divides the liver into right and left lobes and the falciform ligament divides the left lobe into medial and lateral segments.

The normal hepatic parenchyma has a relatively high density prior to contrast enhancement; higher than that of muscle and higher or equal in density to the spleen. On images taken without intravenous contrast medium, the hepatic veins and portal veins are seen as branching, low density structures coursing through the liver. As CT is a sectional technique, some of these branches may be seen as round or oval low-density areas, which should not be confused with metastases (Fig. 5.9). After contrast enhancement, the veins opacify to become similar or higher in density than the surrounding parenchyma. Because the normal intrahepatic bile ducts are not visible and hepatic vessels opacify with contrast medium, the normal hepatic parenchyma after contrast shows either uniform density,

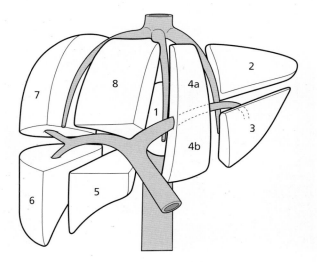

Fig. 5.8 The liver is divided anatomically into eight segments each of which has its own independent vascular supply and biliary drainage.

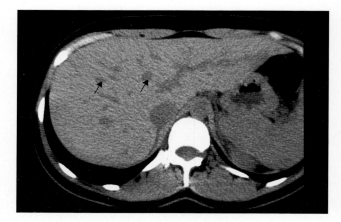

Fig. 5.9 CT scan of normal liver showing unopacified veins (arrows), which should not be confused with metastases.

or shows the veins clearly opacified against a background of uniform density. The region of the porta hepatis is recognizable as the entrance and exit points of the major vessels and bile ducts. The biliary system distal to the right and the left hepatic ducts can be identified, but the smaller intrahepatic bile ducts are not visible in the normal patient.

MRI of the liver

Magnetic resonance imaging is used as a problem-solving technique to give additional information to ultrasound and CT. It is, however, an excellent technique for demonstrating primary and secondary tumours and is often used if hepatic surgery is contemplated. Axial sections give images akin to CT (Fig. 5.10), but images can also be obtained in the coronal and sagittal planes. Intravenous contrast is used to improve visualization and help characterize lesions. New liver specific agents are being developed: some are taken up by hepatocytes and some by the reticulo-endothelial cells. Malignant tumours do not normally possess hepatocytes or reticulo-endothelial cells, so there is heightened contrast between tumour and normal liver.

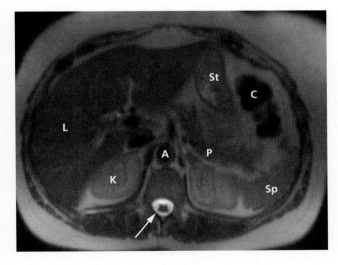

Fig. 5.10 Normal T2-weighted MRI scan of the upper abdomen. The liver parenchyma (L) shows intermediate signal intensity. The CSF has high signal intensity (arrow). A, aorta; C, splenic flexure of colon; Sp, spleen; St, stomach; P, pancreas; K, kidney.

Liver masses

Ultrasound, CT and MRI are all good methods of deciding whether a mass is present. Modern imaging techniques can go a long way to predicting the nature of the mass though occasionally the definitive diagnosis depends on biopsy. This, however, should not be undertaken in a potentially resectable lesion without discussion with a hepatic surgeon as seeding along the biopsy tract may compromise the surgical field.

Malignant liver neoplasms

Metastases, notably from carcinoma of the stomach, colon, pancreas, lung and breast are much more common than primary tumours (hepatoma and malignant lymphoma, both of which can be multifocal).

Metastases are often multiple, situated peripherally and of variable size. At ultrasound, they may show increased echogenicity (Fig. 5.11a) or, more usually, decreased echogenicity compared with the surrounding parenchyma (Fig. 5.11b). At times, they show a complex echo pattern and when they undergo central necrosis they may even resemble cysts. A metastasis may have an echogenic centre giving an appearance described as a target lesion (Fig. 5.11c). Some metastases have an echo pattern virtually identical to that of the surrounding parenchyma, which means they cannot be identified at sonography. At CT, metastases are seen as rounded areas, usually lower in density than the contrast-enhanced surrounding parenchyma (Fig. 5.12a). Most are well demarcated from the adjacent parenchyma. Intense contrast enhancement is sometimes seen within the tumour, or immediately surrounding it – a useful differentiating feature, which is not seen with cysts. Some metastases, notably carcinoid, are hypervascular and appear as high-density areas on arterial phase images (Fig. 5.12b). MRI is an excellent method of demonstrating metastases, which typically have a signal lower than normal liver on a T1-weighted scan and a high signal intensity on a T2-weighted scan (Fig. 5.13). Various intravenous contrast agents may be used to aid their visualization.

Primary carcinomas of the liver, which include hepatocellular carcinoma and cholangiocarcinoma, are usually solitary but they may be multifocal. Their CT, ultrasound and MRI features are similar to metastatic neoplasms (Fig. 5.14).

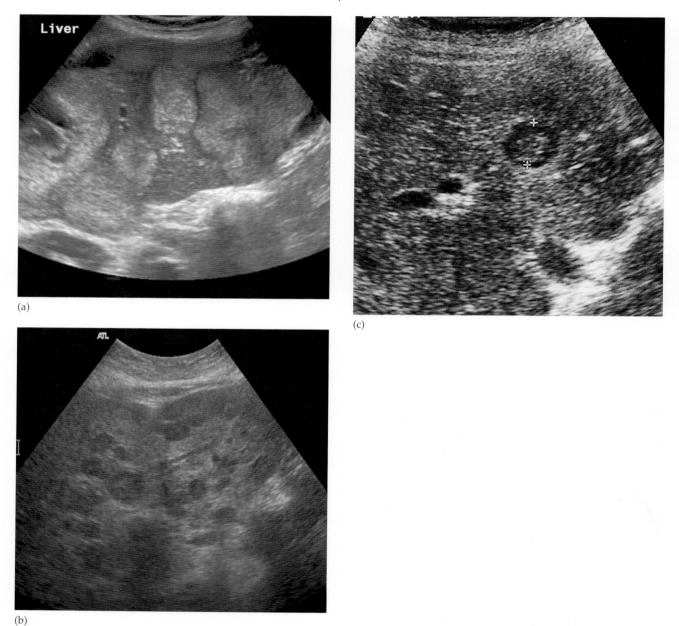

(a)

(b)

(c)

Fig. 5.11 Ultrasound of liver metastases. (a) Multiple hyperechoic metastases scattered throughout the liver. (b) Multiple metastases appearing as well-defined round hypoechoic lesions scattered throughout the liver. (c) The cursors indicate a metastasis showing reduced echogenicity, but with an echogenic centre known as a target lesion.

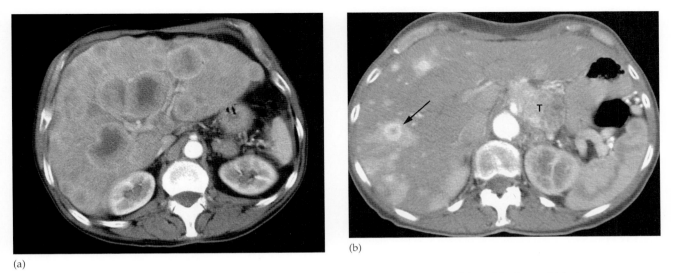

(a)

(b)

Fig. 5.12 CT scan of liver metastases. (a) There are a large number of low-density lesions in both lobes of the liver, which show enhancement around their edges. The patient had carcinoma of the bronchus. (b) Vascular metastases (arrow) due to a carcinoid tumour (T) appearing as areas of high density on this arterial-phase image.

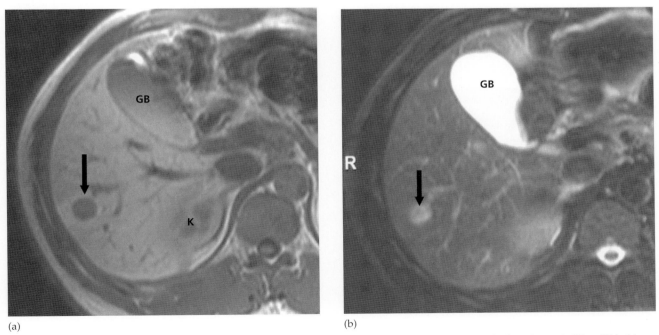

(a)

(b)

Fig. 5.13 Liver metastasis on MRI. (a) T1-weighted MRI showing a solitary low signal intensity focus in the liver (arrow). GB, gall bladder; K, kidney. (b) T2-weighted MRI (with fat saturation) showing the same metastasis. This is of higher signal intensity than the normal liver parenchyma. However, the signal intensity is not as bright as a haemangioma or cyst.

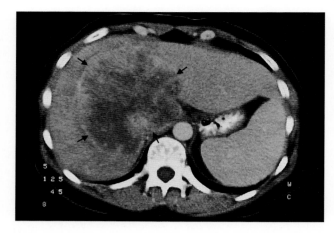

Fig. 5.14 Hepatoma. The CT scan shows a large mass of variable density (arrows).

Benign liver masses

Benign masses are encountered fairly frequently in the general population. Most are cysts, some are haemangiomas. Focal nodular hyperplasia and adenomas are rare but can closely resemble malignant masses. MRI can be very helpful in differentiating benign from malignant lesions.

Liver cysts

Simple cysts of the liver may be single or multiple, and are usually congenital in origin; some are due to infection. Multiple hepatic cysts occur in adult polycystic disease, which not only affects the kidneys but may also involve the liver and other organs. These cysts are variable in size and are scattered through the liver.

At ultrasound, liver cysts show the typical features of cysts elsewhere in the body, namely sharp margin, no echoes within the lesion, and intense echoes from the front and back walls with acoustic enhancement deep to the larger cysts (see Fig. 5.4, p. 183).

At CT, cysts show very well-defined margins and have attenuation values similar to that of water (Fig. 5.15a). It is

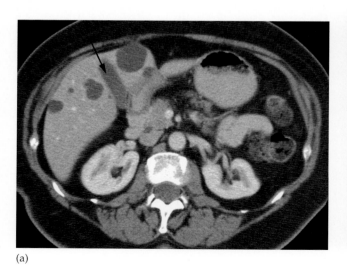

(a)

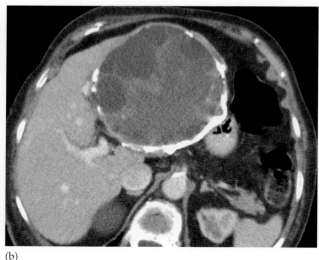

(b)

Fig. 5.15 Liver cysts on CT. (a) Simple cysts. CT shows several well-defined low attenuation lesions of near water density. Note their density is equivalent to the bile in the gall bladder (arrowed). (b) Complex cyst. CT scan showing a multilocular hydatid cyst with calcification in its wall.

often not possible to characterize small lesions, and with lesions below 1 cm in diameter it may be difficult to distinguish cyst from neoplasm.

At MRI, the features are similar to those found at CT. Cysts have the expected signal intensity of water, namely low signal on a T1-weighted scan and high signal on a T2-weighted scan.

Cysts due to echinococcus (hydatid) disease may be single or multiple; a few show calcified walls. Daughter cysts may be seen within a main cyst at both ultrasound and CT (Fig. 5.15b). Unless these features are present, hydatid cysts may prove indistinguishable from simple cysts at both ultrasound and CT.

Occasionally metastases can have a cystic appearance.

Haemangiomas of the liver

The detection of one or more haemangiomas of the liver is a common incidental finding and rarely requires treatment.

Occasionally, they can cause significant haemorrhage, especially following trauma, and therefore percutaneous biopsy should be avoided if possible. Haemangiomas are typically well-defined, peripheral echogenic masses at ultrasound (Fig. 5.16a). At CT, there is usually a characteristic enhancement pattern characterized by sequential contrast opacification beginning as nodular or globular areas of enhancement at the periphery, proceeding toward the centre over time until the density increases to become similar to that of the surrounding liver (Fig. 5.16b).

Magnetic resonance imaging shows uniform very high intensity on T2-weighted images (Fig. 5.17), a characteristic that is shared with benign cysts, but which is very unusual with malignant neoplastic lesions.

Adenoma and focal nodular hyperplasia

Both of these conditions appear as hypervascular masses on arterial phase both on CT and MRI (Fig. 5.18).

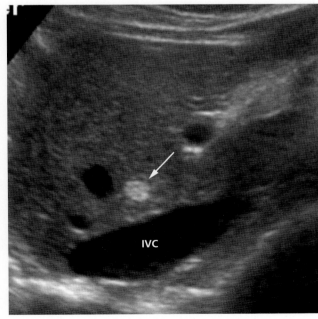

(a)

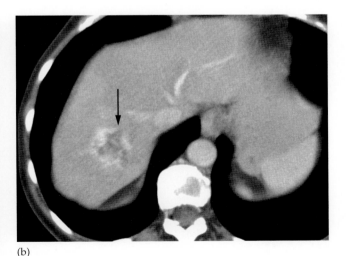

(b)

Fig. 5.16 Haemangioma (incidental finding). (a) Ultrasound scan shows an echogenic mass in the right lobe of the liver (arrow). IVC, inferior vena cava. (b) CT scan, in another patient, after intravenous contrast enhancement shows a low density lesion in the right lobe of the liver (arrow) with peripheral nodular enhancement, characteristic of a haemangioma.

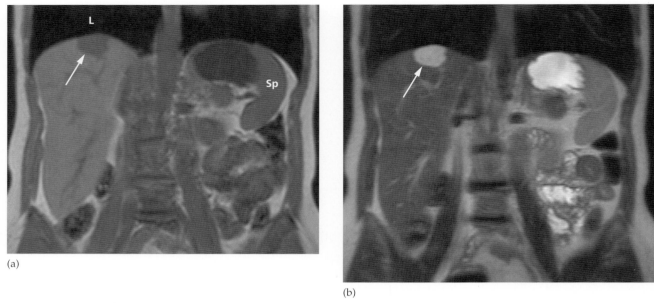

Fig. 5.17 MR images of a haemangioma. (a) Low signal intensity focus (arrow) on a coronal T1-weighted image. (b) High signal intensity focus (arrow) on a coronal T2-weighted image. L, right lung base; Sp, spleen.

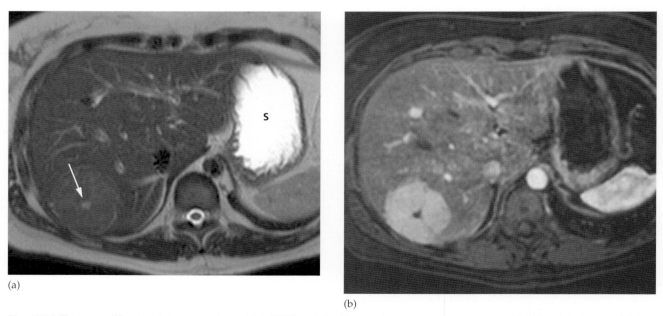

Fig. 5.18 MR images of focal nodular hyperplasia. (a) Axial T2-weighted image demonstrates a mass in the right lobe of the liver which is isointense to normal liver with a hyperintense central scar (arrow). S, stomach. (b) An axial TI-weighted image, post contrast, demonstrates avid enhancement of the mass with sparing of the central scar on this arterial phase image. These features are characteristic of focal nodular hyperplasia (FNH).

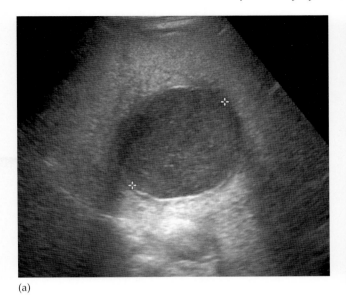

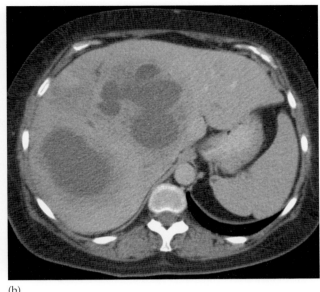

(a)

(b)

Fig. 5.19 Liver abscess. (a) Ultrasound scan showing an area of mixed echogenicity in the liver. (b) CT in another patient showing multifocal areas of low attenuation. Compared to the liver cysts (Fig. 5.15a), they are not nearly as well circumscribed.

Liver abscess

Abscesses appear somewhat similar to cysts but usually they can be distinguished (Fig. 5.19). Hepatic abscesses tend to have fluid centres, with walls that are thicker, more irregular and more obvious than those of simple cysts. Although the CT attenuation values in the centre of an abscess may be the same as water, usually they are higher. At ultrasound, a layer of necrotic debris may be seen within the abscess. Occasionally, chronic abscesses calcify.

Abscesses cannot usually be distinguished from necrotic tumours at either ultrasound, CT or MRI, but the clinical situation should aid in making the distinction. Aspiration and drainage are invariably undertaken in any case of suspected abscess and are conveniently performed under ultrasound guidance.

Cirrhosis of the liver and portal hypertension

In portal hypertension the pressure in the portal venous system is elevated due to obstruction of the flow of blood in the portal or hepatic venous systems. Cirrhosis of the liver is by far the most frequent cause. Other causes include

occlusion of the hepatic veins (Budd–Chiari syndrome) and thrombosis of the portal vein, particularly following infection of the umbilical vein in the neonatal period or secondary to pancreatitis.

Because the portal venous pressure is raised, blood flows through anastomotic channels, known as portosystemic anastomoses, to enter the vena cavae, bypassing the liver. These collateral channels may be found in various sites, but the most important are varices at the lower end of the oesophagus and in the upper abdomen (Fig. 5.20). The collateral channels can be shown with colour-flow Doppler ultrasound.

The signs of cirrhosis of the liver at CT and ultrasound are reduction in size of the right lobe of the liver and irregularity of the surface of the liver, together with splenomegaly. Ascites may be present as well. The texture of the liver at ultrasound may be diffusely abnormal; at CT, the parenchyma appears normal until late in the disease.

Patency of the splenic, portal and hepatic veins can be assessed with Doppler ultrasound, CT or MRI.

As a last resort for the treatment of bleeding varices the percutaneous procedure known as TIPSS (transjugular intrahepatic portosystemic shunt) is undertaken. In this

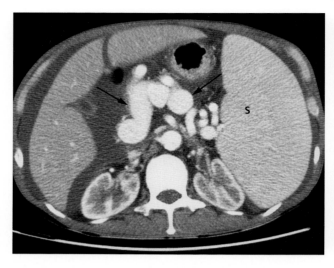

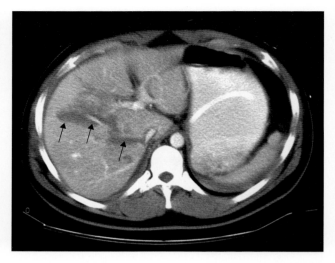

Fig. 5.20 Varices on CT due to portal hypertension. There is marked enhancement of multiple serpinginous vessels in the upper abdomen (arrows), extending into the splenic hilum. There is splenomegaly and ascites. S, spleen.

Fig. 5.21 Liver trauma. Computed tomography scan showing laceration in the right lobe of the liver (arrows). A nasogastric tube is present in the stomach.

procedure, a connection between the portal and systemic venous system is created by placing a stent connecting a large hepatic and portal vein within the liver (see Chapter 15, p. 450).

Liver trauma

Trauma to the liver is the commonest abdominal injury that leads to death. Parenchymal lacerations are the most frequent injury and they are often accompanied by subcapsular and intrahepatic haematomas (Fig. 5.21). Ultrasound has become part of the standard assessment of patients who give a history of abdominal trauma and are hypotensive or unable to give an accurate history due to impaired consciousness. Focused Assessment with Sonography for Trauma (FAST scan) is a rapid bedside examination which examines four areas for free fluid:
- perihepatic and hepato-renal space
- perisplenic
- pelvis
- pericardium.

As a rapid, non-invasive, bedside test, ultrasound has significant advantages over diagnostic peritoneal lavage (DPL) and CT scanning for the evaluation of free intraperitoneal fluid. The average time to perform a FAST in the hands of an experienced operator is 2–3 minutes. Computed tomography scanning, however, is more sensitive and specific, and lacerations and haematomas are recognized as low density areas relative to the contrast-enhanced parenchyma. Leakage of contrast indicates active bleeding.

Fatty infiltration of the liver

Fatty infiltration of the liver, whilst not normal, is a relatively frequent finding, particularly in those with hypercholesterolaemia, obesity, diabetes or those who take alcohol to excess. Fatty infiltration may involve the whole liver, or it may just involve individual subsections. In some patients it is a benign process (non-alcoholic fatty liver disease), whilst in others it can proceed to cirrhosis (non-alcoholic steato-hepatitis).

Fatty infiltration leads to a reduction in the attenuation of the affected parenchyma causing low density on CT scans (Fig. 5.22). The vessels are then seen as relatively high-attenuation structures against a background of low-density parenchyma, even on images taken without intravenous contrast medium. On ultrasound, the liver parenchyma shows increased echogenicity, the so-called bright liver,

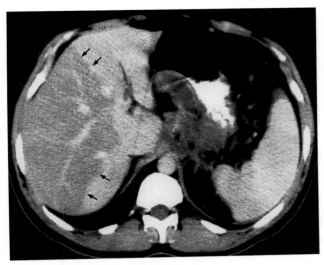

Fig. 5.22 Fatty degeneration of the liver shown by CT as a large focal area of reduced attenuation in the right lobe of the liver (arrows).

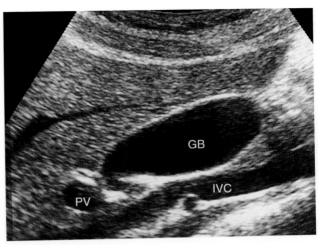

Fig. 5.23 Ultrasound of normal gall bladder. Note the thin wall and absence of echoes from within the gall bladder. GB, gall bladder; IVC, inferior vena cava; PV, portal vein.

in which the echogenicity of the liver is similar to that of the central echo-complex of the kidney. MRI can be very helpful in problem cases because fat gives a characteristic set of signals.

BILIARY SYSTEM

The gall bladder and bile duct system can be demonstrated by a variety of imaging techniques. Ultrasound is the initial method of imaging because it is the simplest test for showing gall stones, diseases of the gall bladder and excluding bile duct dilatation. Occasionally, radionuclide imaging using hepatobiliary agents is used as a functional assessment to exclude biliary obstruction.

Gall stones, gall bladder wall thickening and dilatation of the common bile duct are also visible at CT, but as ultrasound provides better information it is used as the primary method of examination for these problems.

Imaging techniques

Ultrasound of the gall bladder and bile ducts

As the gall bladder is a fluid-filled structure, it is parti-

cularly amenable to sonographic examination. Because it is important that the gall bladder should be full of bile, the patient is asked to fast in order to prevent gall bladder contraction, but no other preparation is necessary. The normal gall bladder wall is so thin that it is sometimes barely perceptible (Fig. 5.23). *Gall bladder wall thickening* suggests either acute or chronic cholecystitis. *Gall stones* greater than 1 or 2 mm in size can usually be identified at ultrasound examination. It is usually impossible to diagnose cystic duct obstruction with ultrasound; the cystic duct is too small to identify and the stones that impact in it are often too small to see.

Ultrasound is the initial investigation for demonstrating the *bile ducts*. The common hepatic or common bile duct can be visualized in almost all patients; it is seen as a small tubular structure lying anterior to the portal vein in the porta hepatis and should not measure more than 7 mm in diameter (Fig. 5.24) unless the patient has had a cholecystectomy when it may be larger. The lower end of the common bile duct is often obscured by gas in the duodenum.

The normal intrahepatic biliary tree is of such small caliber that only small portions a few millimetres long may be seen at ultrasound.

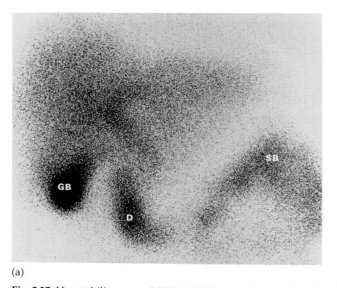

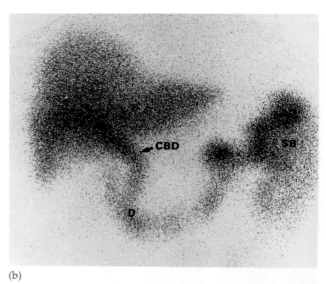

(a)   (b)

Fig. 5.27 Hepatobiliary scan. (a) Normal IDA scan. There is obvious filling of the gall bladder. Activity is also present in the duodenum and small bowel. (b) Cystic duct obstruction. The IDA scan in this patient with acute right upper quadrant pain shows the duct system but no filling of the gall bladder. CBD, common bile duct; D, duodenum; GB, gall bladder; SB, small bowel.

across an obstruction if this cannot be achieved endoscopically at ERCP.

Hepatobiliary radionuclide scanning

Iminodiacetic acid (IDA) pharmaceuticals labelled with ^{99m}Tc are excreted by the liver following intravenous injection and may be used for imaging the bile duct system. Hepatic excretion occurs despite relatively high serum bilirubin levels, and, therefore, these agents can be used when the patient is jaundiced, even with serum bilirubin levels of up to 250 µmol/L (15 mg%). All that is required is that the patient fasts for 4 hours prior to the injection of the radionuclide. Normally, the gall bladder, common bile duct, duodenum and small bowel are all seen within the first hour, confirming the patency and integrity of both the cystic duct and the common bile duct. The main use of this technique is in patients with suspected biliary leak following biliary surgery. Excretion of the radionuclide tracer from the biliary tree into the peritoneal cavity is diagnostic of a leak. The technique may also be used in acute cholecystitis (with non-filling of the gall bladder in cases of an impacted stone in the cystic duct, Fig. 5.27) or in children, when biliary atresia is suspected.

Gall stones and cholecystitis

Gall stones are a frequent finding in adults, particularly middle-aged females. Together with accompanying chronic cholecystitis, they are a major cause of recurrent upper abdominal pain. The presence of stones within the gall bladder does not necessarily mean the patient's pain is due to gall stones. In the appropriate clinical setting, however, identification of gall stones may be sufficient for many surgeons to take action.

Some 20% of gall stones contain sufficient calcium to be visible on plain film (Fig. 5.28). They vary greatly in size and shape and, typically, have a dense outer rim with a more lucent centre. Calcified sludge within the gall bladder is also known as 'milk of calcium' bile.

At ultrasound, gall stones are seen as strongly echogenic foci within the dependent portion of the gall bladder. Acoustic shadows are usually seen behind stones, because most of the ultrasound beam is reflected by the stones and only a little passes on through the patient (Fig. 5.29). The presence of an acoustic shadow is an important diagnostic feature for confirming stones in the gall bladder or common bile duct. Acoustic shadowing is not seen with polyps. The

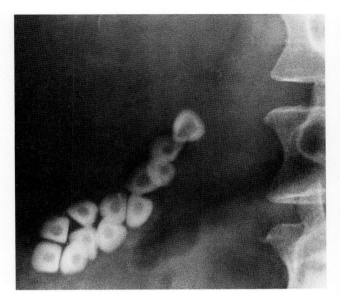

Fig. 5.28 Radio-opaque gall stones. Plain film showing multiple faceted stones with lucent centres.

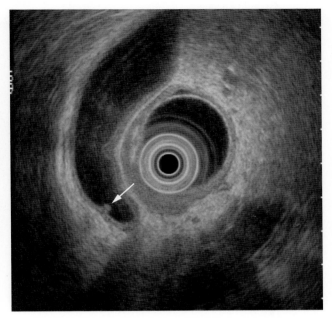

Fig. 5.30 Endoscopic ultrasound showing a small polyp in the gall bladder with no acoustic shadow (arrow).

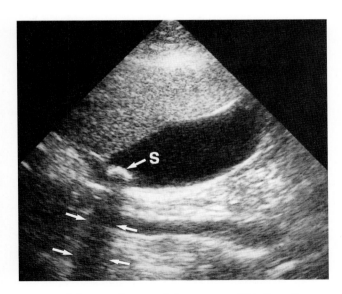

Fig. 5.29 Gall stone. Ultrasound shows a stone (S) in the gall bladder. The arrows point to the acoustic shadow behind the stone.

vast majority of polyps are small (Fig. 5.30), measuring only a few millimetres and are not neoplasms but aggregations of cholesterol.

Although ultrasound is very accurate at diagnosing gall stones, it is much less reliable for detecting stones in the common bile duct which are better demonstrated with MRCP.

Cholecystitis

In acute cholecystitis ultrasound will usually detect gall stones, inflammatory debris, gall bladder wall thickening and a rim of fluid adjacent to the gall bladder (Fig. 5.31a). On CT, the gall bladder wall is thickened and there is surrounding inflammatory change seen as stranding in the adjacent fat (Fig. 5.31b). In acute cholecystitis, pain is often localized to the gall bladder. In chronic cholecystitis, the gall bladder is often contracted and thick-walled.

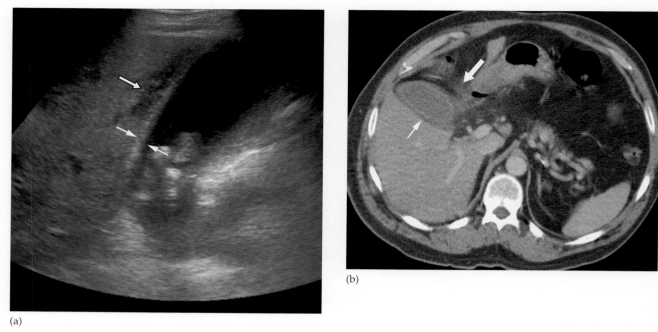

(a)   (b)

Fig. 5.31 Acute cholecystitis. (a) Ultrasound showing a thick oedematous gall bladder wall indicated by the thin arrows. There is also evidence of fluid adjacent to the gall bladder indicative of acute inflammation (thick arrow). (b) CT scan of acute cholecystitis shows a thick-walled gall bladder with adjacent oedema and inflammatory change as evidenced by a surrounding low attenuation rim (thin arrow) and lack of clarity (stranding) in the adjacent fat (thick arrow).

Box 5.1 Major causes of biliary obstruction

- Impacted stone in the common bile duct
- Carcinoma of the head of the pancreas
- Carcinoma of the ampulla of Vater
- Cholangiocarcinoma

Jaundice

Clinical examination and biochemical tests often permit the cause of jaundice to be diagnosed. Imaging tests may, however, be required when there is doubt as to the nature of the jaundice. The basis of this distinction is that dilated biliary ducts are a feature of jaundice from biliary obstruction. Imaging is used to determine the site (e.g. distal CBD or hilar obstruction) and, if possible, the cause of obstruction (see Box 5.1).

Dilatation of the intra- and extrahepatic biliary system can be identified at ultrasound (Fig. 5.32a), CT (Fig. 5.32b) and

MRI. Ultrasound is the more available test and is usually the first test to be performed. Dilated intrahepatic biliary ducts are seen at ultrasound as serpentine structures paralleling the portal veins, a finding known as 'the double-channel sign'. The common bile duct lies just in front of the portal vein and is dilated when more than 7 mm in diameter. Ultrasound is good for demonstrating the level of obstruction and sometimes the specific cause for biliary obstruction can be seen, e.g. a stone impacted within the common bile duct (Fig. 5.33) or a mass in the pancreatic head. More often, the cause cannot be seen, mainly because overlying gas in the duodenum obscures the lower end of the common bile duct and further imaging is required depending on the ultrasound findings. For suspected stone disease or a hilar stricture, MRCP is often more helpful than CT in delineating the biliary tree and, conversely, CT is more often used for further evaluation and staging of a distal obstruction secondary to an underlying pancreatic malignancy. Substantial dilatation of the common hepatic and common bile ducts

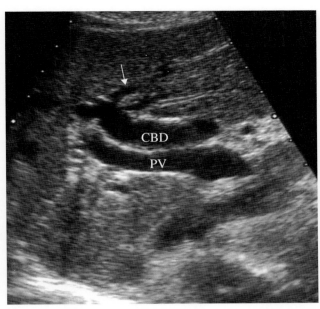

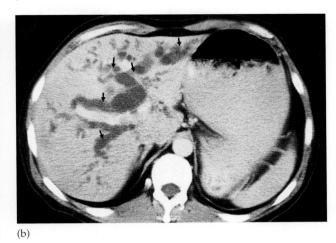

(b)

(a)

Fig. 5.32 Dilated biliary ducts. (a) Longitudinal ultrasound scan showing a dilated common bile duct (CBD) measuring 11 mm in diameter lying in front of the portal vein (PV). Normally the duct is much smaller than the accompanying vein. A dilated intrahepatic duct is arrowed. (b) CT scan showing dilated intrahepatic ducts (arrows) in the liver.

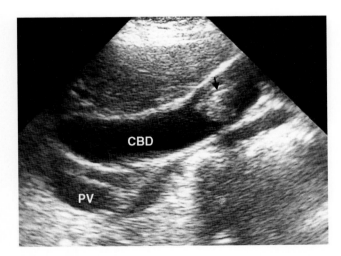

Fig. 5.33 Stones in the common bile duct (CBD). The common bile duct is dilated measuring 2 cm in diameter and a large stone (arrow) is seen in its lower portion. PV, section through portal vein.

may be present with only minimal dilatation of the intrahepatic ducts; the intrahepatic biliary tree may not dilate at all within the first 48 hours following obstruction.

Once a diagnosis has been established, the patient usually undergoes biliary decompression at ERCP. If this fails, or there is a hilar stricture present then decompression is performed at PTC. Occasionally, patients who are well enough may go straight to surgery to remove an underlying malignancy if it is thought that complete resection is possible and there is no metastatic disease.

PANCREAS

Computed tomography is now the mainstay for imaging the pancreas. A major advantage of CT over transabdominal ultrasound is that it can image the pancreas regardless of the amount of bowel adjacent to it, whereas the ultrasound beam is absorbed by gas in the gastrointestinal tract. This has led to the development of endoscopic ultrasound, which is routinely used in the diagnosis (including

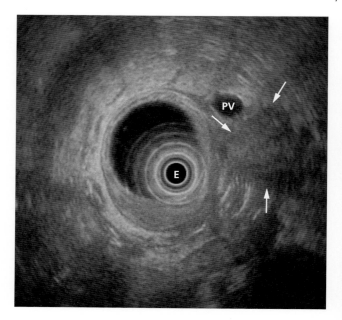

Fig. 5.34 Endoscopic ultrasound (E) showing mass in the pancreas (arrow heads) which involves the portal vein (PV).

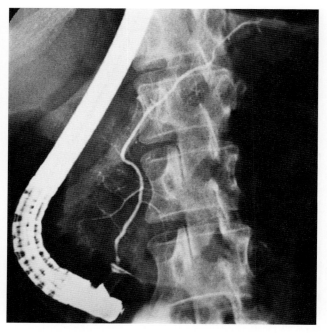

Fig. 5.35 Endoscopic retrograde pancreatography. The pancreatic duct has been cannulated from the endoscope in the duodenum. Contrast has been injected to demonstrate a normal duct system.

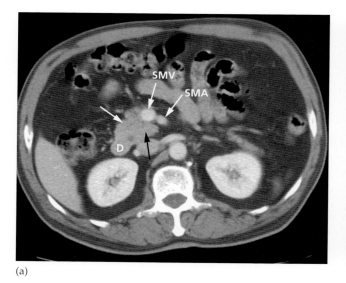

(a)

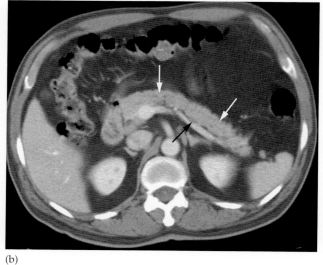

(b)

Fig. 5.36 CT of normal pancreas. Note that several sections may be needed to display the pancreas. (a) The head (white arrow) nestling between the second part of the duodenum (D) and the superior mesenteric vessels (SMA and SMV). The uncinate process lies anterior to the IVC (black arrow). (b) CT taken 3 cm higher, showing the body and part of the tail (white arrows). Note the splenic vein, which lies posterior to the body of pancreas (black arrow).

biopsy) of pancreatic disease and staging in patients with pancreatic cancer (e.g. involvement of the superior mesenteric artery precludes a surgical cure) (Fig. 5.34). Magnetic resonance imaging, ERCP (Fig. 5.35) and arteriography, are used in selected cases.

The normal pancreas is an elongated retroperitoneal organ surrounded by a variable amount of fat (Fig. 5.36). The head nestles in the duodenal loop (for CT scanning, the duodenum is opacified by an oral contrast agent) and the uncinate process folds behind the superior mesenteric artery and vein; these vessels form a useful landmark to help identify the head of the pancreas. The body of the pancreas lies in front of the superior mesenteric artery and vein, and passes behind the stomach, with the tail situated near the hilum of the spleen. The splenic vein, which can be a surprisingly large structure, is another very useful landmark. Lying behind the pancreas, it joins the superior mesenteric vein posterior to the neck of the pancreas to form the portal vein.

In most people, the pancreas runs obliquely across the retroperitoneum, being higher at the splenic end. Because of this oblique orientation, CT shows different portions of the pancreas on the various sections. The normal pancreas shows a feathery texture, corresponding to pancreatic lobules inter-spersed with fat. Atrophy is a common feature of ageing. At ultrasound, the pancreas gives reasonably uniform echoes of medium to high level compared to the adjacent liver (Fig. 5.37). The pancreatic duct may be seen, with the normal lumen being no more than 2 mm in diameter.

Pancreatic masses

The usual causes of masses in, or immediately adjacent to, the pancreas are: carcinoma of the pancreas, neoplasm of the adjacent lymph nodes, focal pancreatitis, pancreatic abscess and pseudocyst formation. Occasionally, congenital cysts may be seen.

Most neoplasms of the pancreas are *adenocarcinomas*, two-thirds of which occur in the head of the pancreas. Tumours arising in the head may obstruct the common bile duct giving rise to jaundice, and are, therefore, sometimes diagnosed when relatively small. Tumours arising in the body and tail have to be fairly large to give rise to signs or symptoms, pain being the cardinal symptom. As the pancreas is so variable, measurements have not proved useful in diagnosing masses. The important sign of carcinoma of the pancreas at both CT and ultrasound is, therefore, a focal mass within or deforming the outline of the gland

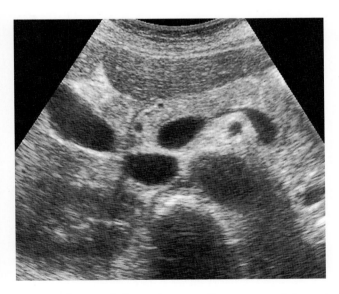

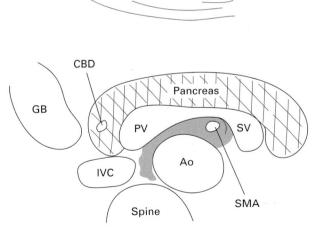

Fig. 5.37 Ultrasound of normal pancreas (transverse scan). Ao, aorta; CBD, common bile duct; GB, gall bladder; IVC, inferior vena cava; PV, portal vein; SMA, superior mesenteric artery; SV, splenic vein.

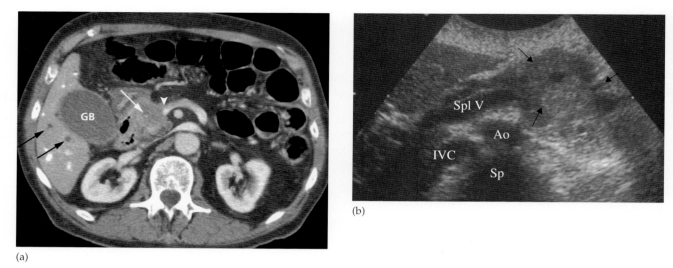

(a)

(b)

Fig. 5.38 Carcinoma of the pancreas. (a) CT scan showing a focal mass in the head of the pancreas (white arrow), which involves the portal/mesenteric vein confluence (arrow head) and may preclude curative surgery (compare with endoscopic ultrasound image Fig. 5.34, performed in the same patient). Note the dilated intrahepatic bile ducts (black arrows) and distended gall bladder (GB). (b) Ultrasound. Transverse scan showing a large mass in the body of the pancreas (arrows). Ao, aorta; IVC, inferior vena cava; Sp, spine; Spl V, splenic vein.

(Fig. 5.38). On contrast-enhanced CT, the tumour appears of lower density compared to the normal pancreatic tissue (Fig. 5.38a). The main pancreatic duct may be dilated distal to an obstructing tumour mass and can be identified on all imaging modalities.

Staging investigations attempt to identify potentially resectable tumours. Most are irresectable at presentation: the presence of liver metastases, lymphadenopathy, retroperitoneal invasion, tumour encasement of arteries and veins are contraindications to surgery.

The presence of pancreatic *endocrine secreting tumours*, of which insulinoma is the commonest example, is suggested by clinical presentation and biochemical investigations. These tumours are difficult to detect as they are usually small and do not deform the pancreatic contour. They may be seen on ultrasound, CT or MRI as small round masses within the pancreas (Fig. 5.39a). Sometimes selective angiography is required, where they stand out from the rest of the pancreas by virtue of their hypervascularity (Fig. 5.39b). Special somatostatin receptor radionuclide scans (Octreoscan) may also demonstrate the tumour and any metastases.

Acute pancreatitis

Acute pancreatitis causes abdominal pain, fever, vomiting and leucocytosis, together with elevation of the serum amylase. The findings at CT and ultrasound vary with the amount of necrosis, haemorrhage and suppuration (Fig. 5.40). The pancreas is usually enlarged, often diffusely and may show irregularity of its outline, caused by extension of the inflammatory process into the surrounding retroperitoneal fat: features that are well seen at CT. There may be low-density areas at CT and echo-poor areas at sonography, representing oedema and focal necrosis within or adjacent to the pancreas.

The diagnosis of pancreatitis is usually made on clinical and biochemical grounds; the purpose of imaging is to assess the severity of the disease and to demonstrate complications:

• The pancreas may be necrotic and non-viable if it does not enhance at CT after intravenous contrast.

• An abscess appears as a localized fluid collection, which may contain gas.

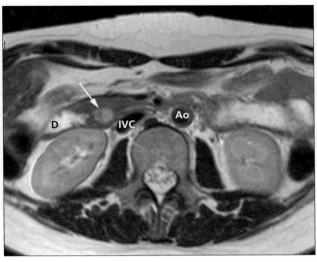

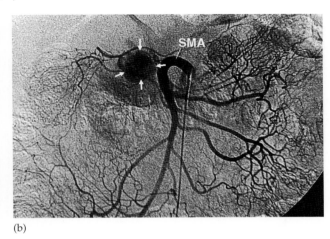

(a)

(b)

Fig. 5.39 Insulinoma. (a) Axial T2-weighted MRI demonstrating a 1.5 cm insulinoma in the uncinate process of the pancreas (arrow). (b) Selective superior mesenteric angiogram in another patient showing the tumour as a vascular blush (arrows). SMA, superior mesenteric artery. D, duodenum; IVC, inferior vena cava; Ao, aorta.

• Vascular complications are serious and these include splenic vein thrombosis, arterial erosion and the formation of a pseudoaneurysm.
• *Pseudocysts* are a complication of acute pancreatitis in which tissue necrosis leads to a leak of pancreatic secretions, which are then contained in a cyst-like manner within and adjacent to the pancreas. They can be well demonstrated by CT (or ultrasound) as thin- or thick-walled cysts containing fluid (Fig. 5.41). They vary in size from very small to many centimetres in diameter. Many pseudocysts resolve in the weeks following an attack of acute pancreatitis. Some persist and may need surgical or percutaneous drainage. Both CT and ultrasound are excellent methods of following such cysts and determining the best approach to treatment.

Chronic pancreatitis

Chronic pancreatitis results in fibrosis, calcifications, and ductal stenoses and dilatations. Pseudocysts are seen with chronic pancreatitis just as they are in the acute form. The calcification in chronic pancreatitis is mainly due to small calculi within the pancreas; they are often recognizable on plain films (see old Fig. 3.17, p. 129) and ultrasound, but are particularly obvious at CT (Fig. 5.42a). The gland may enlarge generally or focally. Focal enlargement is rare and is then often indistinguishable from carcinoma. Conversely, the pancreas may atrophy focally or generally. Atrophy is a non-specific sign; it is frequently seen in normal elderly people and also occurs distal to a carcinoma. The pancreatic duct may be enlarged and irregular, a feature that is visible at CT, and particularly striking at ultrasound.

ERCP is occasionally used to try and document chronic pancreatitis and exclude carcinoma. The generalized irregular dilatation of the duct system seen with chronic pancreatitis is very well demonstrated. MRCP can be used as an alternative non-invasive method (Fig. 5.42b).

Pancreatic trauma

Trauma to the pancreas is uncommon but serious. Injuries to other structures are frequent, so CT is the best method of investigation. In addition to lacerations and haematomas, the release of pancreatic enzymes into the surrounding tissues leads to traumatic pancreatitis and tissue necrosis.

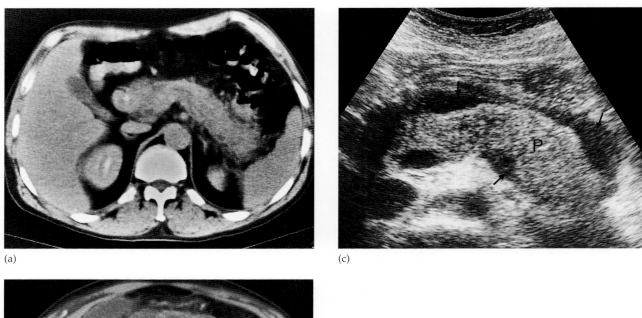

(a)

(c)

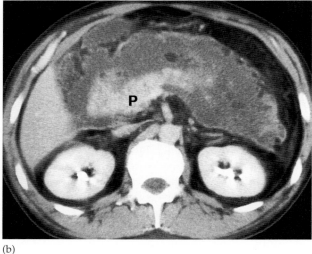

(b)

Fig. 5.40 Acute pancreatitis. (a) CT scan showing diffuse enlargement of the pancreas with ill-defined edges. (b) CT scan showing considerable inflammation around the pancreas (P). (c) Ultrasound. Transverse scan showing a swollen pancreas (P) with some fluid around the pancreas (arrows).

The features here are similar to other forms of acute pancreatitis (see above), including the subsequent development of pseudocysts.

SPLEEN

Imaging the spleen is, in many respects, similar to imaging the liver. At ultrasound, the spleen has a homogeneous appearance with the same echo-density as the liver. CT and MRI are excellent ways to examine the spleen; normal CT images are shown in the appendix.

The commonly encountered splenic masses are cysts, including hydatid cysts (Fig. 5.43), abscesses and tumours; lymphoma (Fig. 5.44) is much commoner than metastases, which are rare in the spleen.

Many conditions cause enlargement of the spleen but cause no change in splenic texture on ultrasound, or any change in density on a CT scan. These conditions include lymphoma, portal hypertension (see Fig. 5.20, p. 192),

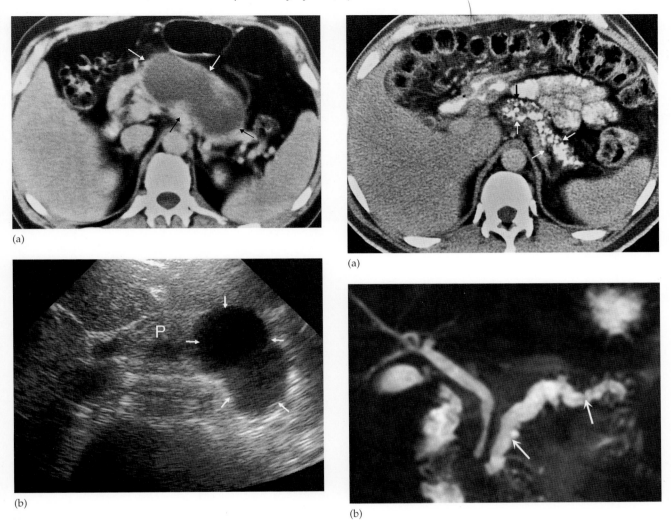

(a)

(b)

Fig. 5.41 Pancreatic pseudocyst. (a) CT scan showing large cyst arising within the pancreas (arrows). (b) Ultrasound (transverse scan). The arrows indicate a pseudocyst arising from the body of the pancreas. P, pancreas. Same patient as Fig. 5.40c, 6 weeks later.

(a)

(b)

Fig. 5.42 Chronic pancreatitis. (a) CT scan showing numerous small areas of calcification within the pancreas (arrows). (b) Magnetic resonance cholangiopancreatography (MRCP) showing a normal biliary duct system but irregular dilatation of the pancreatic duct (arrows).

chronic infection and various blood disorders, e.g. hae-molytic anaemias and leukaemia. As the appearance of the enlarged spleen in all these conditions is similar, imaging does little except confirm the presence of splenomegaly.

Splenic infarction, which may occur secondary to severe pancreatitis, pancreatic carcinoma, sickle cell or trauma,

is well demonstrated on CT as either focal or complete loss of normal enhancement following intravenous contrast (Fig. 5.45).

Splenic trauma

The spleen is the most commonly injured organ in blunt

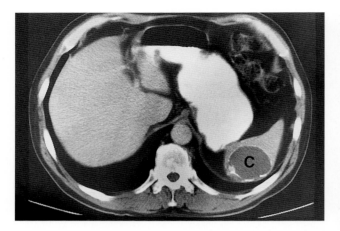

Fig. 5.43 Hydatid cyst. CT showing a cyst (C) in the spleen with calcification in its walls.

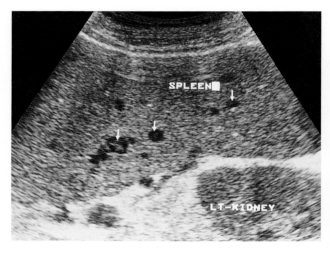

Fig. 5.44 Lymphoma. Ultrasound showing an enlarged spleen with several hypoechoic areas within it. Some of these are arrowed.

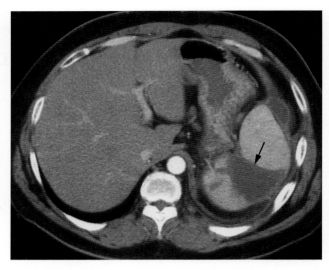

Fig. 5.45 Splenic infarction. CT with contrast demonstrates a wedge-shaped non-enhancing segment of spleen, consistent with infarction (arrow).

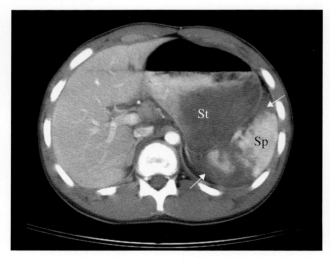

Fig. 5.46 Ruptured spleen on CT. The spleen is shattered with low-density blood (arrows) adjacent to the fragments. Sp, spleen; St, stomach.

abdominal trauma and lacerations, contusions or haematomas may result. Rupture may be delayed until some time after the injury. *Splenic injury* may be detected by ultrasound, but CT is a superior method of investigation, as not only does it demonstrate better the damage to the spleen, but it can also show intraperitoneal blood and visualize injuries to other abdominal organs, particularly the adjacent liver and left kidney (Fig. 5.46). In patients

with splenic laceration, consideration should be given to selective arterial embolization. This may allow some preservation of splenic function, which would be lost if the patient underwent surgery and splenectomy.

6

Urinary Tract

The four basic examinations of the urinary tract are ultrasound, intravenous urography (IVU), computed tomography (CT) and radionuclide examinations. Magnetic resonance imaging (MRI), arteriography and studies requiring catheterization or direct puncture of the collecting systems are limited to selected patients. Fluorodeoxyglucose positron emission tomography (FDG-PET)/CT is still under investigation as an imaging tool in the urinary tract, as there are currently several limitations due to excretion of the tracer in the renal tract and poor uptake in many urologic malignancies.

Ultrasound, CT and MRI are essentially used for anatomical information; the functional information they provide is limited. The converse is true of radionuclide examinations where functional information is paramount. The IVU provides both functional and anatomical information.

IMAGING TECHNIQUES

Ultrasound

Ultrasound is the first-line investigation in most patients, providing anatomical information without requiring ionizing radiation or the use of intravenous contrast medium. The main uses of ultrasound are to:
- Investigate patients with symptoms thought to arise from the urinary tract.
- Demonstrate the size of the kidneys and exclude hydronephrosis in patients with renal failure.

Diagnostic Imaging, 6th Edition. By Peter Armstrong, Martin Wastie and Andrea Rockall. Published 2009 by Blackwell Publishing. ISBN: 978-1-4051-7039.

- Diagnose hydronephrosis, renal tumours, abscesses and cysts including polycystic disease.
- Assess and follow-up renal size and scarring in children with urinary tract infections.
- Assess the bladder and prostate.

Normal renal ultrasound (Fig. 6.1)

At ultrasound, the kidneys should be smooth in outline. The parenchyma surrounds a central echodense region, known as the central echo complex (also called the renal sinus), consisting of the pelvicaliceal system, together with surrounding fat and renal blood vessels. In most instances, the normal pelvicaliceal system is not visible within the renal

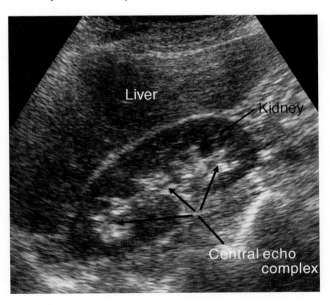

Fig. 6.1 Normal ultrasound of the right kidney.

sinus. The renal cortex generates homogeneous echoes that are of equal reflectivity or less reflective than those of the adjacent liver or spleen, and the renal pyramids are seen as triangular hypoechoic areas adjacent to the renal sinus. During the first 2 months of life, cortical echoes are relatively more prominent and the renal pyramids are disproportionately large and strikingly hypoechoic.

The normal adult renal length, measured by ultrasound, is 9–12 cm. Renal length varies with age, being maximal in the young adult. There may be a difference between the two kidneys, normally less than 1.5 cm. A kidney with a bifid collecting system is usually 1–2 cm larger than a kidney with a single pelvicaliceal system. Minor changes in size occur in many conditions (see Boxes 6.1 and 6.2).

Normal ureters are not usually visualized due to overlying bowel gas. The urinary bladder should be examined in the distended state: the walls should be sharply defined and barely perceptible (Fig. 6.2). The bladder may also be assessed following micturition, to measure the postmicturition residual volume of urine.

Box 6.1 Small kidneys

Diagnosis		*Imaging*
Unilateral but may be bilateral	Chronic pyelonephritis	Focal scars and dilated calices
	Tuberculosis	See p. 238
	Obstructive atrophy	Dilatation of all calices with uniform loss of renal parenchyma
	Renal artery stenosis or occlusion	Outline may be smooth or scarred, but the calices appear normal
	Hypoplasia	Very rare; kidneys may be smooth or irregular in outline with fewer calices
		Calices may be clubbed
	Radiation nephritis	
Always bilateral	Chronic glomerulonephritis of many types	Usually no distinguishing features. In all these conditions the kidneys may be small with smooth outlines and normal pelvicaliceal system
	Hypertensive nephropathy	
	Diabetes mellitus	
	Collagen vascular diseases	
	Analgesic nephropathy	Calices often abnormal (see p. 240)

Box 6.2 Enlarged kidneys

Diagnosis		*Imaging*
Always unilateral	Compensatory hypertrophy	Opposite kidney small or absent
May be unilateral or bilateral	Bifid collecting system	Diagnosis obvious from abnormalities of collecting systems
	Renal mass	
	Hydronephrosis	
	Lymphomatous infiltration	May show obvious masses; the kidneys may, however, be large but otherwise unremarkable
	Renal vein thrombosis	
Always bilateral	Polycystic disease	Characteristic imaging appearance (Fig. 6.52, p. 247)
	Acute glomerulonephritis	Non-specific enlargement
	Amyloidosis	Non-specific enlargement (rare)

Minor degrees of enlargement occur in many conditions. Only those conditions that give rise to easily recognized enlargement are listed here.

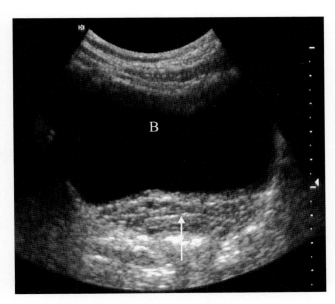

Fig. 6.2 Normal ultrasound of the full bladder (B). Note the smooth thin bladder wall. The vagina lies posteriorly (arrow).

Box 6.3 Main indications for urography

Intravenous urography or CT urography
- When detailed demonstration of the pelvicaliceal system and ureters are required
- Suspected ureteric injury, e.g. following pelvic surgery or trauma
- Assessment of acute ureteric colic

CT urography
- Investigation of renal calculi
- Investigation of haematuria
- Characterization of a renal mass
- Staging and follow-up of renal carcinoma
- To delineate renal vascular anatomy (e.g. suspected renal artery stenosis or prior to live related kidney donation)
- To diagnose or exclude renal trauma

Urography

Urography is the term used to describe the imaging of the renal tract using intravenous iodinated contrast medium. The traditional intravenous urogram or IVU has largely been replaced by a combination of ultrasound and CT urography. CT has the advantage of being highly sensitive for the detection of stones including those which may be radiolucent on plain film, allows the characterization of renal lesions, the detection of ureteric lesions and demonstrates the surrounding retroperitoneal and abdominal tissues. In addition, CT overcomes the overlap of superimposed tissues which can cause difficulty when interpreting the traditional IVU.

The principles of both techniques are similar. Firstly, 'non-contrast' imaging of the renal tract is required, in order to identify all renal tract calcifications. In some cases, where the clinical question relates to renal calculi, the non-contrast CT may be sufficient (known as the CT KUB). However, where a renal mass is suspected or a possible ureteric or bladder mass is suspected, then the non-contrast study is

followed by the injection of iodinated contrast medium, with images being obtained at specific time intervals in order to demonstrate the nephrogram (contrast within the kidneys) and the urogram (contrast within the ureters and bladder). The CT IVU may be reformatted in the coronal plane, in order to have a similar appearance to a traditional IVU. The main indications for urography are listed in Box 6.3.

Contrast medium and its excretion

Urographic contrast media are highly concentrated solutions of organically bound iodine. A large volume, e.g. 100 ml, is injected intravenously and is carried in the blood to the kidneys, where it passes into the glomerular filtrate. The contrast medium within the glomerular filtrate is concentrated in the renal tubules and then passes into the pelvicaliceal systems.

Adverse reactions to intravenous contrast media are discussed in Chapter 1, p. 5.

Patients are allowed to drink up to 500 mL of fluid in the 4 hours before IVU or CT but should not eat. It is particularly important not to fluid-restrict patients with impaired renal function before they are given contrast medium, as this may predispose to contrast medium-induced nephrotoxicity.

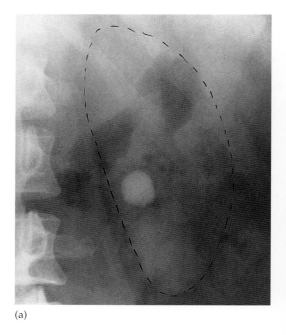

(a)

(b)

Fig. 6.3 (a) A rounded calcification is seen overlying the left kidney in the anteroposterior plain film. (b) Post contrast film in the same patient. As the contrast medium and the calculus have the same radiographic density, the calculus is hidden by the contrast medium.

Intravenous urogram

The plain film

Identify all calcifications. Decide if they are in the kidneys by relating them to the renal outlines during inspiration and expiration or oblique views or tomograms where necessary. Calcifications seen in the line of the ureters or bladder must be reviewed with post contrast scans, to determine whether the calcification lies in the renal tract. Note that calcification can be obscured by contrast medium and stones are missed if no plain film is taken (Fig. 6.3). The major causes of urinary tract calcification include calculi, diffuse nephrocalcinosis, localized nephrocalcinosis (e.g. TB or tumours)

and prostatic calcification. *Look at the other structures on the film.* Include a review of the bones and other soft tissues, just as you would on any plain abdominal film.

Films taken after injection of contrast medium

Kidneys

1 *Check that the kidneys are in their normal positions* (Fig. 6.4). The left kidney is usually higher than the right.
2 *Identify the whole of both renal outlines.* If any indentations or bulges are present they must be explained.
  • *Local indentations* (Fig. 6.5). The renal parenchymal width should be uniform and symmetrical, between 2

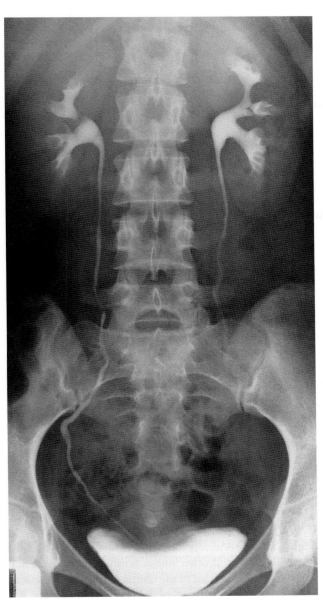

Fig. 6.4 Normal intravenous urography. Full-length 15 minute film. Note that the bladder is well opacified. The whole of the right ureter and part of the left ureter are seen. Often, only a portion of the ureter is visualized owing to peristalsis emptying certain sections. The bladder outline is reasonably smooth. The roof of the bladder shows a shallow indentation from the uterus.

and 2.5 cm. Minor indentations between normal calices are due to persistent fetal lobulations. All other local indentations are scars.
• *Local bulges of the renal outline*. A bulge of the renal outline may be due to a mass or a cyst, which often displaces and deforms the adjacent calices. An important normal variant causing a bulge of the outline is the so-called splenic hump (Fig. 6.6).
3 *Measure the renal lengths*. The normal length of the adult kidney at IVU is between 10 and 16 cm. These figures are higher than those for renal size measured on ultrasound mainly due to radiographic magnification of the image.

Calices

The calices should be evenly distributed and reasonably symmetrical. The shape of a normal calix is 'cupped' and when it is dilated it is described as 'clubbed' (Fig. 6.7). The normal 'cup' is due to the indentation of the papilla into the calix. Caliceal dilatation has two basic causes: destruction of the papilla or obstruction (see Box 6.4).

Box 6.4 Causes of dilated calices

Due to obstruction, with dilatation down to a specific point of hold-up
• Within the lumen
  ○ calculus
  ○ blood clot
  ○ sloughed papilla
• Within the wall of the collecting system
  ○ intrinsic pelviureteric junction obstruction
  ○ transitional cell tumour
  ○ infective stricture (e.g. tuberculosis or schistosomiasis)
• Extrinsic compression
  ○ retroperitoneal fibrosis
  ○ pelvic tumour, e.g. cervical, ovarian or rectal carcinoma
  ○ aberrant renal artery or retrocaval ureter

Due to papillary atrophy or destruction
• Reflux nephropathy
• Papillary necrosis
• Tuberculosis

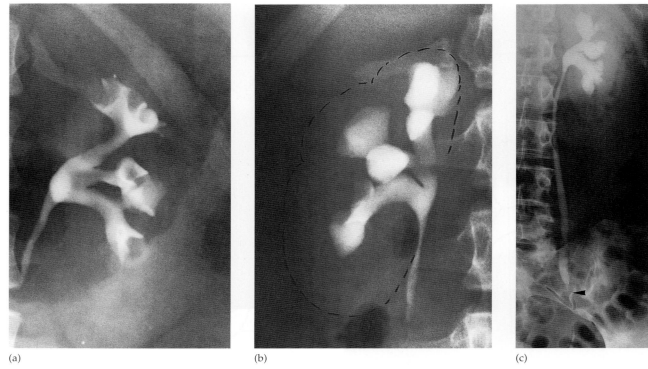

(a)   (b)   (c)

Fig. 6.7 The calices. (a) Normal calices. Each calix is 'cup-shaped'. (b) Many of the calices are clubbed. There is scarring of the parenchyma of the upper half of the kidney indicating that the diagnosis is chronic pyelonephritis. (c) All the calices are dilated, the dilatation of the collecting system extending down to the point of obstruction (arrow), in this case owing to a malignant retroperitoneal lymph node.

MDCT, it is possible to reconstruct the axial CT slices into very thin axial sections of 1–2 mm. Viewing the thin section images increases the ability to detect very small stones and allows reconstruction of coronal and sagittal images of diagnostic quality (see Fig. 6.22, p. 224). Occasionally, it may be difficult to differentiate a small calcified phlebolith from a non-obstructing ureteric stone, particularly if the ureter is not distended above the stone. In this case, correlation with a post contrast CT IVU may be necessary. The appearance of the other organs, including liver, spleen, pancreas, adrenal glands and the GI tract should be assessed. In cases where the CT is being performed for suspected acute renal colic, alternative causes of pain should be sought, such as appendicitis. The bones should be viewed on bone window settings.

CT after injection of contrast medium

Corticomedullary phase. At approximately 35–40 seconds following the start of the contrast injection, the only parts of the renal tract which have enhanced are the renal arteries and renal cortex. Thus, there is a marked difference in the attenuation of the cortex and the medulla (Fig. 6.8b). There is no contrast medium in the collecting system, which therefore has a low attenuation. This early stage of enhancement is particularly useful for evaluation of the renal arteries, which may be reformatted as a CT angiogram, as well as for the evaluation of highly vascular renal tumours.

Nephrographic phase. Later images, at approximately 90 seconds, demonstrate uniform opacification of the renal parenchyma. There is homogeneous opacification of the

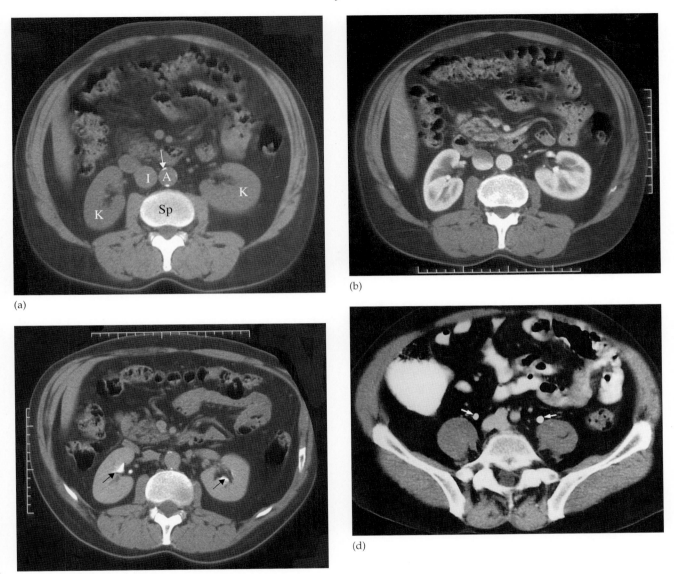

Fig. 6.8 Normal CT of kidneys and bladder. (a), (b) and (c) showing the same level through the renal hilum. (a) Before the intravenous contrast has been given. Note the calcification in the wall of the aorta (arrow). A, aorta; I, inferior vena cava; K, kidney; Sp, spine. (b) Forty seconds after intravenous contrast infusion, demonstrating the corticomedullary phase, with marked enhancement of the renal cortex. (c) Ten minutes following the contrast infusion, demonstrating homogeneous opacification of parenchyma and dense opacification of the pelvicaliceal system (arrows). (d) Section through the pelvis showing the ureters (arrows) after contrast has been given.

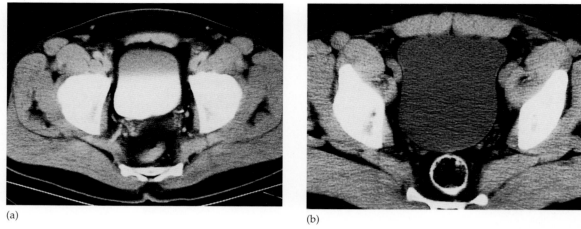

(a)   (b)

Fig. 6.9 (a) CT section through opacified bladder in a male patient shows that the bladder wall is too thin to be seen. Note the layering of contrast medium. (b) Section through bladder without contrast opacification. The bladder wall can be identified as a thin line.

cortex and the medulla, the 'homogeneous nephrogram' phase and some contrast medium is seen in the renal pelves. There is usually a clearly visible difference in the density of normal renal tissue and a tumour.

Urographic phase. At delayed phase imaging, obtained at approximately 10–15 minutes after contrast injection, the pelvicaliceal system, ureters and bladder should contain contrast. The pelvicaliceal system should show cupped calices with uniform width of renal parenchyma from calix to renal edge, and the renal sinus fat that surrounds the pelvicaliceal system should be clearly visualized. The ureters are seen in cross-section as dots lying on the psoas muscles (Fig. 6.8d). They will not necessarily be seen at all levels because peristalsis obliterates the lumen intermittently. The bladder has a smooth outline and stands out against the pelvic fat; its wall is thin and of reasonably uniform diameter. Contrast medium opacification of the urine in the bladder is variable depending on how much contrast medium has reached the bladder. The contrast medium is heavier than urine and, therefore, the dependent portion is usually more densely opacified (Fig. 6.9). Curved reformats of the ureters may be used to display the urographic phase (Fig. 6.10).

MRI

Magnetic resonance imaging gives similar anatomical information to CT, with the advantage of being able to obtain scans directly in the coronal, sagittal and oblique planes, in addition to the axial plane. It is generally used in selected circumstances, e.g. to demonstrate renal artery stenosis or inferior vena caval extension of renal tumours or to clarify problems not solved by ultrasound or CT. It is also used to assess the extent of bladder or prostate cancer prior to consideration for surgery. Calcification is not visible on MRI, which is one of the main disadvantages of the technique for renal tract imaging.

Normal MRI (Fig. 6.11)

As with CT and ultrasound, the renal contours should be smooth. Corticomedullary differentiation is best seen on T1-weighted images and immediately following intravenous contrast enhancement with gadolinium. The renal collecting systems, ureters and bladder are best seen on T2-weighted images, as the fluid returns a high signal intensity (Fig. 6.12). A heavily T2-weighted

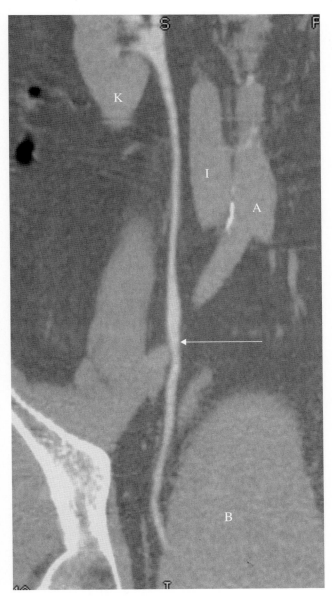

Fig. 6.10 CT reformat. This is the same patient as in Fig. 6.8a–c. The ureter (arrow) has been reformatted in the coronal plane. A, aorta; I, inferior vena cava; K, kidney; B, bladder.

image may be used to acquire an MR urogram. Some normal variants are well demonstrated on MRI: fetal lobulation is seen as an undulating renal contour but with uniform cortical thickness on coronal images (Fig. 6.6b); a column of Bertin (which is normal renal parenchyma that may look mass-like) may be distinguished from a mass, as it has the same signal characteristics as the rest of the kidney on all sequences. The renal vasculature is best demonstrated following intravenous gadolinium and may be displayed using three-dimensional software (Fig. 6.13).

Radionuclide examination

Radionuclide techniques for studying the kidneys include:
1 The renogram which measures renal function.
2 Scans of renal morphology (DMSA scan). The advent of CT and ultrasound has reduced the need for such scans. They are now used mainly for evaluating renal scarring (see Fig. 6.43, p. 241).
3 The presence of reflux in children may be diagnosed using the technique of indirect voiding cystography. A radionuclide tracer is infused into the bladder via a catheter. The child then voids whilst being imaged by the gamma camera. The presence of reflux can be detected if tracer activity is seen to rise up into one or both of the ureters at the time of micturition (Fig. 6.14).

Renogram (Fig. 6.15)

If substances which pass into the urine are labelled with a radionuclide and injected intravenously, their passage through the kidney can be observed with a gamma camera.

The two agents of choice are ^{99m}Tc DTPA (diethylene triamine pentacetic acid) and ^{99m}Tc MAG-3 (mercaptoacetyl triglycine). DTPA is filtered by the glomeruli and not absorbed or secreted by the tubules, whereas MAG-3 is both filtered by the glomeruli and secreted by the tubules.

The gamma camera is positioned posteriorly over the kidneys and a rapid injection of the radiopharmaceutical is given. Early images show the major blood vessels and both kidneys. Subsequently, activity is seen in the renal parenchyma and by 5 minutes the collecting systems should

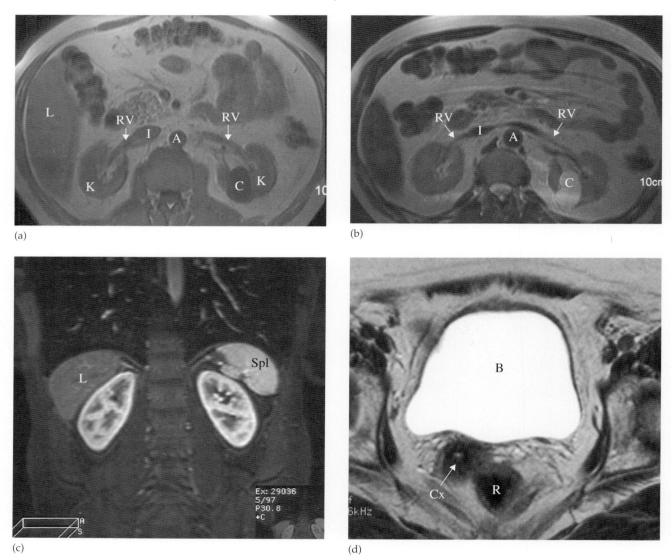

(a)

(b)

(c)

(d)

Fig. 6.11 MRI of the kidneys. (a) T1-weighted and (b) T2-weighted images in the axial plane at the level of the renal hila. Note the simple cyst in the left kidney, which returns a low signal on T1- and a high signal on T2-weighted images. (c) Coronal image of the kidneys, in a different patient, following intravenous gadolinium infusion. (d) Normal bladder (B) on a T2-weighted image. The bladder wall is thin and smooth. A, aorta; C, cyst; Cx, cervix; I, inferior vena cava; K, kidney; L, liver; R, rectum; RV, renal vein; Spl, spleen.

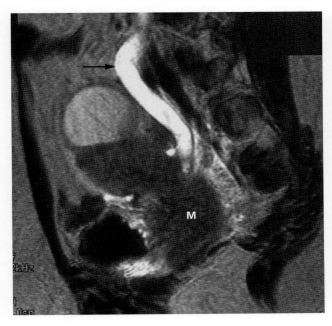

Fig. 6.12 T2-weighted MRI showing a dilated ureter, due to obstruction by a pelvic mass (M).

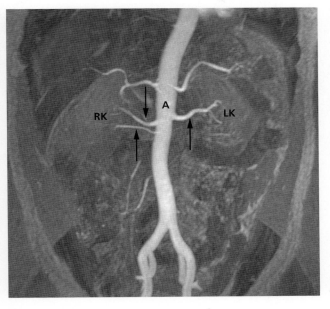

Fig. 6.13 Magnetic resonance angiogram of normal renal arteries, displayed coronally (arrows). There are two renal arteries supplying the right kidney (RK) and one supplying the left kidney (LK). A, aorta.

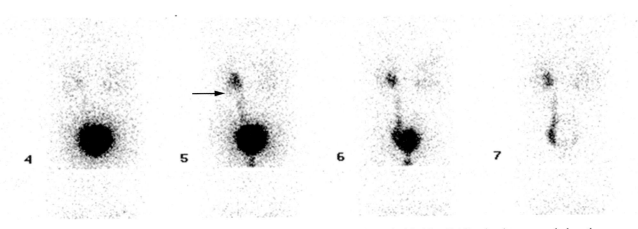

Fig. 6.14 Indirect voiding cystogram (posterior view). Tracer has been instilled into the bladder. Voiding has been recorded on the gamma camera, starting at image 5. There is immediate reflux into the left ureter (arrow). The bladder is virtually empty on the final image, 7.

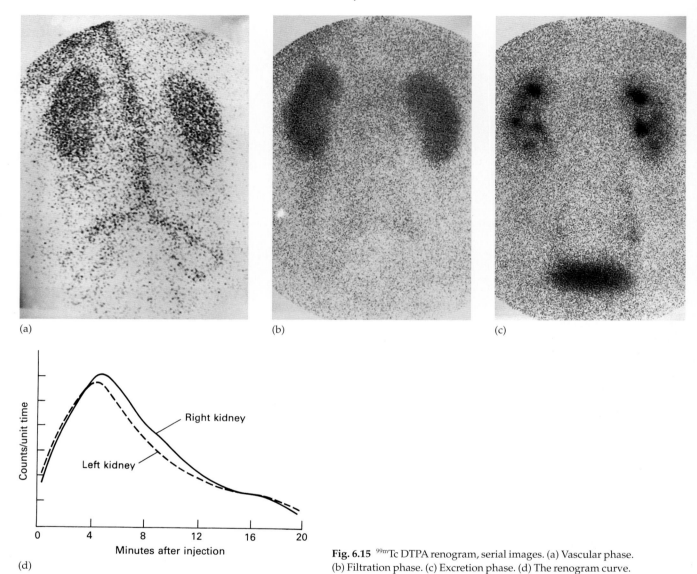

(a)

(b)

(c)

(d)

Fig. 6.15 ^{99m}Tc DTPA renogram, serial images. (a) Vascular phase.
(b) Filtration phase. (c) Excretion phase. (d) The renogram curve.

be visible. Serial images over 20 minutes show progressive excretion and clearance of activity from the kidneys. Quantitative assessment with a computer enables a renogram curve to be produced and the relative function of each kidney calculated.

The main indications for a renogram are:

- Measurement of relative renal function in each kidney – this may help the surgeon decide between nephrectomy or more conservative surgery.
- Investigation of urinary tract obstruction, particularly pelviureteric junction obstruction.
- Investigation of renal transplants.

Special techniques

Retrograde and antegrade pyelography

The techniques of retrograde and antegrade pyelography (the term pyelography means demonstrating the pelvicaliceal system and ureters) involve direct injection of contrast material into the pelvicaliceal system or ureters through catheters placed via cystoscopy (retrograde pyelography) or percutaneously into the kidney via the loin (antegrade pyelography). The indications are limited to those situations where the information cannot be achieved by less invasive means, e.g. IVU, CT or MRI to confirm a possible transitional cell carcinoma in the renal pelvis or ureter.

Voiding cystourethrogram (micturating cystogram) and videourodynamics (see Fig. 6.61, p. 252)

In voiding cystourethrography, the bladder is filled with iodinated contrast medium through a catheter and films are taken during voiding. The entire process is observed fluoroscopically to identify vesicoureteric reflux. The bladder and urethra can be assessed during voiding to demonstrate strictures or urethral valves.

Videourodynamic examination combines voiding cystourethrography with bladder pressure measurements, which necessitate bladder and rectal pressure lines. It is useful in the investigation of incontinence to distinguish detrusor instability from sphincter weakness (stress incontinence). The test is also helpful in patients with obstructive symptoms, mainly elderly men, to differentiate true obstruction from bladder instability, and in patients with a neurogenic bladder.

Urethrography (see Fig. 6.60, p. 252)

The urethra is visualized during voiding cystourethrography. For full visualization of the male urethra, however, an ascending urethrogram with contrast medium injection via the external urethral meatus is necessary. The usual indications for the examination are the identification of urethral strictures and to demonstrate extravasation from the urethra or bladder neck following trauma.

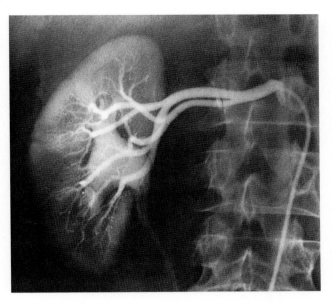

Fig. 6.16 Normal selective right renal arteriogram. Note that not only are the arteries well shown but there is also an excellent nephrogram. The renal pelvis and ureter are opacified because of a previous injection of contrast.

Renal arteriography

Renal arteriography is performed via a catheter introduced into the femoral artery by the Seldinger technique (see p. 438). Selective injections are made into one or both renal arteries (Fig. 6.16). It is mainly used to confirm the CT or MRI findings of vascular anatomy prior to renal surgery and to confirm renal artery stenosis prior to percutaneous balloon angioplasty.

URINARY TRACT DISORDERS

Urinary calculi

Urinary calculi may be asymptomatic; the imaging of calculi causing urinary obstruction is described below (p. 225).

Most urinary calculi are calcified and show varying density on plain x-ray examinations. Many are uniformly calcified but some, particularly bladder stones, may be laminated. Only pure uric acid and xanthine stones are

Chapter 6

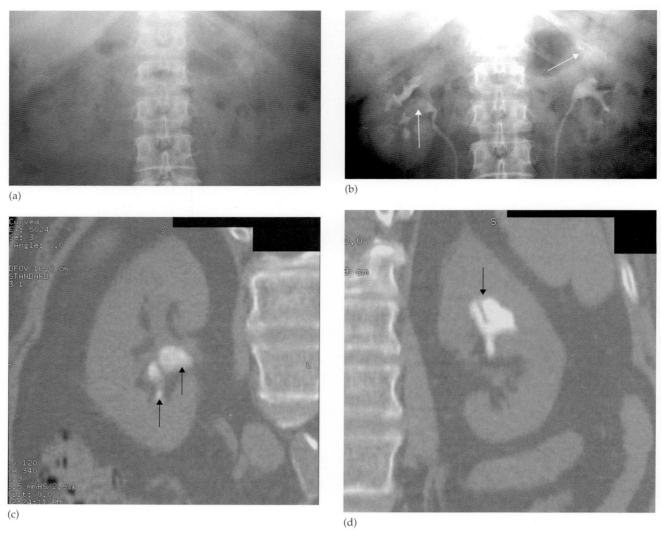

(a)

(b)

(c)

(d)

Fig. 6.17 (a) Intravenous urography (IVU) control film. Renal stones are not visible on the right and very poorly visualized on the left. (b) IVU following intravenous contrast. Filling defects are seen in the right lower calix and pelvis and in the left upper pole calices (arrows). (c) and (d) CT of the kidneys in the same patient with no contrast medium, reformatted in the coronal plane, demonstrating the renal stones in both the right (c) and left (d) kidneys (arrows).

radiolucent on plain radiography, but they can be identified at CT or ultrasound (Fig. 6.17).

Small renal calculi are often round or oval; the larger ones frequently assume the shape of the pelvicaliceal system and are known as staghorn calculi (Fig. 6.18).

Plain film examination of the urinary tract is more sensitive than ultrasound for detecting opaque renal and ureteric calculi. It is essential to examine the preliminary film of an IVU carefully, because even large calculi can be completely hidden within the opacified collecting system

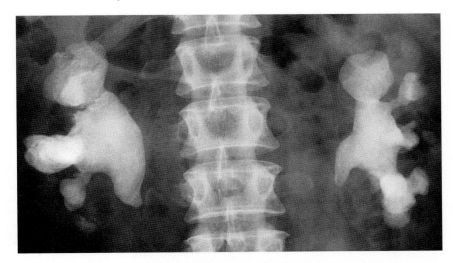

Fig. 6.18 Plain film showing a calcified staghorn calculus in each kidney.

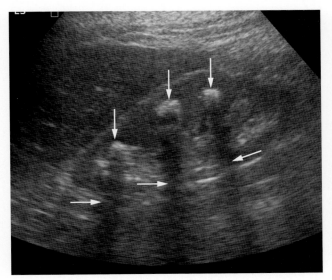

Fig. 6.19 Ultrasound of stones in right kidney. The stones (vertical arrows) appear as bright echoes. Note the acoustic shadows behind the stones (horizontal arrows).

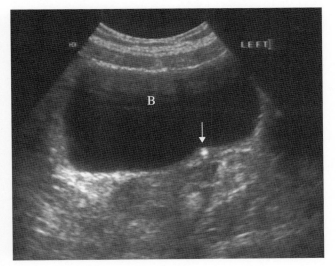

Fig. 6.20 Ultrasound of the bladder (B), demonstrating a stone lodged at the left vesicoureteric junction (arrow). In this case, no acoustic shadow was seen.

once contrast medium has been given (see Fig. 6.3, p. 210). Stones in the ureters may be partly obscured where they overlie the vertebral transverse processes or the sacrum.

Most renal calculi of more than 5 mm in size are readily seen at ultrasound, but smaller calculi may be missed, particularly if they are located within the renal sinus, where they may be obscured by echoes from the surrounding fat. Stones, regardless of their composition, produce intense echoes and cast acoustic shadows (Fig. 6.19). Staghorn calculi, filling the caliceal system, cast very large acoustic shadows, which may even mask an associated hydronephrosis. Stones in the ureters cannot be excluded on

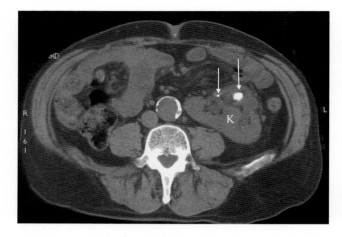

Fig. 6.21 Non-contrast enhanced CT in a patient with crossed fused ectopia, a renal anatomical variant (K). Multiple stones were demonstrated (arrows), allowing accurate planning of his lithotripsy treatment.

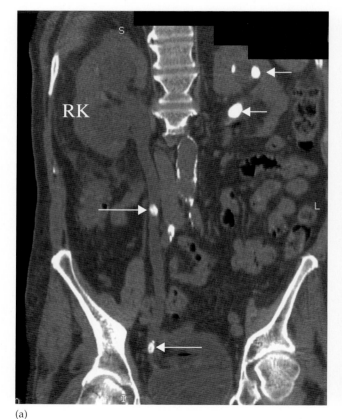

(a)

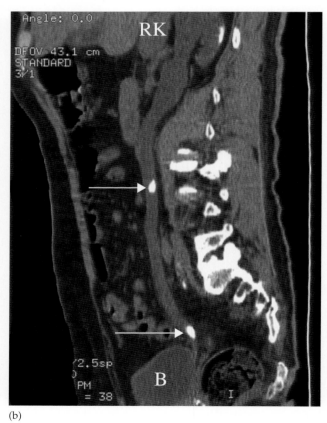

(b)

Fig. 6.22 Non-contrast enhanced CT reformatted in the coronal (a) and the sagittal plane (b), demonstrating a hydronephrotic right kidney (RK) and two stones in the dilated right ureter (long arrows). The patient also has kidney stones in the left pelvicaliceal system (short arrows).

ultrasound, although stones lodged at the vesicouteric junction may be demonstrated (Fig. 6.20). Stones in the bladder, or in bladder diverticula, are well demonstrated on ultrasound.

CT, when performed without intravenous contrast medium, is exquisitely sensitive for the detection of calculi. It is used in place of IVU for the detection and precise anatomical localization of stones prior to treatment in most centres (Figs 6.21 and 6.22). If a stone is obstructing a ureter, the dilated ureter can usually be followed down to the level of the stone, below which the ureter is undistended. In some cases, particularly if a small ureteric stone is not causing obstruction and the ureter is not dilated, it can be difficult to be certain if a calcification lies within or outside the ureter. In these cases, the use of intravenous contrast media and delayed phase imaging can be very helpful to delineate the line of the ureter.

Nephrocalcinosis

Nephrocalcinosis is the term used to describe focal or diffuse calcification within the renal parenchyma (Fig. 6.23). Diffuse nephrocalcinosis:
• May be associated with hypercalcaemia and/or hypercalciuria, notably hyperparathyroidism and renal tubular acidosis.
• May be associated with widespread papillary necrosis and medullary sponge kidney (a congenital condition with dilated collecting tubules in which small calculi can form) in the presence of normal calcium metabolism.

Urinary tract obstruction

The principal feature of obstruction is dilatation of the pelvicaliceal system and ureter. All the affected calices are dilated to approximately the same degree; the degree depends on the chronicity, with more marked dilatation seen more often in long-standing obstruction. The obstructed collecting system is dilated down to the level of the obstructing pathology and demonstrating this level is a prime objective of imaging (see Fig. 6.7c, p. 214). Ultrasound and urographic examination play major roles when evaluating urinary tract

obstruction and CT urography has overtaken IVU for the investigation of obstruction (Fig. 6.22). Radionuclide studies show typical changes, but are rarely the primary imaging procedures.

Ultrasound in urinary tract obstruction

Dilatation of the pelvicaliceal system is demonstrated sonographically as a multiloculate fluid collection in the central echo-complex, caused by pooling of urine within the distended pelvis and calices (Fig. 6.24a). As the distension becomes more severe, the dilated calices can resemble multiple renal cysts, but dilated calices, unlike cysts, show continuity with the renal pelvis (Fig. 6.24b). With prolonged obstruction, thinning of the cortex due to atrophy will be seen.

Proximal ureteric dilatation can frequently be identified, but overlying bowel often obscures dilatation of the mid and distal ureter. If the obstruction is at the level of the vesicoureteric junction, the distal ureter can usually be visualized. It follows, therefore, that while some causes of obstruction are identifiable, e.g. carcinoma of the bladder or a stone at the vesicoureteric junction, it is often not possible to determine the cause of urinary tract obstruction at ultrasound examination. Ultrasound may demonstrate a pelvic mass, such as a uterine or ovarian mass, causing external compression of the collecting system.

Intravenous urogram in urinary tract obstruction

In some centres, the IVU remains the primary imaging modality in patients with suspected acute obstruction, which is usually caused by a calculus. Plain films may demonstrate the calculus responsible for the obstruction. However, as parts of the ureter overlie the transverse processes of the vertebrae and the wings of the sacrum, the calculus may be impossible to see on plain film. Following injection of intravenous contrast medium, a film of the renal tract is taken at approximately 15 minutes. If the urogram is normal, with contrast seen in normal, undistended ureters bilaterally, then this effectively rules out ureteric colic as the cause of acute pain. If one of the ureters is obstructed, then a dense nephrogram will be seen

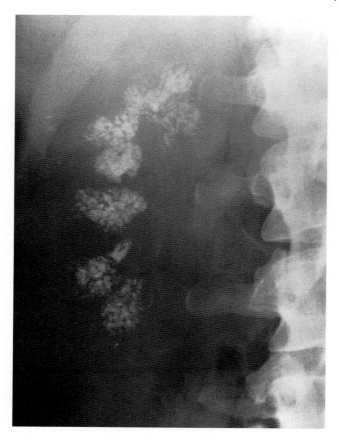

Fig. 6.23 Nephrocalcinosis. There are numerous calcifications in the pyramids of both kidneys (the left kidney is not illustrated).

CT in urinary tract obstruction

Computed tomography is now widely used to evaluate urinary tract obstruction (Figs 6.22 and 6.26). In acute obstruction, non-contrast enhanced CT sensitively demonstrates calculi and the unopacified, dilated collecting system can frequently be traced down to the point of obstruction (Fig. 6.22). Non-contrast CT is often used in acute ureteric colic, as an alternative to IVU, in patients with an allergy to intravenous contrast medium. CT also has the advantage of demonstrating possible alternative causes of acute abdominal pain, such as appendicitis. Chronic obstruction by tumour, either within the renal collecting system or by an external tumour causing compression, may be visualized directly on CT or MRI and staging of the tumour can be performed during the same investigation.

Causes of obstruction to the ureters and pelvicaliceal systems

There are many causes of obstruction to the urinary tract, which may arise at any level from the pelvicaliceal system down to the urethra (see Box 6.4, p. 211).

Causes within the lumen of the urinary tract

Calculi are by far the commonest cause of obstruction of the urinary tract. The imaging techniques are described above. A sloughed papilla in papillary necrosis is a rare cause of ureteric obstruction. The diagnosis can be suspected when other papillae still within the kidney show signs of papillary necrosis (see Fig. 6.44, p. 242). Blood clot within the collecting system needs to be differentiated from other causes such as stones or a tumour (see Fig. 6.38, p. 237).

Causes arising in the wall of the collecting system

A *transitional cell carcinoma* (TCC) (see Fig. 6.39, p. 237) within the ureter or the bladder in the region of the vesicoureteric junction may cause obstruction (a TCC in the pelvicaliceal system rarely causes obstruction). Ureteric tumours may be seen as a filling defect on IVU or as a point of obstruction with no visible mass. Ureteric TCCs are well demonstrated by pyelography, either retrograde

and opacification of the pelvicaliceal system and ureter on the obstructed side takes much longer. Delayed films are, therefore, an essential part of any IVU where the level of obstruction is not shown on the routine films. In time, the collecting system and the level of obstruction can usually be demonstrated (Fig. 6.25).

Obstruction can be intermittent and between attacks the IVU may be normal. If, however, the urogram is performed during an attack of colic (the so-called emergency urogram) the level of obstruction is usually demonstrated.

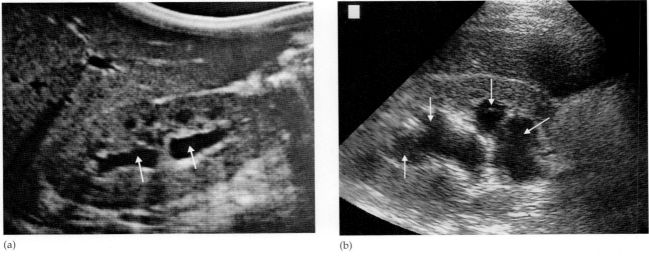

(a)
(b)

Fig. 6.24 Dilatation of the pelvicaliceal system. (a) Longitudinal ultrasound scan of right kidney showing spreading of the central echo-complex of the dilated collecting system (arrows). (b) Here the dilatation of the calices is greater (arrows).

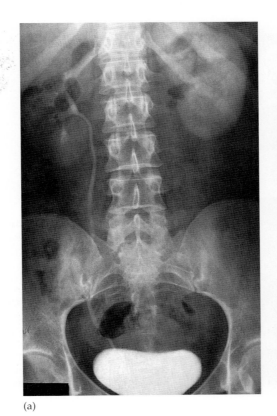

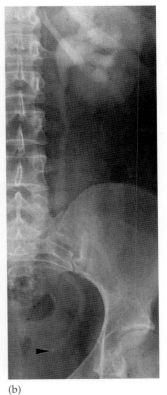

Fig. 6.25 Acute ureteric obstruction from a stone in the lower end of the left ureter. (a) A film taken 30 minutes after the injection of contrast medium. There is obvious delay in the appearance of the pyelogram on the left. The left kidney shows a very dense nephrogram which is characteristic of acute ureteric obstruction. (b) A film taken 23 hours later shows opacification of the obstructed collecting system down to the obstructing calculus (arrow).

(a)
(b)

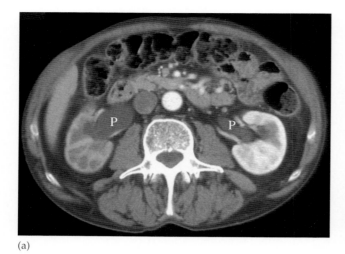

(a)

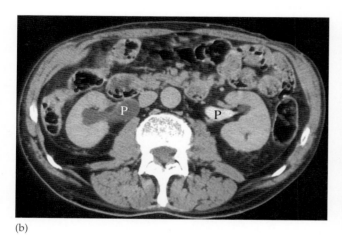

(b)

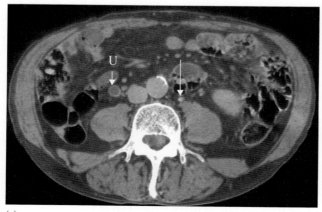

(c)

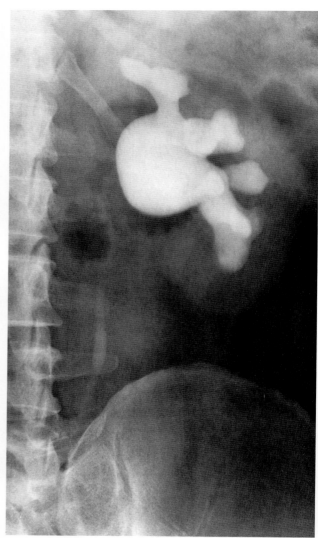

Fig. 6.27 Intrinsic pelviureteric junction obstruction. The pelvicaliceal system is considerably dilated, but the ureter from the pelviureteric junction onward is normal in caliber.

Fig. 6.26 (a) CT at the corticomedullary phase of enhancement. There is obstruction of the right kidney with dilatation of the pelvicaliceal system (P, renal pelvis), reduced cortical enhancement and some loss of cortical thickness, suggesting that the obstruction may be longstanding. (b) Computed tomography at the delayed phase of enhancement. Intravenous contrast is seen in the left renal pelvis but not in the obstructed right renal pelvis. (c) Computed tomography through the dilated right ureter (U), in the same patient as (a) and (b). Note the normal left ureter (long arrow).

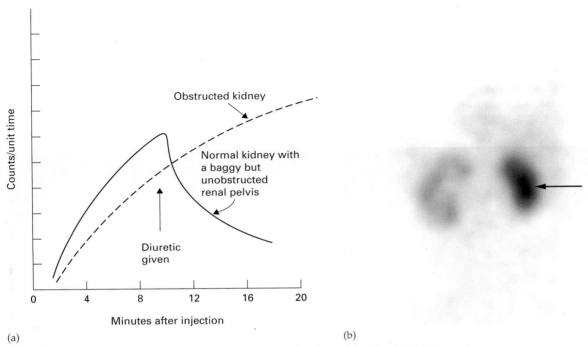

Fig. 6.28 (a) Diuretic renogram comparing pelviureteric junction obstruction (dotted line) with a 'baggy' but otherwise normal renal pelvis (continuous line). Frusemide was given at 10 minutes and in the case of the 'baggy' pelvis resulted in rapid washout of radioactivity from the kidney. (b) The post diuretic renogram image demonstrates washout of tracer on the unobstructed side and accumulation of tracer in the dilated renal pelvis on the obstructed side (arrow).

or antegrade. Computed tomography, particularly MDCT, may also be used to demonstrate pelvicaliceal and ureteric tumours, particularly on the delayed 'urographic' images, when the pelvicaliceal system and ureter are filled with contrast medium. Carcinoma of the bladder causing ureteric obstruction can usually be identified on IVU, ultrasound, CT or MRI, though cystoscopy is the best method of establishing the diagnosis.

Infective strictures of the collecting systems are mostly due to tuberculosis or schistosomiasis. In the case of tuberculosis there is usually other imaging evidence to suggest the diagnosis (see Fig. 6.42, p. 240).

Congenital intrinsic pelviureteric junction (PUJ) obstruction

In this disorder, peristalsis is not transmitted across the pelviureteric junction. The disease may present at any age but it is usually discovered in children or young adults. The diagnosis depends on identifying dilatation of the pelvis and calices, with an abrupt change in caliber at the pelviureteric junction (Fig. 6.27). Often, the ureter cannot be identified at all. If it is seen, it will be either narrow or normal in size.

Pelviureteric junction obstruction can be difficult to distinguish on IVU from an otherwise normal, unobstructed dilated renal pelvis – the so-called baggy pelvis. This distinction can be made by giving a diuretic intravenously. In PUJ obstruction, the induced diuresis causes further dilatation of the pelvicaliceal system and the patient develops loin pain, whereas a baggy system drains. Similarly, a diuretic can be given during a renogram (Fig. 6.28). If there is obstruction, the radionuclide accumulates within the kidney and renal pelvis, whereas with a 'baggy' pelvis there is rapid washout of the radionuclide from the suspect kidney.

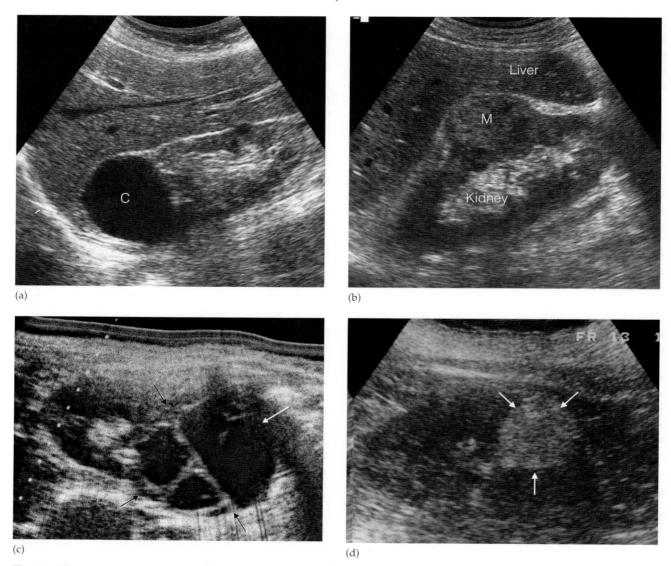

Fig. 6.30 Ultrasound in renal masses. (a) Cyst (C) showing sharp walls and no echoes arising within the cyst. Note the acoustic enhancement behind the cyst. (b) Tumour showing echoes within a solid mass (M). (c) Complex mass due to cystic renal cell carcinoma. The arrows point to the edge of the mass. Note the thick septa within the mass. (d) Angiomyolipoma. This incidental finding shows the typical appearance of a small echogenic mass (arrow). Same patient as in Fig. 6.32b.

CT and MRI of renal masses

Increasingly, renal masses are detected incidentally as part of a CT scan undertaken for a different purpose. In addition, CT has proved very useful for characterizing indeterminate renal masses identified on ultrasound. Computed tomography may be used to differentiate cysts from tumours, to diagnose angiomyolipomas, and to stage renal carcinoma (Fig. 6.32). Renal masses may be characterized on MRI, but MRI is usually reserved for solving specific problems.

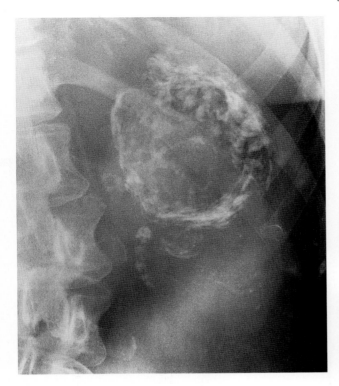

Fig. 6.31 Partially calcified renal cell carcinoma.

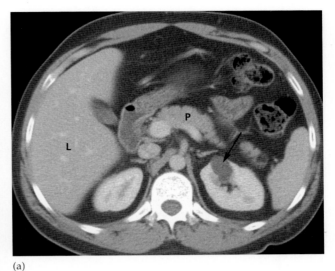

(a)

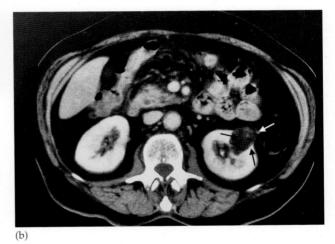

(b)

Fig. 6.32 CT of benign renal masses. (a) Cyst in left kidney (arrow) showing a well-defined edge, imperceptible wall and uniform water density. The cyst shows no enhancement. It was an incidental finding. L, liver; P, pancreas. (b) Angiomyolipoma (same patient as in Fig. 6.30d) with a small mass (arrows) of fat density.

At CT, a typical *simple renal cyst* is a spherical mass with an imperceptible wall (Fig. 6.32a). The interior of the cyst is homogeneous with attenuation values similar to water. The margins between the cyst and the normal renal parenchyma are sharp. When all of these criteria are met, the diagnosis of simple cyst is certain and there is no need to proceed further. On MRI, a simple cyst appears as a well-defined rounded mass with a homogeneous high signal intensity on T2-weighted images and low signal on T1-weighted images, with no enhancement post gadolinium enhancement (see Fig. 6.11, p. 218). *Angiomyolipomas* are usually incidental findings. They are benign tumours, which rarely cause problems, although, on occasion, they cause significant retroperitoneal haemorrhage. At CT and MRI, their fat content allows a confident diagnosis (Fig. 6.32b).

Renal cell carcinomas are approximately spherical and often lobulated (Fig. 6.33). The attenuation value of renal tumours on scans without intravenous contrast enhancement is often fairly close to that of normal renal parenchyma, but focal necrotic areas may result in areas of low density, and stippled calcification may be present in the interior of the mass as well as around the periphery. Following intravenous contrast administration, renal cell carcinomas enhance, but not to the same degree as the

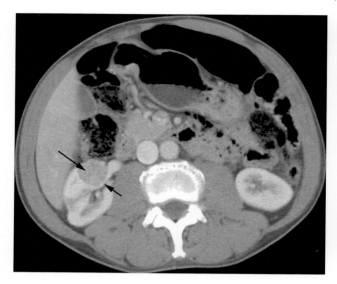

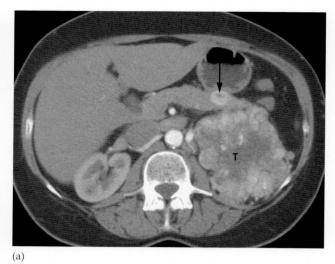

(a)

Fig. 6.33 Renal cell carcinoma. The mass in the right kidney (long arrow) shows substantial enhancement and is invading the anterior wall of the right renal vein (short arrow).

normal parenchyma, and they are inhomogeneous in their enhancement pattern. The CT diagnosis of renal carcinoma is usually sufficiently accurate so that preoperative biopsy is rarely performed.

Diagnostic difficulty arises with indeterminate cystic masses. The degree and appearance of any solid component within the cyst influences the risk of the lesion being malignant. Depending on the clinical circumstance and on the imaging appearances, the clinician may opt to follow-up the lesion on imaging or may decide to proceed to surgery, on the assumption that the lesion is likely to be malignant. In some centres, indeterminate renal lesions are further evaluated with percutaneous biopsy under CT guidance, but this is not currently a widespread practice.

Staging of renal cell carcinoma is usually undertaken with CT, the current method of choice (Fig. 6.34). CT shows local direct spread, can demonstrate enlargement of draining lymph nodes in the retroperitoneum, diagnose liver, adrenal and pancreatic metastases and show tumour growing along the renal vein into the inferior vena cava. The renal vein and IVC are particularly well demonstrated on sagittal and coronal views on MRI (Fig. 6.35), as well as on sagittal and coronal reformats of

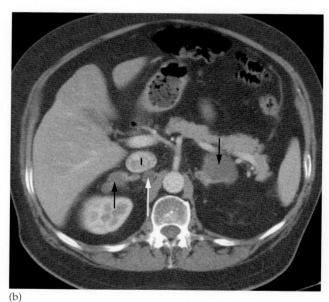

(b)

Fig. 6.34 Staging renal carcinoma. CT scan showing a large tumour (T) in the left kidney from renal cell carcinoma and an enhancing metastasis (arrow) in the pancreas. (b) In another patient, there are bilateral adrenal metastases (black arrows) and a nodal metastasis (white arrow). I, inferior vena cava.

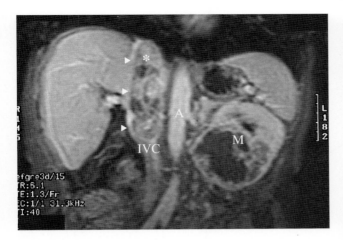

Fig. 6.35 Coronal MRI scan showing a huge left renal carcinoma (M) with tumour extending into the inferior vena cava (IVC) via the left renal vein (not seen on the view). The caval extension of tumour (arrowheads) extends to the top of the IVC (*). A, aorta.

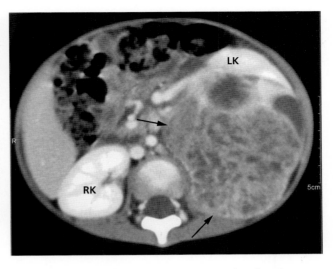

Fig. 6.36 Wilms' tumour. A large heterogeneously enhancing mass arises from the posterior aspect of the left kidney (arrows). The remainder of the left kidney (LK) parenchyma lies anteriorly. RK, right kidney.

MDCT images. These additional scan planes help to demonstrate the anatomical relations of the mass to the renal hilar vessels and may help in planning partial resections of the kidney.

Wilms' tumour is the likely diagnosis in a child with a renal mass (Fig. 6.36). These lesions are frequently large and may contain stippled calcifications.

Urothelial tumours

Almost all tumours that arise within the collecting systems of the kidneys are *transitional cell carcinomas*. The tumours sometimes occur in multiple sites and, therefore, both pelvicaliceal systems and ureters should be carefully scrutinized. Although bladder tumours may be demonstrated, these are better evaluated at cystoscopy.

In some centres, the IVU plays an important role in demonstrating the 'upper tracts' (pelvicaliceal system and ureters). *Filling defects* within the renal pelvis and ureters should be looked for. In the pelvicaliceal system, TCCs are seen as lobulated or, very occasionally, as fronded filling defects projecting into the lumen (Fig. 6.37a). It is easy to confuse

such tumours with overlying gas shadows on an IVU, and tomography or ultrasound may be required to solve the problem. The differential diagnosis of a filling defect in the collecting systems on IVU includes calculi and blood clot. Most urinary stones contain visible calcification, and virtually all calcified filling defects are stones. However, radiolucent calculi can cause a diagnostic problem and CT plays an important role in confirming or ruling out 'radiolucent' calculi (see Fig. 6.17, p. 222). The diagnosis of blood clot as the cause of a filling defect rests on knowing that the patient has severe haematuria and noting the smooth outline of the filling defect (Fig. 6.38). Sometimes the distinction between tumour and clot is difficult. If clot is a possibility, then follow-up to check for resorption of the clot may be helpful.

At ultrasound, TCCs can be difficult to see because they blend with the renal sinus fat, although large tumours can usually be demonstrated as a central mass within the sinus (Fig. 6.37b). Ultrasound may help to differentiate between a radiolucent stone and tumour, as the calculus demonstrates acoustic shadowing.

CT urography demonstrates thickening of the wall of the ureter at the site of a urothelial tumour. The ureter

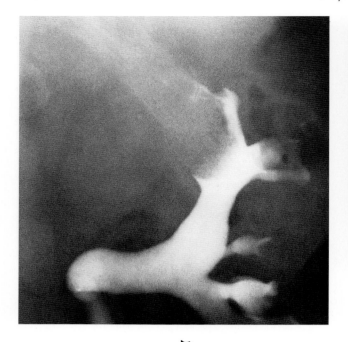

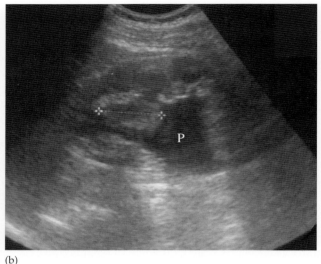

(b)

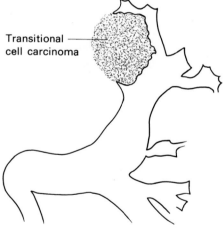

Transitional cell carcinoma

(a)

Fig. 6.37 (a) Filling defect in an upper calix due to transitional cell carcinoma. (b) Ultrasound, in a different patient, demonstrating a tumour mass (between the cursors) projecting into the renal pelvis (P).

is often obstructed at the level of a TCC (Fig. 6.39). If this is the case, then no contrast may be seen in the ureter on the 10 minute delayed phase CT images. Three-dimensional reformatting of the collecting system may be undertaken, to demonstrate the location and extent of the tumour prior to surgery. Tumour staging may be done at the same time.

In some cases, where there is an equivocal appearance on CT urography, antegrade or retrograde pyelography may also be used to demonstrate the tumour.

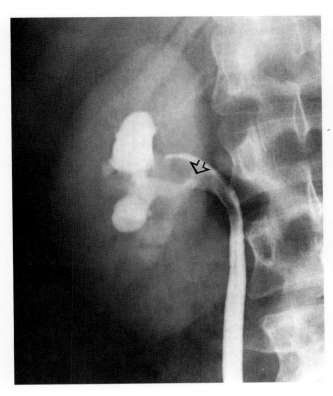

Fig. 6.38 Filling defect due to blood clot in the pelvis and upper ureter (arrow).

Acute infections of the upper urinary tracts

Acute pyelonephritis

Acute pyelonephritis is usually due to bacterial infection from organisms that enter the urinary system via the urethra. Anatomical abnormalities such as stones, duplex systems complicated by obstruction or reflux, obstructive lesions and conditions such as diabetes mellitus all predispose to infection. In adults, only selected patients require imaging.

Most patients with acute urinary tract infection do not require urgent imaging investigations. In patients presenting with signs of infection associated with pain, particularly if the symptoms are not settling with antibiotics, ultrasound and plain films may diagnose underlying stones, obstruction or abscess formation. In acute pyelonephritis, the ultrasound

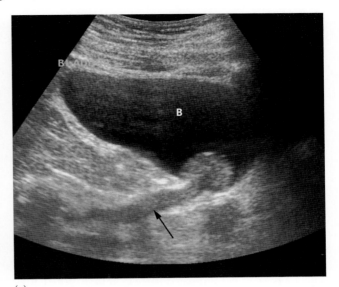

(a)

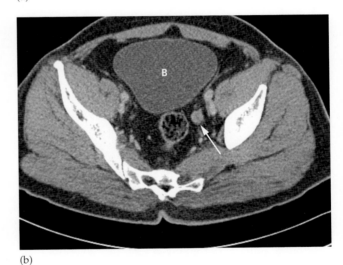

(b)

Fig. 6.39 Transitional cell carcinoma. (a) Ultrasound demonstrates a polypoid mass arising at the vesicoureteric junction in the bladder, extending up the ureter (arrow). (b) CT in the same patient demonstrates thickening and enhancement of the left ureter (arrow). B, bladder.

is either normal or demonstrates diffuse or focal swelling of the kidney, with diminished echoes due to cortical oedema. In some cases, if the pain is severe, an IVU or CT KUB may be done to demonstrate or rule out acute ureteric colic.

Following resolution of the acute episode, imaging of the renal tract is undertaken in women with recurrent infections or after a single confirmed urinary tract infection in men. Ultrasound of the kidneys may demonstrate underlying obstruction or stones. The bladder is imaged while full, to rule out a bladder stone, and then following micturition in order to demonstrate residual urine, which could account for recurrent infection. Urography may be performed if there is a suspected duplex system complicated by obstruction or reflux.

Investigation of the renal tract is indicated in all children with a confirmed urinary tract infection. The aim is to identify an abnormality, such as reflux, which could lead to renal damage, if left untreated (see Fig. 6.14, p. 219). Ultrasound is used to measure the size of the kidneys, to identify any stones or scarring and to demonstrate or rule out hydronephrosis or hydroureter. The bladder is assessed for post-micturition residual urine. Many hospitals do a DMSA radionuclide scan of the kidneys to demonstrate scarring. Micturating cystography is performed in male (and in some female) children to look for vesicoureteric reflux and urethral valves.

Renal and perinephric abscesses

Ultrasound is the initial imaging investigation in most suspected renal abscesses, although in patients who are very unwell CT is often the first imaging investigation.

Intrarenal abscesses (Fig. 6.40) may have thick walls and show both cystic and solid components recognizable at both ultrasound and CT, but may just look like a simple cyst. With CT, it is possible to see enhancement of the wall of the abscess following intravenous contrast injection.

Simple cysts may become secondarily infected, in which case the ultrasound and CT features resemble those of a simple cyst, but the wall may be a little thicker and there will frequently be a layer of echogenic debris in the dependent portion of the cyst.

Perinephric abscesses may conform to the shape of the underlying kidney. The CT and sonographic characteristics are variable, usually showing both solid and cystic

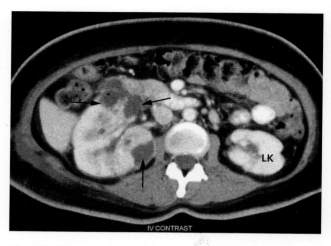

Fig. 6.40 CT scan with intravenous contrast demonstrates multiple low attenuation fluid collections in the right renal cortex, consistent with multiple renal abscesses (arrows). LK, left kidney.

elements (Fig. 6.41). The cystic portions frequently contain internal echoes at ultrasound owing to debris. As most perinephric abscesses are secondary to an infective focus within the kidney, an underlying renal abnormality is often demonstrable.

Pyonephrosis

Pyonephrosis only occurs in collecting systems that are obstructed. Ultrasound is the most useful imaging modality for pyonephrosis. In addition to showing the dilated collecting system, it may demonstrate multiple echoes within the collecting system from infected debris.

Tuberculosis

Urinary tuberculosis follows blood-borne spread of *Mycobacterium tuberculosis*, usually from a focus of infection in the lung.

The tubercle bacilli infect the cortex of the kidneys and may cause tiny cortical granulomas, which rupture through capillaries into the renal tubules and involve other portions of the urinary and genital systems.

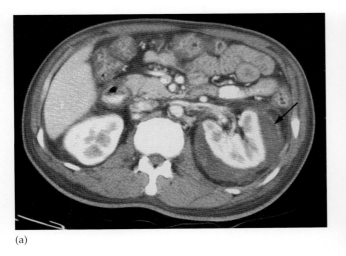

(a)

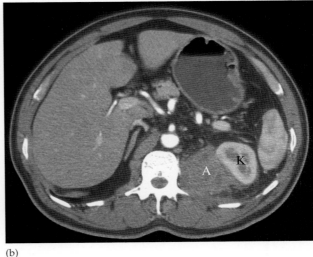

(b)

Fig. 6.41 Perinephric abscess. (a) CT scan showing loculated fluid (arrow) with a thick enhancing wall surrounding the left kidney. (b) An abscess collection (A) lies posterior to the left kidney (K), with the enhancing kidney displaced anteriorly by the collection.

In the early stages of the disease, the ultrasound and IVU may be normal. There are various signs that develop in the later stages that are best seen on IVU:

• Calcification is common (Fig. 6.42). Usually, there are one or more foci of irregular calcification, but in advanced cases with long-standing tuberculous pyonephrosis the majority of the kidney and hydronephrotic collecting system may be calcified, leading to a so-called autonephrectomy. Calcification implies healing but does not mean that the disease is inactive.

• The earliest change on the post contrast films is irregularity of a calix. Later, a definite contrast-filled cavity may be seen adjacent to the calyx.

• Strictures of any portion of the pelvicaliceal system or ureter may occur, producing dilatation of one or more calices (Fig. 6.42). The multiplicity of strictures is an important diagnostic feature.

• If the bladder is involved, the wall is irregular because of inflammatory oedema; advanced disease causes fibrosis resulting in a thick-walled small volume bladder. Multiple strictures may be seen in the urethra.

Ultrasound may demonstrate calcifications and pelvicaliceal dilatation and cavities, but the appearances are non-specific. CT can sensitively demonstrate early calcifications, small cavities and extrarenal spread.

Chronic pyelonephritis (reflux nephropathy)

Chronic pyelonephritis or reflux nephropathy refers to the late appearances of focal or diffuse scarring of the kidney, thought to be due to reflux of infected urine from the bladder into the kidneys, leading to destruction and scarring of the renal substance. Most damage occurs in the first years of life. The severity of reflux diminishes as the child gets older and may have ceased by the time the diagnosis of reflux nephropathy is made (see Fig. 6.14, p. 219). The condition is often bilateral and asymmetrical.

The signs of reflux nephropathy are (Fig. 6.43):

• *Local reduction in renal parenchymal width (scar formation).* The distance between the calix and the adjacent renal outline is usually substantially reduced and may be as little as 1 or 2 mm. The upper and lower calices are the most susceptible to damage from reflux. Intravenous urography, DMSA radionuclide scans and ultrasound are all useful for demonstrating cortical scars.

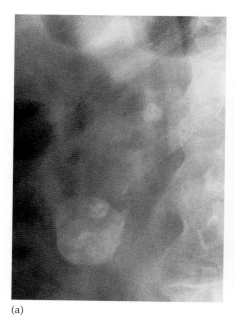

(a)

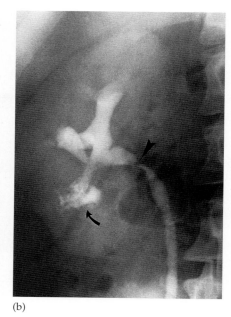

(b)

Fig. 6.42 (a) Renal parenchymal calcification from tuberculosis on plain film. (b) In another patient, after contrast, there is irregularity of the calices (curved arrow) and stricture formation of the pelvis (arrow head).

• *Dilatation of the calices in the scarred areas.* The dilatation is the result of atrophy of the pyramids.
• *Overall reduction in renal size* partly from loss of renal substance and partly because the scarred areas do not grow.
• *Dilatation of the affected collecting system* from reflux may be seen.
• *Vesicoureteric reflux* may be demonstrated at micturating (voiding) cystography.

Papillary necrosis (Fig. 6.44)

In papillary necrosis, part or all of the renal papilla sloughs and may fall into the pelvicaliceal system. These necrotic papillae may remain within the pelvicaliceal system, sometimes causing obstruction, or they may be voided. There are a number of conditions with strong associations with papillary necrosis. The most frequent are:
• high analgesic intake
• diabetes mellitus
• sickle cell disease
• infection, but usually only with very severe infections or infection with obstruction.

The IVU is currently the established modality for demonstrating papillary necrosis, although CT urography is gaining acceptance. The pattern of destruction of the papilla takes many forms; the disease is usually patchy in distribution and severity. If the papilla is only partially necrotic, contrast can be seen tracking around or into it. If the papilla is totally sloughed the calix appears spherical, having lost its papillary indentation. When sloughed, the papilla may then be seen as a filling defect in a spherical calix or it may have passed down the ureter, often causing obstruction as it does so.

The necrotic papilla can calcify prior to sloughing. A sloughed, calcified papilla within the collecting system may closely resemble a urinary calculus.

Renal trauma

The kidney and the spleen are the most frequent internal abdominal organs to be injured. Blunt trauma, particularly road traffic accidents and contact sports, are the mechanisms of injury in well over three-quarters of patients, the remainder being caused by penetrating injury. Loin pain and haematuria are the major presenting features.

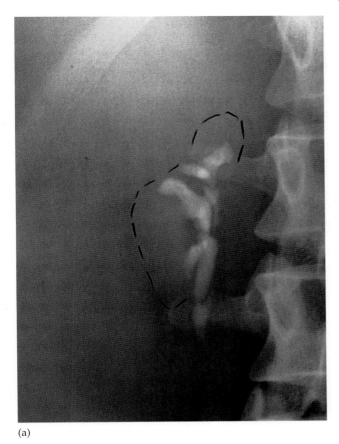

(a)

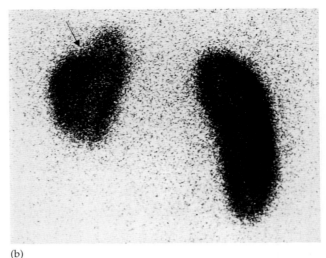

(b)

Fig. 6.43 Reflux nephropathy (chronic pyelonephritis).
(a) Intravenous urography showing a severely shrunken kidney
with multiple scars and clubbed calices. (b) DMSA scan (posterior
view) showing shrunken left kidney with a focal scar in upper pole
(arrow).

The indications for imaging tests depend on the clinical features and surgical approach. Computed tomography is the preferred investigation as it has the advantage that it can not only demonstrate the kidneys but can also show or exclude damage to other abdominal structures (Fig. 6.45). Computed tomography can:

• Demonstrate the presence or absence of perfusion to the injured kidney.

• Ensure that the opposite kidney is normal.

• Show the extent of renal parenchymal damage.

• Demonstrate injuries to other organs, a feature of great importance in penetrating injury, where other organs are frequently lacerated.

The appearances depend on the extent of injury. Minor injury (contusion and small capsular haematomas) produces swelling of the parenchyma, which compresses the calices.

If the kidney substance is torn, the renal outline is irregular and the calices are separated. Large subcapsular and extracapsular blood collections may be present and extravasation of contrast may be seen. Retroperitoneal haemorrhage may displace the kidney. Fragmentation of the kidney is a serious event, often, although by no means always, requiring nephrectomy or surgical repair. If thrombosis or rupture of the renal artery occurs, there will be no nephrogram. Renal infarction is a very serious condition demanding urgent restoration of blood flow or nephrectomy.

Hypertension in renal disease

Most patients with hypertension have essential, or primary, hypertension. However, renal disease may account for hypertension in a small percentage of patients. Renal con-

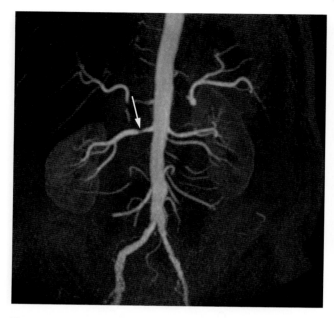

Fig. 6.46 Renal artery stenosis (right) demonstrated on a magnetic resonance angiogram (arrow). There is post-stenotic dilatation beyond the stenosis. The right kidney is small in size.

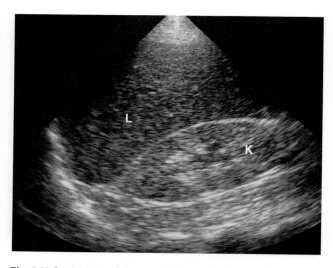

Fig. 6.48 Intrinsic renal disease. Ultrasound of right kidney (longitudinal scan). The kidney is small and the cortical echoes are increased and therefore the central echo is less obvious. Normally, the liver is more echo-reflective than the renal cortex. L, liver; K, kidney.

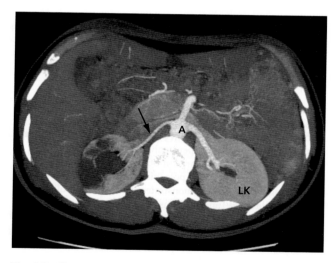

Fig. 6.47 Chronic pyelonephritis secondary to stones on computed tomography angiography. The right kidney is smaller than the left and contains multiple cystic areas following chronic infection from stone disease. The right renal artery is small in caliber (arrow). A, aorta; LK, left kidney.

nephrogram persists for up to 24 hours without visible caliceal filling.

Congenital anomalies of the urinary tract

Congenital variations in the anatomy of the urinary tract are frequent. Only the more common anomalies are discussed here (congenital pelviureteric junction obstruction is discussed on p. 229).

Bifid collecting systems

Bifid collecting systems (Fig. 6.49) are the most frequent congenital variations. The condition may be unilateral or bilateral. The two ureters may join at any level between the renal hilum and the bladder or may insert separately into the bladder. Sometimes just the pelvis is bifid, an anomaly of no importance. At the other extreme, the two ureters may be separate throughout their length and have separate openings into the bladder. The ureter draining

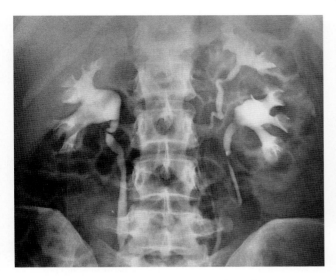

Fig. 6.49 Bifid collecting system. There is a bifid collecting system on the left with the two ureters joining at the level of the transverse process of L5. Note that the left kidney is larger than the right.

the upper moiety may drain outside the bladder, e.g. into the vagina or urethra, producing incontinence if the opening is beyond the urethral sphincter. Such ureters, known as *ectopic ureters*, are frequently obstructed (Fig. 6.50) and lead to dilatation of the entire moiety; the dilated lower ureter may prolapse into the bladder, forming a *ureterocele*. The ureterocele causes a smooth filling defect in the bladder on IVU, and on ultrasound may be seen as a cystic structure within the bladder at the position of the vesicoureteric junction.

Ectopic kidney

During fetal development the kidneys ascend within the abdomen. An ectopic kidney results if this ascent is halted. They are usually in the lower abdomen and rotated so that the pelvis of the kidney points forward. The ureter is short and travels directly to the bladder. In some cases, both kidneys lie on the same side of the pelvis and are fused (see Fig. 6.21, p. 224). Chronic pyelonephritis, hydronephrosis and calculi are all more common in ectopic kidneys, but

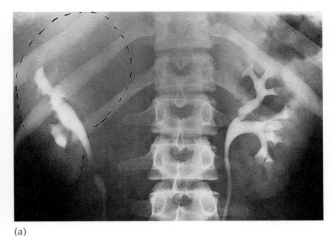

(a)

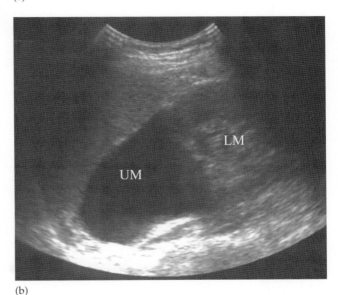

(b)

Fig. 6.50 (a) Obstructed ectopic ureter. There is a bifid collecting system on the right. The upper moiety is obstructed and dilated causing deformity of the lower moiety. The obstructed moiety does not opacify. (b) Ultrasound, in a different patient, showing a dilated upper moiety, with no remaining renal parenchyma (UM). The lower moiety appears normal (LM).

ectopic kidneys are often incidental findings of no consequence to the patient, except as a cause of diagnostic confusion with other causes of lower abdominal masses; the diagnosis can be made on ultrasound in most cases.

Horseshoe kidney

The kidneys may fail to separate, giving rise to a horseshoe kidney. Almost invariably it is the lower poles that remain fused (Fig. 6.51).

The anomaly may be an incidental finding and of no significance, but pelviureteric junction obstruction to the collecting systems and calculi formation are both fairly common.

Inherited cystic disease of the kidneys

There are many varieties of cystic renal disease varying from simple cysts, which may be single or multiple, to complex renal dysplasias. The most frequent complex dysplasia encountered in clinical practice is autosomal dominant polycystic kidney disease. This is a familial disorder which, although inherited, usually presents between the ages of 35 and 55 years with hypertension, renal failure or haematuria, or following the discovery of bilaterally enlarged kidneys.

The reason for the late presentation is that the cysts are initially small and do not cause trouble for a long time. The diagnosis is readily made at ultrasound, as well as on CT (Fig. 6.52). The liver and pancreas may also contain cysts and these organs are routinely examined in such patients. Early diagnosis of autosomal dominant polycystic kidney disease is now possible using ultrasound, when only a few cysts are present. Ultrasound screening is usually offered at the age of 18 to the offspring of those with the disease.

Renal agenesis

In renal agenesis, the opposite kidney, providing it is normal, will show compensatory hypertrophy. Complete absence of blood flow and function on the affected side will be shown on radionuclide studies, and no renal tissue can be identified with ultrasound or CT examination.

Bladder

The bladder is well demonstrated on all imaging modalities. At ultrasound, the simplest routine method of imaging, the bladder lumen should be free of echogenic structures and its wall should be of uniform thickness (see

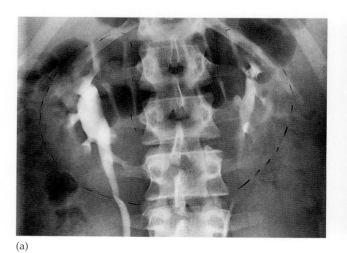
(a)

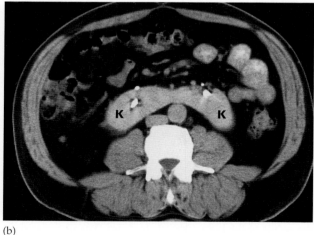
(b)

Fig. 6.51 Horseshoe kidneys. (a) The two kidneys are fused at their lower poles. The striking feature is the alteration in the axis of the kidneys: the lower calices are closer to the spine than the upper calices. The kidneys are rotated so that their pelves point forward and the lower calices point medially. The medial aspects of the lower poles cannot be identified. (b) CT scan of a different patient, following intravenous contrast enhancement, showing fusion of the lower poles of the kidneys. K, kidney.

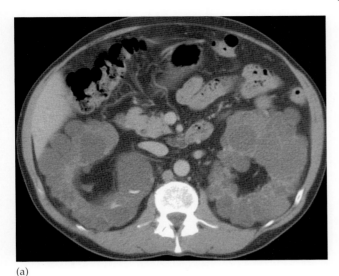

(a)

(b)

Fig. 6.52 Advanced polycystic disease in adults. (a) CT scan, taken after intravenous contrast enhancement, showing that both kidneys are greatly enlarged and almost entirely replaced by cysts of variable size. (b) Coronal T2-weighted MRI in another patient demonstrates multiple bilateral renal cysts as well as a few cysts in the liver. L, liver; S, spleen.

Fig. 6.2, p. 209). When the bladder is distended, the wall should be less than 3 mm thick. The volume of the bladder may be calculated by measuring the dimensions of the bladder.

Bladder tumours (Fig. 6.53)

The bladder is the most frequent site for neoplasms in the urinary tract. Almost all are transitional cell carcinomas of varying degrees of malignancy. They vary in shape: some are delicate fronded papillary lesions, some are sessile irregular masses, and others form flat, plaque-like growths that infiltrate widely. On ultrasound examination, bladder tumours are seen as soft tissue masses protruding into the fluid-filled bladder or as localized bladder wall thickening, but the technique is poor for detecting extravesical spread. Intravenous urography is less sensitive than ultrasound in detecting small bladder masses, but if the mass is large enough, a filling defect in the bladder may be seen. Gas and faeces in the sigmoid colon or rectum, projected over the bladder outline on IVU may closely resemble a bladder neoplasm. Ultrasound can be used to confirm an intravesical mass. On rare occasions, there is visible calcification on the surface of the tumour.

The nature and extent of a tumour in the bladder is best observed at cystoscopy. The main role of urography is to demonstrate any other lesions in the upper tracts (pelvicaliceal systems and ureters), as transitional cell carcinomas are often multifocal.

On CT and MRI, a bladder tumour is seen as a soft tissue mass projecting from the wall or a focal thickening of the bladder wall (Fig. 6.53). As the diagnosis is best established by cystoscopy and biopsy, the roles of CT and MRI are to stage the tumour. No imaging technique is very reliable for assessing the depth of invasion within the muscle of the bladder, but CT and MRI can determine spread of tumour beyond the bladder wall and assess lymph node involvement (Fig. 6.53d).

Bladder diverticula (Fig. 6.54)

Bladder diverticula may be congenital in origin but are usually the consequence of chronic obstruction to bladder

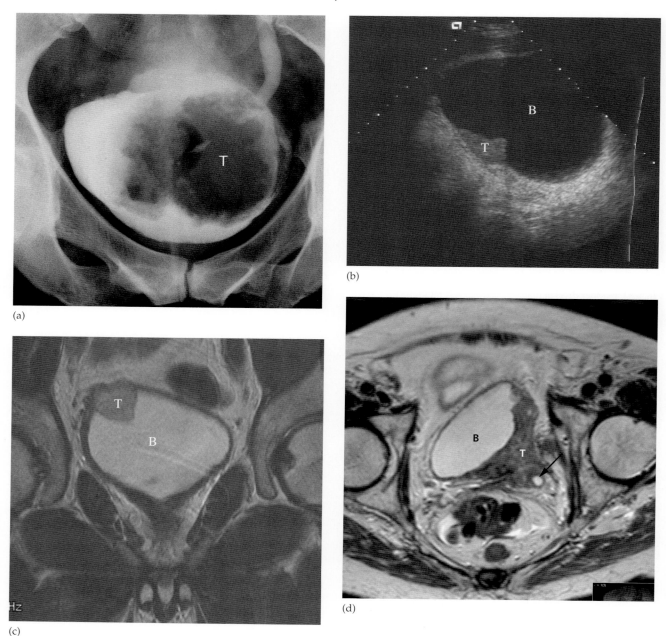

Fig. 6.53 Bladder neoplasm. (a) There is a large filling defect in the left side of the bladder from a transitional cell carcinoma. Note the obstructive dilatation of the left ureter. (b) Ultrasound scan from a different patient showing a small tumour within the bladder. (c) T2-weighted coronal MR image of the bladder tumour seen on ultrasound (b). (d) Advanced stage bladder tumour arising from the left bladder wall and extending into the perivesical fat. Note the obstructed left ureter (arrow). B, bladder; T, tumour.

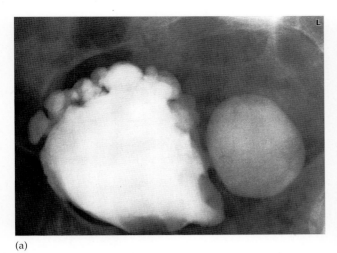

(a)

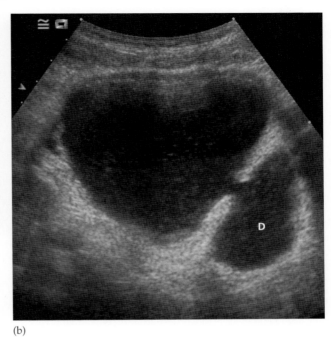

(b)

Fig. 6.54 Bladder diverticula. (a) Cystogram showing numerous out-pouchings from the bladder with a very large diverticulum projecting to the left. (b) Ultrasound of a large diverticulum in a different patient. B, bladder; D, diverticulum.

outflow. Because of urinary stasis, diverticula predispose to infection and stone formation and tumours may, on occasion, arise within them. Most diverticula fill at urography and cystography. They are readily demonstrated at ultrasound, CT and MRI. When large, diverticula may deform the adjacent bladder or ureter.

Bladder calcification

The most frequent cause of calcification in the bladder is calculi. Such calculi are frequently large and laminated. Calcification in the wall of the bladder is rare. When seen, it is usually due to schistosomiasis or bladder tumour.

Neurogenic bladder

There are two basic types of neurogenic bladder (attempts to correlate these types with specific neurological lesions have not been satisfactory):
• The large atonic smooth-walled bladder with poor or absent contractions and a large residual volume.

• The hypertrophic type, which can be regarded as neurologically induced bladder outflow obstruction. In this condition, the bladder is of small volume, has a very thick, grossly trabeculated wall and shows marked sacculation (Fig. 6.55). The ureters and pelvicaliceal systems may be dilated.

Full assessment of neuropathic bladder dysfunction requires voiding cystourethrography combined with pressure measurements, so-called videourodynamics.

Trauma to the bladder and urethra

A direct blow to the distended bladder may result in intraperitoneal bladder rupture: contrast introduced into the bladder will leak out into the peritoneal cavity.

Extraperitoneal rupture of the bladder may be part of an extensive injury such as occurs with fractures of the pelvis. A common site of rupture is at the bladder base, in which case the bladder shows elevation and compression from extravasated urine and haematoma.

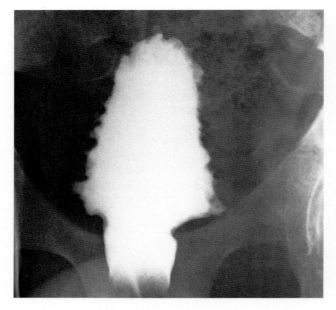

Fig. 6.55 Neurogenic bladder. The outline of the bladder is very irregular due to trabeculation of the bladder wall. The bladder has a small volume with an elongated shape. This appearance has been described as a 'Christmas tree bladder'. There is a balloon catheter in the dilated posterior urethra.

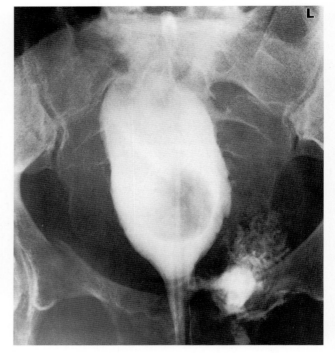

Fig. 6.56 Rupture of the base of the bladder. Cystogram showing extravasation of contrast into the extraperitoneal space on the left, and deformity of the bladder due to surrounding haematoma and urine. There is a fracture of the right pubic bone.

Rupture of the bladder may be revealed sonographically by the presence of a perivesicular fluid collection but the actual site of a tear will not be seen.

Cystography remains the best way of demonstrating the actual site of leakage from the bladder (Fig. 6.56). If there is any suspicion of associated damage to the urethra, an ascending urethrogram with a water-soluble contrast medium may show rupture of the urethra with exravasation of contrast medium into the adjacent tissues. The urethrogram should be performed before passing the catheter into the bladder for the cystogram.

Computed tomography may demonstrate fresh haematomas within the pelvis (which are of high density) or urine collections (which are of low density). It also demonstrates the associated fractures, some of which may not be apparent on plain radiographs.

Prostate and urethra

Prostatic enlargement

Prostatic enlargement is very common in elderly men. It is usually due to benign hypertrophy but may be due to carcinoma. The diagnosis of enlargement is made by digital rectal examination.

Prostatic ultrasound uses a transducer designed to be introduced into the rectum. Transrectal ultrasound (TRUS) can show the overall size of the prostate and can diagnose relatively small masses within its substance (Fig. 6.57). Unfortunately, ultrasound cannot distinguish benign from malignant disease when confined to the prostate, except on the basis that masses in the peripheral zone are likely to be malignant and those in the central zone are more likely to be benign.

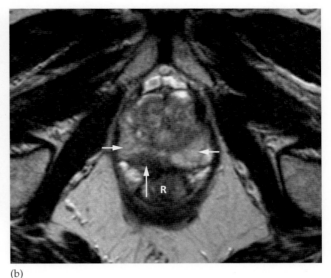

(a)

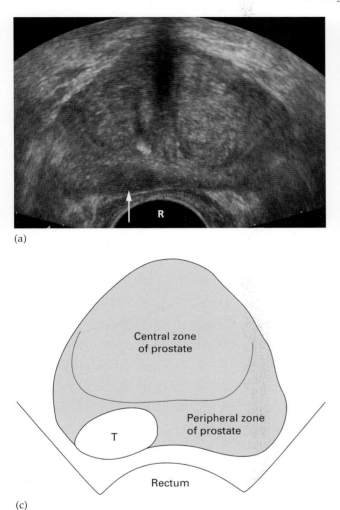

(b)

(c)

Fig. 6.57 Early prostate cancer. (a) Prostate carcinoma shown by transrectal ultrasound. The tumour is seen as a low echogenic ovoid mass in the right peripheral zone (arrow). (b) Axial T2-weighted MRI of the same patient. The peripheral zone is of high signal intensity (short arrows) and the tumour is of low signal intensity (long arrow). (c) Diagram of the prostate gland and the tumour (T). R, rectum.

Transrectal ultrasound-guided biopsy is used extensively for the diagnosis of prostatic carcinoma. Antibiotic prophylaxis is given prior to introducing the biopsy needle, which is positioned within a needle guide along the transrectal ultrasound probe. Usually six to twelve biopsies are then obtained, one from each area of the gland, as well as from any suspicious areas.

Computed tomography does not demonstrate the internal structure of the prostate as well as TRUS or MRI. However, in cases of known prostatic carcinoma, it is helpful in determining the extent of local spread as well as lymph node metastases.

Magnetic resonance imaging is used to assess early stage prostate cancer in patients being considered for radical surgery or radiotherapy. Tumour in the peripheral zone is seen as a relatively low signal mass within the normal high signal of the peripheral zone on T2-weighted images (Fig. 6.57). MRI is used to demonstrate extracapsular tumour spread, to show invasion of the seminal vesicles, and to demonstrate possible lymph node metastases (Fig. 6.58).

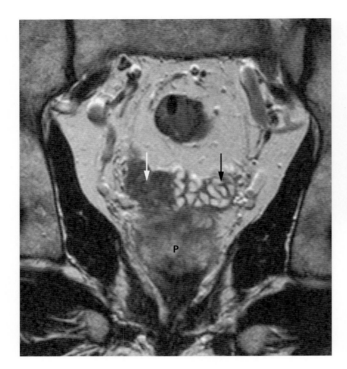

Fig. 6.58 Coronal T2-weighted MRI of the prostate gland (P) demonstrating invasion of the right seminal vesicle by carcinoma of the prostate (white arrow). Note the normal left seminal vesicle (black arrow).

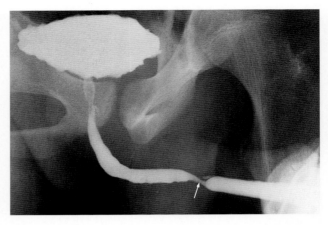

Fig. 6.60 Urethral stricture. An ascending urethrogram showing a stricture in the penile urethra (arrow). The patient had gonorrhoea.

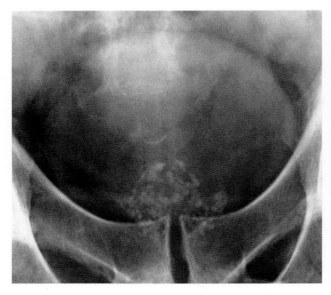

Fig. 6.59 Prostatic calcification. Numerous calculi just above the pubic symphysis are present in the prostate.

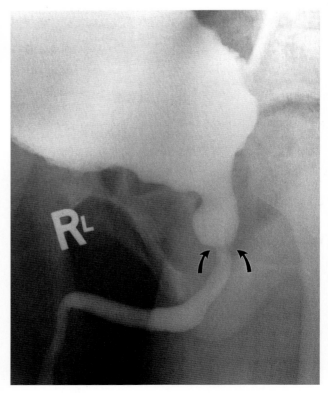

Fig. 6.61 Posterior urethral valves in a 6-year-old boy. On this micturating (voiding) cystogram the site of the valves is arrowed. The presence of the valves is recognized by dilatation of the posterior urethra. Note the irregular outline of the thick-walled bladder due to chronic obstruction.

Prostatic calcification

Prostatic calcification is due to numerous prostatic calculi (Fig. 6.59). It is so common that it can be regarded as a normal finding in older men. It shows no correlation with the symptoms of prostatic hypertrophy nor any relation to prostatic carcinoma. Flecks of calcification of varying size, approximately symmetrical about the midline, are seen just inferior to the bladder.

Bladder outflow obstruction

The most frequent cause of bladder outflow obstruction is enlargement of the prostate. Other causes include bladder tumours, urethral strictures and, in male infants or boys, posterior urethral valves. As discussed above, patients with neurological deficit may have neurogenic obstruction to bladder emptying. Regardless of the cause, ultrasound can demonstrate all the imaging signs of bladder outflow obstruction, which are:

- Increased trabeculation and thickness of the bladder wall, often with diverticula formation.
- Residual urine in the bladder after micturition.
- Dilatation of the collecting systems.

Urethral stricture (Fig. 6.60)

The majority of urethral strictures are due to previous trauma or infection. Post-traumatic strictures are usually in the proximal penile urethra – the most vulnerable portion of the urethra to external trauma. Such strictures are usually smooth in outline and relatively short. Inflammatory strictures, which are usually gonococcal in origin, may be seen in any portion of the urethra, but are usually found in the anterior urethra. Urethral strictures are imaged by urethrography (see p. 221).

Posterior urethral valves (Fig. 6.61)

Congenital valves in the posterior urethra in boys are the commonest cause of bladder outflow obstruction in male

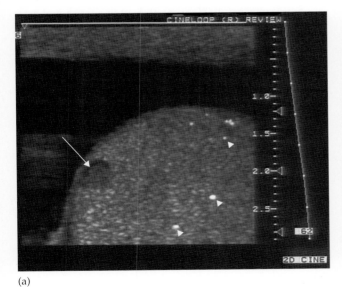

(a)

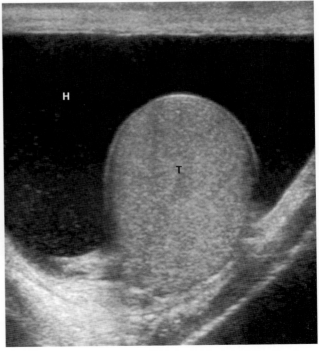

(b)

Fig. 6.62 (a) Ultrasound of testis demonstrating a small seminoma (arrow). Several very bright echogenic specks of microcalcification are seen (arrowheads). (b) A hydrocoele is demonstrated (H) surrounding an otherwise normal testis (T).

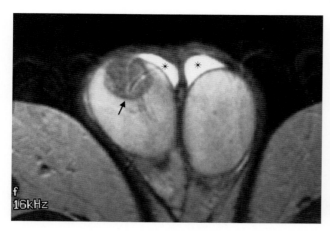

Fig. 6.63 Magnetic resonance imaging of seminoma (arrow) in the right testis. The two testes are well demonstrated. The high signal adjacent to both testes is normal fluid between the layers of the tunica vaginalis (*).

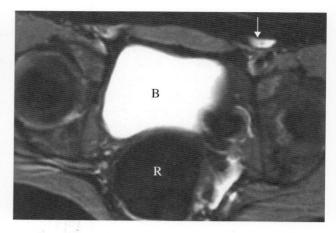

Fig. 6.64 Magnetic resonance imaging of undescended left testis (arrow). The testis lies in the region of the inguinal canal and appears of very high signal on the T2-weighted image with fat saturation. B, bladder; R, rectum.

children. The diagnosis may be first suspected at antenatal ultrasound, when there is bilateral hydronephrosis. After birth, ultrasound confirms bilateral hydronephrosis and hydroureters and a thick-walled bladder. Urethral valves cannot be demonstrated by retrograde urethrography as there is no obstruction to retrograde flow. They are easily demonstrated at micturating cystourethrography, where substantial dilatation of the posterior urethra is seen which terminates abruptly in a convex border formed by the valves.

Scrotum and testes

The scrotal contents are usually imaged with ultrasound, but MRI is occasionally used.

The two main indications for scrotal ultrasound are scrotal swelling or scrotal pain.

In patients with *scrotal swelling*, it is essential to differentiate between an intratesticular cause, such as sus-

pected testicular tumour, and an extratesticular cause, such as varicocele, hydrocele or infection (such as epididymitis or epididymo-orchitis) (Fig. 6.62). Benign epididymal cysts are common and can be readily distinguished from testicular tumours on ultrasound examination.

Doppler ultrasound can be used for patients with acute *testicular pain and/or swelling* to distinguish between testicular torsion, in which testicular perfusion is dramatically decreased, and acute epididymitis/orchitis in which testicular perfusion is normal or increased.

Magnetic resonance imaging can produce highly detailed images of the scrotal contents (Fig. 6.63) and is used in those cases where ultrasound does not provide sufficient information.

Ectopic testis in the inguinal canal, the commonest site, can be diagnosed by ultrasound. In those few cases where the ectopic testis lies within the abdomen, or where the ultrasound is inconclusive, MRI is the investigation of choice (Fig. 6.64).

7

Female Genital Tract

Ultrasound, computed tomography (CT) and magnetic resonance imaging (MRI) have important roles to play in gynaecological disease. Because of its ease and ready availability, ultrasound is usually the first and principal examination. Magnetic resonance imaging is now routinely used in evaluation of several gynaecologic malignancies, CT being reserved for staging the distant extent of malignant disease. Positron emission tomography may be used in the management of gynaecologic malignancy. Conventional radiology plays almost no part – the major exception being hysterosalpingography. Ultrasound is used extensively in obstetric practice and is a key aspect of ante-natal care.

Normal appearances

Ultrasound

Ultrasound of the pelvis can be carried out in two ways: either by scanning through the abdominal wall or transvaginally with a specialized ultrasound probe inserted directly into the vagina. With the transvaginal route the pelvic organs are nearer the ultrasound probe, so image quality is much improved. The patient is scanned with an empty bladder.

When abdominal scanning is undertaken, it is essential for the patient to have a full bladder to act as an acoustic 'window' through which the pelvic structures can be seen. Scans are usually made in the longitudinal and transverse planes.

On a midline longitudinal or transverse scan the *vagina* can be recognized as a tubular structure, with a central linear echo arising from the opposing vaginal surfaces (Fig. 7.1). The *uterus* lies immediately behind the bladder, and the body of the uterus can be seen to be in continuity with the cervix and vagina. The myometrium shows low-level echoes, whereas the endometrial cavity gives an echogenic linear stripe (Fig. 7.2). The precise appearances of the uterus depend on the age and parity of the patient and also on the lie of the uterus. The normal *fallopian tubes* are too small to be visualized sonographically.

The *ovaries* are suspended from the broad ligament and usually lie lateral to the uterus near the pelvic side walls

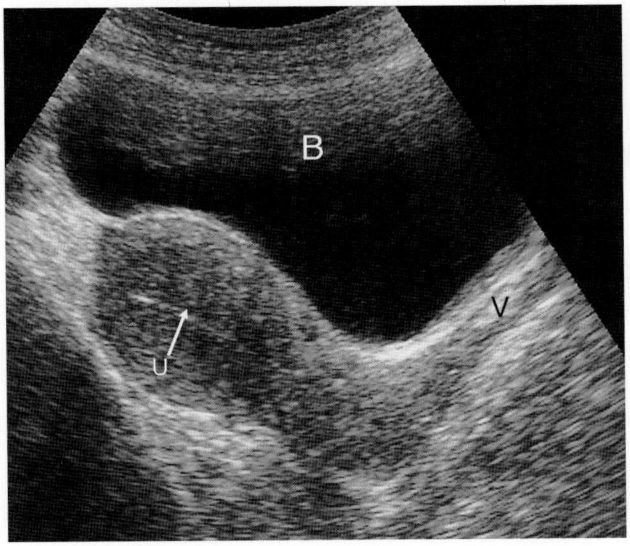

Fig. 7.1 Normal abdominal scan uterus and vagina. Longitudinal section. The central echo of uterus (U) corresponds to the endometrial cavity; the uterus itself has a homogeneous echo texture. V, vagina; B, bladder.

Diagnostic Imaging, 6th Edition. By Peter Armstrong, Martin Wastie and Andrea Rockall. Published 2009 by Blackwell Publishing. ISBN: 978-1-4051-7039.

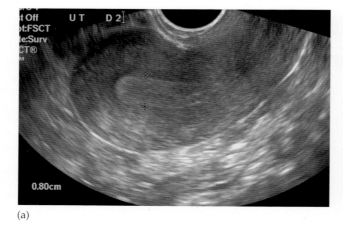

(a)

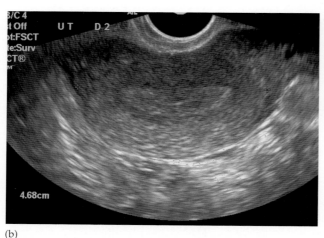

(b)

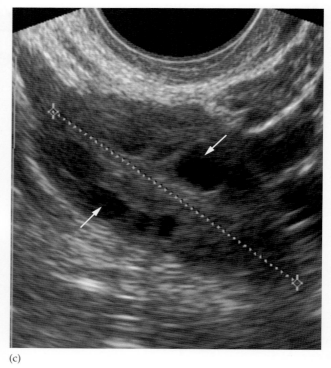

(c)

Fig. 7.2 Normal transvaginal ultrasound scan. (a) Longitudinal section through the uterus. Note the echogenic endometrial stripe between the measurement calipers. (b) Transverse section through the uterus. (c) Normal ovary. Several normal follicles are seen (arrows).

(Fig. 7.2c). During childbearing years, the ovaries measure 2.5–5 cm in greatest diameter, but after the menopause, they atrophy. The endocrine changes occurring during the menstrual cycle have a great effect on the appearance of the ovaries. During the early phase, several cystic structures are seen, representing developing follicles. Around the eighth day of the cycle, one follicle becomes dominant and may reach 2–2.5 cm in diameter prior to ovulation. At ovulation, the follicle ruptures and immediately decreases in size giving rise to the corpus luteum, which degenerates if there is no intervening pregnancy. By observing these changes it is possible to determine whether an infertile woman is ovulating.

CT

The quality of pelvic CT has improved with fast multislice CT systems which allow thin reconstruction, resulting in less movement artefact and high resolution. The diagnostic quality of pelvic scans is also improved with the use of oral and intravenous contrast medium. The vagina is seen as a linear structure between the urethra and rectum. Immediately above the vagina, the *cervix* is seen as a rounded soft tissue structure approximately 3 cm in diameter. The body of the *uterus* (Fig. 7.3) merges with the cervix, its precise appearance depending on the lie of the uterus. The endometrial lining cannot be fully assessed on CT. The fallopian

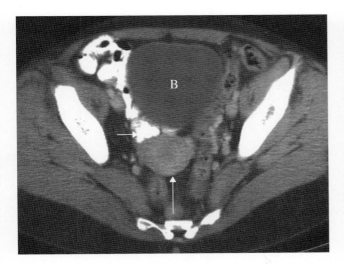

Fig. 7.3 Normal uterus (long arrow) in a 49-year-old patient, on CT, following intravenous contrast enhancement. Note the oral contrast medium within loops of small bowel (short arrow). B, bladder.

tubes and broad ligaments are usually not visible and the ovaries are often not identified. The parametrium is of fat density, the interface with the pelvic musculature being clearly visible. As the peritoneal cavity extends into the pelvis, the uterus may be surrounded by loops of bowel. Oral contrast medium is given 1 hour prior to pelvic imaging to aid the differentiation of bowel loops from adnexal structures. Intravenous contrast medium is given to differentiate between vessels and lymph nodes, and to assess the enhancement pattern of a mass.

MRI

The pelvic anatomy is very well demonstrated because of the excellent soft tissue contrast afforded by MRI. The patient may be given an intravenous muscle relaxant to reduce movement artefacts from bowel. Images are usually taken in the axial and sagittal planes but may be supplemented by oblique images, particularly for the examination of the cervix or endometrium. Axial images give anatomical appearances similar to CT. The sagittal plane shows the vagina and cervix in continuity with the body of the uterus. The cervix is usually low in signal intensity (see Fig. 4.54b, p. 163). On T2-weighted scans, the body of the uterus is

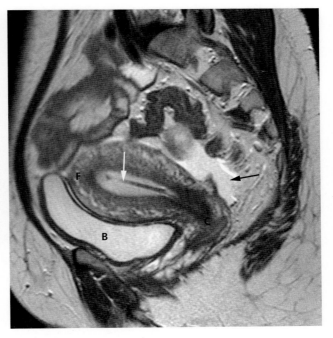

Fig. 7.4 Normal uterus, sagittal T2-weighted MRI. The endometrium, which in this case contains a coil (arrow) returns a high signal intensity. There is some free fluid in the pouch of Douglas (black arrow). This is the same patient as in Fig. 7.19. B, bladder; F, uterine fundus; C, cervix.

easily recognized; the myometrium shows intermediate signal and the endometrium has a high signal (Fig. 7.4). Variations of uterine anatomy are well delineated on MRI (Fig. 7.5). The ovaries are of intermediate signal intensity and often contain multiple high signal follicles on T2-weighted images (Figs 7.5 and 7.6). The broad ligaments can also be identified.

PET/CT

In selected cases, the extent and distribution of gynaecologic cancer may be assessed using fluorodeoxyglucose positron emission tomography (FDG-PET)/CT. This technique is particularly helpful in detecting disease which has metastasized beyond the pelvis (see Fig. 7.9d, p. 261). In addition, some centres are using the technique to assess response to chemotherapy.

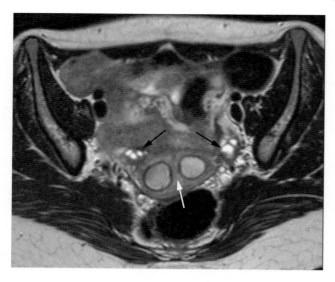

Fig. 7.5 Axial MRI of a septate uterus, an anatomical variant. The endometrial cavity is divided into two compartments by a septum of myometrium (white arrow). Note the normal ovaries bilaterally (black arrows).

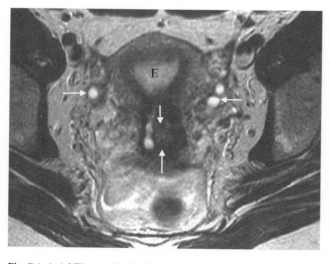

Fig. 7.6 Axial T2-weighted MRI demonstrating normal ovaries (horizontal arrows). The patient has a cervical carcinoma (vertical arrows), resulting in some obstruction of the endocervical canal, with retained secretions seen within the endometrial cavity (E).

Gynaecological pathology

Patients attending for pelvic imaging may present with non-specific symptoms of lower abdominal discomfort or pain, a sensation of bloating, or with abnormal vaginal bleeding or a pelvic mass. Pelvic imaging may also be undertaken for the investigation of infertility. Ultrasound is the initial investigation in most cases.

Pelvic masses

Ultrasound, CT and MRI will be abnormal in virtually any patient in whom a mass can be felt on physical examination. With ultrasound, it is possible to tell whether the mass is cystic or solid. In some cases, the characteristics of the adnexal cyst or mass may indicate whether the lesion is benign in nature or likely to be malignant. However, in many cases, this distinction may not be made on ultrasound alone and MRI may be helpful in further characterization. CT is predominantly used to demonstrate the extent of disease in the abdomen in cases of malignant disease. A limitation of imaging, particularly ultrasound and CT, is that sometimes it is not possible to determine from which organ the mass arises; an ovarian mass which lies in contact with the uterus may appear similar to a mass arising within the uterus and vice versa. MRI, which may be performed in any scan plane, may be used to help make the distinction.

Ovarian masses

Ovarian cysts

Sometimes a follicle or corpus luteum persists as a follicular or corpus luteum cyst, both of which are easily recognized by ultrasound, CT or MRI (Fig. 7.7). Follicular cysts are mostly asymptomatic and regress spontaneously. Corpus luteum cysts are most often seen in the first trimester of pregnancy; they usually resolve, but may rupture or twist. Haemorrhage into both types of cyst may occur and gives a characteristic appearance on ultrasound. The typical features of polycystic ovaries on ultrasound or MRI include large volume ovaries with multiple small follicles arranged around the periphery, forming the appearance of a 'string of pearls' (Fig. 7.8).

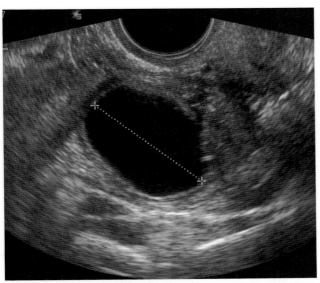

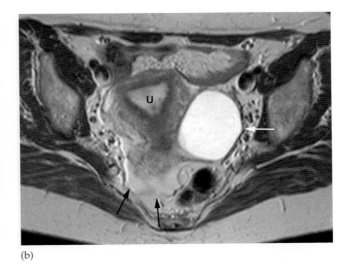

(b)

(a)

Fig. 7.7 Ovarian cyst. (a) Longitudinal ultrasound scan to the right of midline showing a 5 cm cyst in the right ovary with no internal echoes. (b) Axial T2-weighted MRI scan showing a left-sided ovarian cyst with benign features (white arrow). There is a small volume of free fluid in the pouch of Douglas (black arrows). U, uterus.

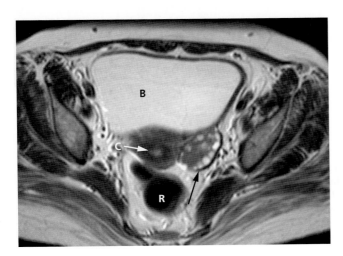

Fig. 7.8 Polycystic ovary. Axial T2-weighted MRI demonstrates the left ovary (black arrow) which is large in size and has multiple small cysts arranged around the periphery of the ovary, in a characteristic 'string of pearls' distribution. B, bladder; C, cervix; R, rectum.

Ovarian tumours

The commonest ovarian tumours are the cystadenoma and the cystadenocarcinoma. Ovarian tumours can be predominantly cystic, solid or a mixture of the two (Fig. 7.9). Those that are cystic may be multilocular. On ultrasound, the recognized features of a benign lesion include a thin cyst wall, thin septations and no significant solid components. The features which are consistent with a malignant lesion include a mixed solid cystic mass with a thick wall and nodular septations with vascularity within the solid components, as shown by Doppler flow. In some cases it is not possible to say whether the mass is benign or malignant unless there is evidence of local invasion or distant spread. MRI may be used to further characterize the mass as benign or malignant prior to deciding on patient management. With disseminated malignancy, deposits within the omentum and ascites may be visible, but omental and peritoneal metastases are frequently difficult to detect due to their small size. FDG-PET/CT may be used to demonstrate the extent of disseminated disease, to aid treatment planning (Fig. 7.9d).

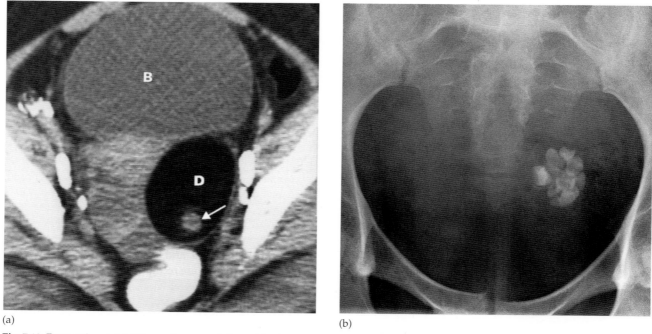

Fig. 7.10 Dermoid cyst. (a) CT scan shows oval-shaped fat density of a dermoid cyst (D) containing calcified material (arrow). B, bladder. (b) Plain film of another patient showing well-developed teeth within the cyst.

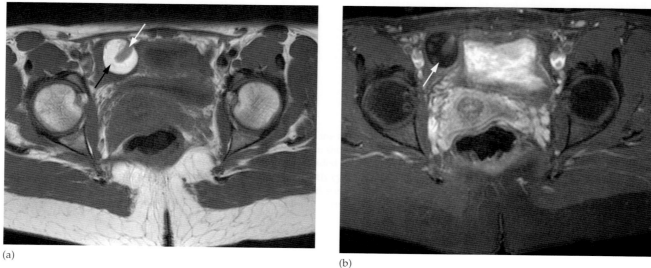

Fig. 7.11 Benign dermoid cyst. (a) Axial T1-weighted MRI demonstrates a complex cyst which contains high signal intensity material, indicating the possible presence of lipid (black arrow). An internal solid component is also seen (white arrow). (b) Axial T1-weighted image with fat saturation demonstrates almost complete drop of signal intensity within the cyst, consistent with the presence of lipid (arrow). This confirms the diagnosis of a dermoid cyst. There was no enhancement of the internal solid component.

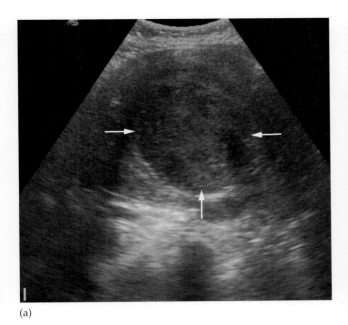

(a)

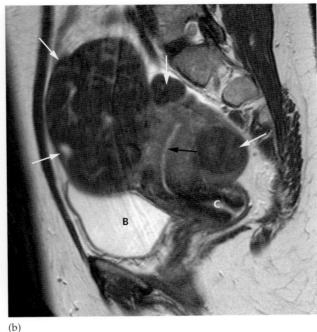

(b)

Fig. 7.12 (a) Transverse ultrasound scan showing a large fibroid in the uterus. Its extent is indicated by the arrows. (b) Sagittal T2-weighted MRI demonstrating several uterine fibroids (white arrows), which are of low signal intensity. The endometrial cavity is normal (black arrow). C, cervix; B, bladder.

heterogeneity of the myometrium. On MRI, there is focal or diffuse thickening of the junctional zone and in some cases, multiple bright projections are seen extending from the endometrium into the myometrium (Fig. 7.13).

Carcinoma of the cervix and body of the uterus

The diagnosis of carcinoma of the cervix is normally made by cytology or biopsy, or by physical examination. Endometrial carcinoma may be suspected on ultrasound when there is widening of the endometrial stripe, but confirmation of the diagnosis is based on histology.

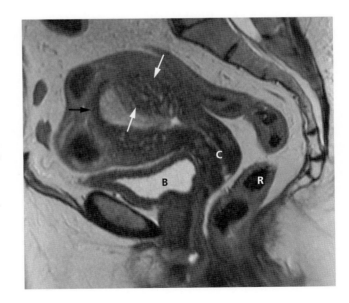

Fig. 7.13 Adenomyosis. Sagittal T2-weighted MRI demonstrates a markedly widened junctional zone containing small cysts (between the white arrows). A normal section of junctional zone is seen in the region of the uterine fundus (black arrow). Two low signal intensity ovoid fibroids are also present in the fundus. B, bladder; C, cervix; R, rectum.

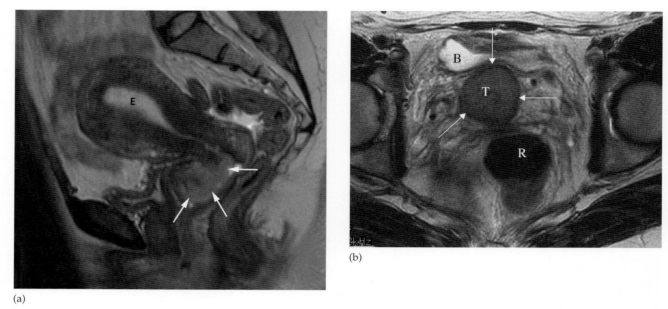

(a)

(b)

Fig. 7.14 Carcinoma of cervix. (a) Sagittal T2-weighted MRI scan showing a tumour confined to the cervix (arrows). (b) Axial T2-weighted MRI in a different patient demonstrating a cervical tumour (T), which is confined to the cervix, with a thin layer of normal, low signal cervical tissue surrounding the tumour (arrows). T, tumour; B, bladder; R, rectum; E, endometrium.

MRI is useful to determine the extent of carcinoma of the cervix pre-operatively, because the extent (or tumour stage) determines whether the patient is managed with surgery, or with radiotherapy and chemotherapy. In essence, the observations to be made are whether the tumour is confined to the cervix (Fig. 7.14) or whether it extends into the parametrium, lymph nodes, rectum, bladder or pelvic side-walls (Fig. 7.15). MRI is very accurate in assessing the local extent of the tumour. CT and MRI also enable detection of dilatation of the ureters in cases where the tumour has caused ureteric obstruction.

Endometrial carcinoma is usually treated by surgical removal of the uterus, ovaries and pelvic lymph nodes. Therefore, the use of imaging to stage the tumour at presentation is limited. MRI can predict the depth of myometrial invasion by tumour (Fig. 7.16), and both CT and MRI can demonstrate lymph node involvement.

Pelvic inflammatory disease

Pelvic inflammatory disease may be due to venereal infection, commonly gonorrhoea, which in the acute stages gives rise to a tubo-ovarian abscess. Pelvic inflammation and abscess formation may also occur following pelvic surgery, childbirth or abortion and may be seen in association with intrauterine contraceptive devices, appendicitis or diverticular disease. The usual imaging technique is ultrasound. Irrespective of the cause of the infection, ultrasound will show a hypoechoic or complex mass in the adnexal region or pouch of Douglas (cul-de-sac) (Fig. 7.17). Blockage of the fallopian tubes may cause a hydrosalpinx, which can be recognized as a hypoechoic adnexal mass, which is often tubular in shape.

The appearance of pelvic inflammatory disease on ultrasound may be indistinguishable from endometriosis and ectopic pregnancy, conditions that both occur in women

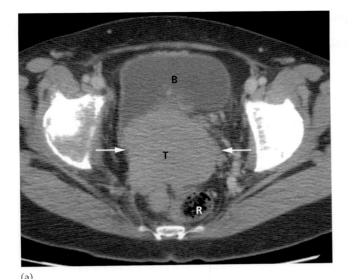

(a)

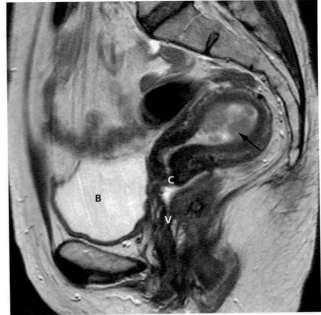

(a)

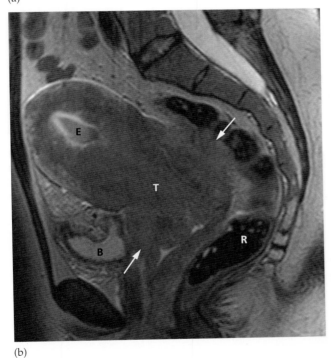

(b)

Fig. 7.15 Advanced carcinoma of cervix. (a) CT scan showing a large tumour of the cervix (T) invading the parametrium (arrows) and extending into the rectum (R) posteriorly. (b) Sagittal T2-weighted MRI of the same patient as (a). Note the tumour extending down the vagina. T, tumour; B, bladder; R, rectum; E, endometrium.

(b)

Fig. 7.16 Endometrial cancer. (a) Sagittal T2-weighted MRI demonstrates a polypoid tumour mass distending the endometrial cavity (arrow). (b) Oblique axial MRI in a different patient. The endometrial tumour mass is invading into the myometrium (arrow). B, bladder; C, cervix; V, vagina.

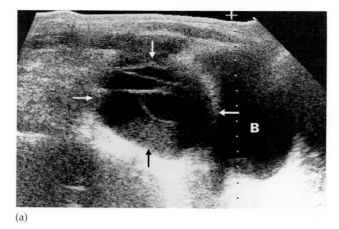

(a)

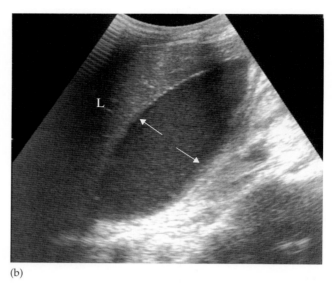

(b)

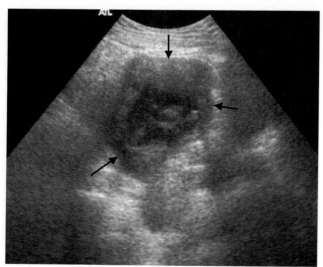

(c)

Fig. 8.5 Pelvic abscess shown by ultrasound in three separate patients. (a) A large complex mass (arrows) just above the bladder (B). This young man had Crohn's disease. (b) A large abscess (arrows) lying directly beneath the liver (L). (c) A large pelvic abscess (arrows). The computed tomography of this patient is illustrated in Fig. 8.6c.

loculations. The gas may take the form of multiple small streaks or bubbles, or it may collect as one large bubble. Air–fluid levels may be present within larger collections. The wall of the abscess often shows enhancement following intravenous contrast administration. Subphrenic abscesses may be difficult to distinguish from pleural empyemas at CT; the peritoneal and pleural cavities are, after all, separated only by the diaphragm, a structure that can be difficult to identify at CT. In such cases, coronal or sagittal reformat of the CT or ultrasound will usually be very helpful because

it can demonstrate the position of the abscess in relation to the diaphragm.

The major diagnostic problems are:
- Distinguishing between abscesses and distended or matted loops of bowel. The distinction at CT can usually be made by opacifying the bowel. With ultrasound, peristalsis of bowel loops can be observed directly.
- It may not be possible to distinguish between infected and uninfected fluid loculations, and needle aspiration may have to be performed.

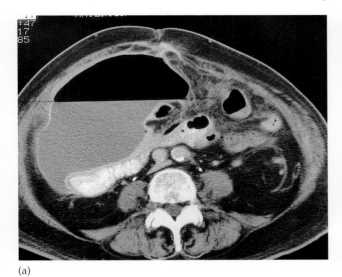

(a)

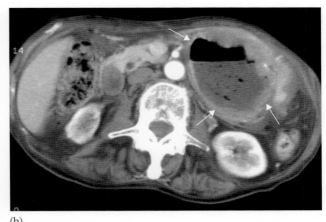

(b)

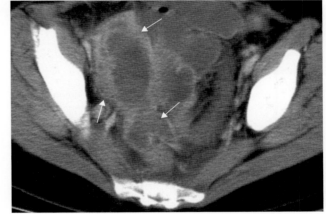

(c)

Fig. 8.6 CT of postoperative intraperitoneal abscesses – three different patients. (a) Large abscess in the right side of the abdomen at the level of the umbilicus. Note the large air–fluid collection with a thin enhancing wall. The abscess displaces adjacent bowel loops (containing air and oral contrast). (b) A typical thick-walled abscess (arrows) containing both air and fluid. (c) A pelvic abscess containing fluid (pus). The ultrasound scan of this patient is illustrated in previous figure (Fig. 8.5c).

MRI appearances

Pelvic abscesses are occasionally assessed on MRI, and usually have the appearance of a complex septate cyst with a thick enhancing wall. MRI may be helpful in delineating fistulous connections between the abscess and other organs, such as the bladder, bowel or vagina (Fig. 8.7).

Radionuclide examinations

If CT and ultrasound have been unsuccessful in locating an abscess, then some of the patient's own white blood cells

can be labelled with ^{99m}Tc or with indium-111, which will accumulate in an abscess (Fig. 8.8).

Retroperitoneum

Computed tomography, MRI and ultrasound all provide information about retroperitoneal structures. Plain films are limited to showing: very large masses or calcification within a mass; the occasional case where gas is seen in an abscess; and the curvilinear calcification of an aortic aneurysm. The discussion in this chapter will be confined to: the adrenal glands; lymphadenopathy; aortic aneurysms; retroperitoneal tumours; haematomas and

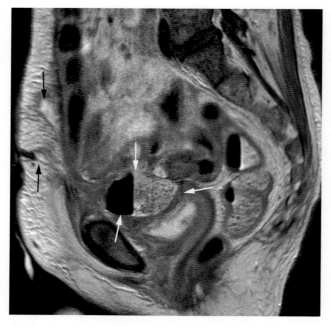

Fig. 8.7 T2-weighted MRI scan in the sagittal plane demonstrates a pelvic abscess (white arrows) containing faecal material and air, which has formed a fistula with the anterior abdominal wall (black arrows).

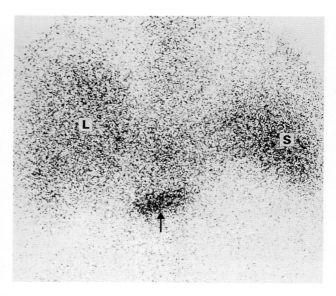

Fig. 8.8 Indium-111-labelled leucocyte scan of an intraperitoneal abscess. This abscess (arrow) followed small bowel surgery with subsequent anastomotic leak. Normal uptake is seen in the liver (L) and spleen (S).

abscesses. The urinary tract and pancreas are covered elsewhere.

When considering the retroperitoneum it is useful to appreciate the anatomy of the anterior and posterior renal fascia which divide the retroperitoneum into three compartments: the anterior pararenal, the perinephric and the posterior pararenal spaces (Fig. 8.9). Infection in one of these compartments tends to be limited to that compartment.

Imaging techniques

Computed tomography

The following normal features should be looked for (Figs 8.9 and 8.10a):
• The complete outline of the aorta and inferior vena cava (IVC) should be clearly visible throughout their

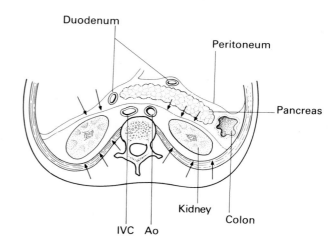

Fig. 8.9 Diagram of anterior (downward pointing arrows) and posterior (upward pointing arrows) renal fascia. Ao, aorta; IVC, inferior vena cava.

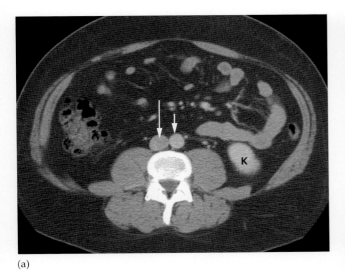

(a)

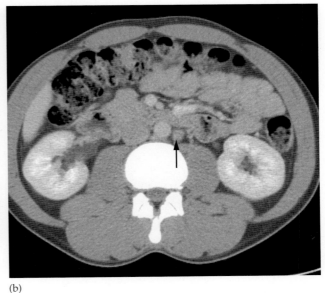

(b)

Fig. 8.10 (a) CT scan of normal retroperitoneum. Note that the aorta (short arrow) and IVC (long arrow) are clearly outlined by fat and that there is a fat-containing space around the vessels. K, kidney. (b) There is a node at the upper limit of normal size in the left para-aortic space (arrow).

lengths. The aorta is round in cross-section and normally measures 2.0–2.5 cm in diameter. CT angiography may be performed, providing three-dimensional views of the aorta and renal vessels which help to plan vascular interventions. The IVC varies in shape from round to oval. Superiorly, the IVC passes through the liver (known as the intrahepatic IVC) before draining into the right atrium.

• There is usually a fat-containing space to the left of the aorta, which is a good area in which to look for lymphadenopathy (Fig. 8.10b). The only structures other than lymph nodes to be seen in this space are the left renal vein and, rarely, a loop of small bowel or an aberrant vessel.

• The psoas muscles are seen as symmetrical, rounded structures outlined anteriorly by fat.

• Both adrenals are well seen in most subjects.

Ultrasound

Retroperitoneal fat, which is very echo-reflective, surrounds the various retroperitoneal structures. The aorta and inferior vena cava are easily identified as hypoechoic tubular structures. Normal adrenal glands are rarely visible in adults. Enlarged lymph nodes can be identified.

Magnetic resonance imaging

Magnetic resonance imaging plays a small part in diagnosing retroperitoneal disorders as it provides few advantages over CT or ultrasound. Characterization of adrenal nodules is often performed on MRI. The ability to display the body in any plane can be an advantage, for example in helping decide whether a mass has arisen in a kidney or in an adrenal gland. However, with the development of multislice CT, multiplanar CT reformats are now available. The ability of MRI to display intravascular spread of tumour can be of value in showing the spread of renal carcinoma into the renal vein, IVC and heart (Fig. 8.11).

Retroperitoneal lymphadenopathy

The normal para-aortic lymph nodes vary in size from invisible up to a short-axis diameter of 1 cm. In the

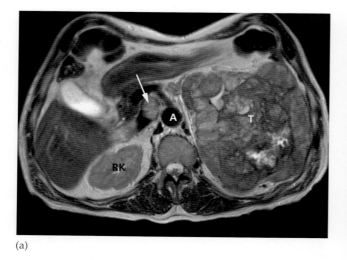

(a)

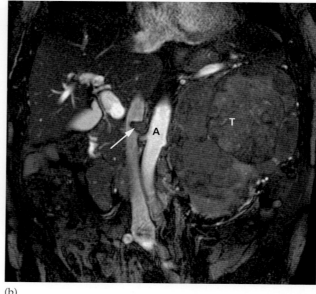

(b)

Fig. 8.11 Renal cell carcinoma invading the inferior vena cava (IVC). (a) T2-weighted MRI demonstrates a very large left renal tumour (T). The tumour has extended along the left renal vein (not shown) and into the IVC (arrow). (b) Coronal MR venogram following gadolinium demonstrates the tongue of tumour tissue in the IVC. A, aorta; RK, right kidney.

retrocrural area, a diameter of 6 mm is the upper limit of normal. Nodal enlargement may occur secondary to inflammatory disease, metastatic tumour deposits and lymphoma. It is often not possible to reliably diagnose the cause of mild nodal enlargement on cross-sectional imaging, as the nodes have the same features and texture, regardless of the cause of enlargement, at CT, ultrasound, and MRI. New techniques such as FDG-PET/CT can be used to identify metastatic nodal tumour deposits. This is of particular importance in the follow-up of patients being treated for lymphoma. An MRI contrast agent that can help distinguish neoplastic nodes from normal or inflammatory nodes is currently under development.

Nodal enlargement of over 2 cm almost always indicates neoplasm, notably lymphoma. Individually enlarged lymphomatous nodes may be seen (Fig. 8.12a), but not infrequently several nodes are matted together to form a lobular mass engulfing the aorta or inferior vena cava

(Fig. 8.12b) and may involve the small bowel mesentery (Fig. 8.12c).

Adrenal glands

The normal adrenal glands are thin, bilobed structures surrounded by fat (Fig. 8.13). The right adrenal gland is situated above the upper pole of the right kidney. The left adrenal gland is usually situated just anterior to the upper pole of the left kidney.

Calcification of the adrenal glands (Fig. 8.14) may follow old intra-adrenal haemorrhage or old healed tuberculosis. Severe destruction and calcification of the adrenal glands may lead to Addison's disease.

Enlargement of the adrenal glands can be recognized at CT and MRI and occasionally on ultrasound. Enlargement may be due to several different pathologies (Box 8.2). CT is the best routine technique for diagnosing adrenal enlarge-

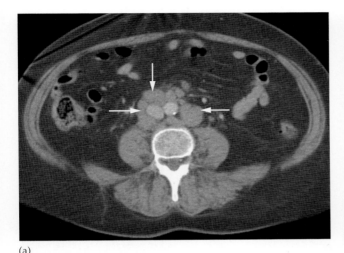

(a)

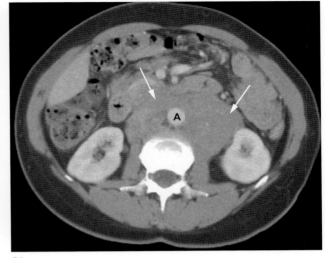

(b)

(c)

Fig. 8.12 Lymphoma. (a) Several enlarged lymph nodes (arrows) are shown surrounding the contrast-enhanced aorta and inferior vena cava. (b) In this case, the para-aortic nodes have become confluent (arrows), forming a lobulated mass around the aorta (A). (c) Extensive nodal disease is seen infiltrating the small bowel mesentery (arrows).

Box 8.2 Causes of adrenal enlargement

- Hyperplasia
- Cortical adenoma
  - Non-functioning
  - Functioning (Conn's or Cushing's)
- Phaeochromocytoma
  - Benign or malignant
- Primary adrenal carcinoma
- Metastasis
- Haemorrhage
- Cyst
- Abscess

ment because it consistently shows the size and shape of the glands.

Functioning adrenal tumours

Patients with tumours producing an excess of hormones will usually have had their endocrine disorder diagnosed clinically and biochemically prior to the imaging examination. CT, or occasionally MRI, is used in this group primarily to localize any tumour. The responsible tumours are usually benign adenomas, but may be carcinomas.

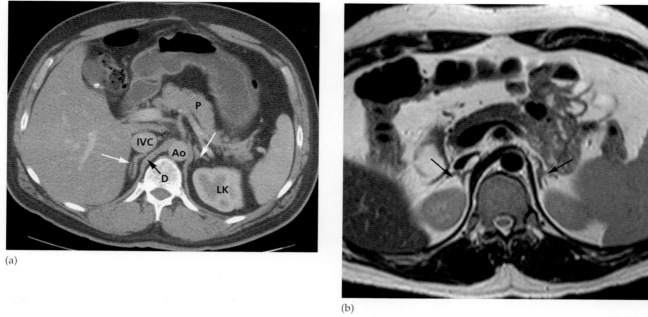

(a)

(b)

Fig. 8.13 Normal adrenal glands. (a) CT scan. Both adrenal glands (white arrows) are visible in this section. Note the different shape of the two glands. Ao, aorta; D, diaphragmatic crus; IVC, inferior vena cava; LK, left kidney; P, pancreas. (b) MRI scan showing the right and left adrenal glands (arrows), which have an intermediate signal intensity on these T2-weighted images.

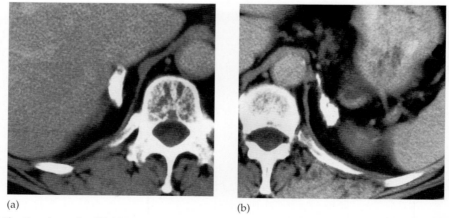

(a)   (b)

Fig. 8.14 Adrenal calcification shown by CT. (a) Heavily calcified right adrenal gland. (b) Heavily calcified left adrenal gland.

An adrenal adenoma appears as a spherical mass arising from one of the adrenal glands. The distinction between pituitary tumour, adrenal adenoma and adrenal hyperplasia as a cause of Cushing's syndrome is usually based on biochemical findings but, on occasions, the precise diagnosis can be in doubt. Adrenal adenomas giving rise to Cushing's syndrome are unilateral and nearly always larger than 2 cm, and can virtually always be localized with CT (Fig. 8.15). Most hyperplastic glands in pituitary-dependent Cushing's syndrome appear normal or are slightly enlarged bilaterally at CT. Aldosteronomas (Conn's tumour) are usually unilateral and usually less than 1 cm in size and may, on occasion, be difficult to identify at imaging.

Phaeochromocytomas are virtually all demonstrable at CT or MRI (Fig. 8.16). Ten per cent are bilateral and, therefore, the opposite adrenal gland must be looked at carefully. They typically enhance avidly following administration of intravenous contrast medium. It should also be remembered that 10% of phaeochromocytomas arise outside the adrenal gland, usually in another retroperitoneal site.

Radionuclide scans can be used to localize functioning adrenal tumours. The only radionuclide in widespread use, now that CT has become the prime method of localizing cortisol and aldosterone-producing tumours, is iodine-123 labelled MIBG (meta-iodo-benzyl guanidine), an agent which is concentrated by phaeochromocytomas (Fig. 8.16c). As already mentioned, the great majority of phaeochromocytomas are single, but a few are multiple, either in both adrenal glands or extra-adrenal in location, and a radioiodine-labelled MIBG scan is an excellent survey technique for finding all sites of phaeochromocytoma.

Non-functioning adrenal masses

In patients with a known underlying malignancy, it is important to distinguish between a small non-functioning adenoma and a small adrenal metastasis. This can pose a major dilemma for patients being staged for a cancer in whom a small adrenal mass (up to 3 cm in diameter) is discovered. The distinction can be made with reasonable specificity on fine-section non-contrast CT, as cortical adenomas typically are of low density (Hounsfield units, HU, less than 10) due to the presence of intracellular lipid, whereas metastases have a HU greater than 10. Special MRI sequences designed to demonstrate intracellular lipid may also be used to make this distinction between adenomas and metastases. Using an MRI sequence called 'chemical shift imaging',

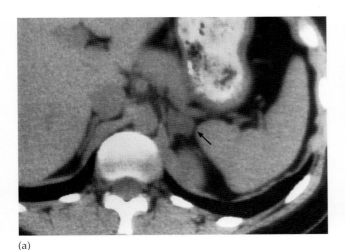

(a)

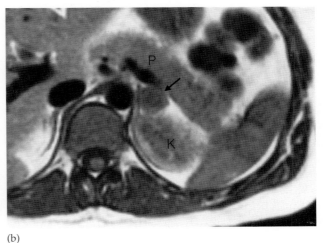

(b)

Fig. 8.15 Functioning adrenal adenoma causing Cushing's syndrome. (a) CT scan showing 2-cm mass in left adrenal gland (arrow). (b) MRI scan (T1-weighted) also showing the lesion (arrow). K, kidney; P, pancreas.

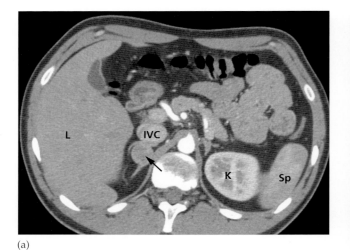

(a)

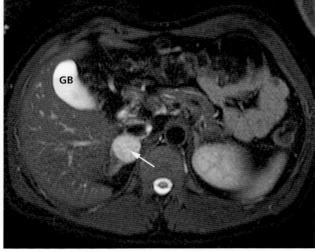

(b)

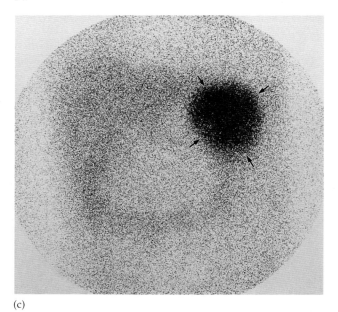

(c)

Fig. 8.16 Phaeochromocytoma. (a) CT scan showing a phaeochromocytoma (arrow) arising in the medial limb of the right adrenal gland. The inferior vena cava, IVC, lies anteriorly. K, kidney; Sp, spleen; L, liver. (b) T2-weighted MRI with fat saturation showing the same phaeochromocytoma as (a) (arrow). GB, gall bladder. (c) Radio-iodine-labelled MIBG scan of a phaeochromocytoma (arrows) in the left adrenal gland.

a diagnosis of a benign cortical adenoma may be made with a high specificity (Fig. 8.17).

Metastases to the adrenal gland are relatively common and may be bilateral (Fig. 8.18). Many different tumours metastasize to the adrenal glands; it is a particular feature of lung carcinoma, and therefore the adrenals are included in CT scans of the chest in patients being staged for bronchial carcinoma.

Non-functioning adenomas larger than 3 cm are very rare, and, therefore, larger adrenal masses in adults are likely to be metastases or, rarely, primary adrenal carcinoma. The malignant adrenal tumour of early childhood is *neuroblastoma*.

Adrenal abscesses and haemorrhage are usually bilateral and are indistinguishable from one another at CT and ultrasound. The clinical features usually suggest the correct diagnosis.

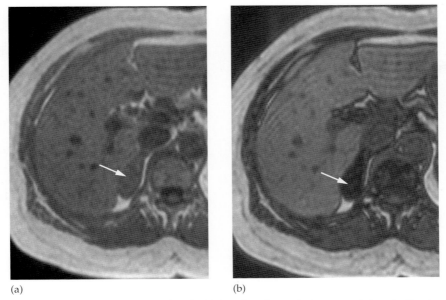

(a)　　　　　　　　　　　　　　　　(b)

Fig 8.17 Adrenal cortical adenoma shown by chemical shift MRI. (a) An adrenal mass is demonstrated on the 'in-phase' image (arrow). (b) There is a marked drop in the signal intensity of the adrenal mass on the 'out-of-phase' image, confirming a benign cortical adenoma (arrow).

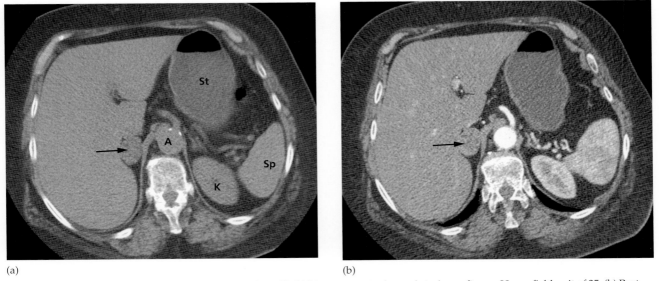

(a)　　　　　　　　　　　　　　　　(b)

Fig. 8.18 CT scan showing a right adrenal metastasis (arrow). (a) Non-contrast enhanced study confirms a Hounsfield unit of 35. (b) Post contrast enhancement characteristics confirmed the presence of a non-adenomatous lesion. K, kidney; A, aorta; Sp, spleen; St, stomach.

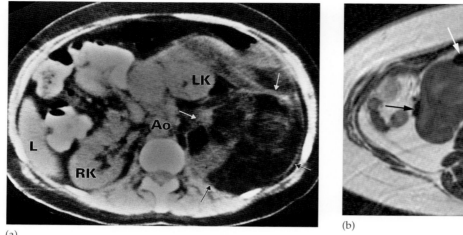

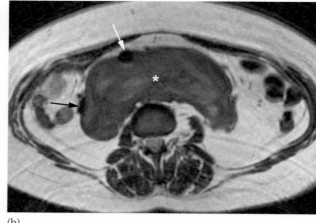

(a)

(b)

Fig. 8.19 Retroperitoneal tumours. (a) Liposarcoma. CT scan showing large partially fatty tumour (arrows) displacing the left kidney forward. The right kidney is normal in position. Ao, aorta; L, liver; LK, left kidney; RK, right kidney. (b) T2-weighted MRI demonstrates an intermediate signal intensity mass arising in the retroperitoneum (*), which is displacing the aorta and inferior vena cava (arrows). A CT-guided percutaneous biopsy confirmed a benign ganglioneuroma.

Retroperitoneal tumours

The term retroperitoneal tumour covers tumours arising primarily in retroperitoneal muscles, fat or connective tissue, the commonest being liposarcoma and fibrosarcoma. All these tumours appear as masses on CT, ultrasound or MRI. Sometimes, the edge of the mass is well defined, but sometimes there is invasion of the adjacent tissue. A lipo-sarcoma (Fig. 8.19a) almost always contains significant amounts of recognizable fat interspersed between strands or masses of soft-tissue density; a combination that permits a specific diagnosis to be made at CT. Tumours of neural origin may also arise in the retroperitoneum (Fig. 8.19b). It is usually not possible to determine the histological nature of the tumour by imaging, unless the mass contains significant amounts of fat.

Aortic aneurysm

Abdominal aortic aneurysms are readily diagnosed at ultra-sound, CT and MRI, although MRI is rarely used for this purpose (Fig. 8.20). Ultrasound is being used increasingly as a screening examination to find asymptomatic aortic aneurysms in older men.

Both CT and ultrasound allow the true maximum diam-eter of the aneurysm to be measured and to identify sepa-rately the wall and any lining thrombus. It is also relatively easy to see any retroperitoneal bleeding from an aneurysm at CT. It is generally held that aneurysms of greater than 5.5 or 6 cm in diameter are in serious danger of rupture, whether or not the patient has had any demonstrable ret-roperitoneal bleeding. Contrast-enhanced CT angiography with reformats in the coronal and sagittal CT planes are often used to plan treatment (Fig. 8.20c).

Aortic aneurysms may also be recognizable on plain films of the abdomen (p. 128), but only if substantial calcification is present in the wall.

Retroperitoneal haematoma

Retroperitoneal bleeding is usually due to trauma or to bleeding from an aortic aneurysm (Fig. 8.21). It is occasion-ally spontaneous in patients with bleeding disorders or in those on anti-coagulant therapy.

The diagnosis is made by CT (Figs 8.21 and 8.22) or MRI, which show a retroperitoneal mass with the characteristics of haematoma.

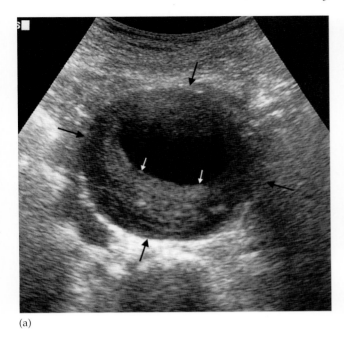

(a)

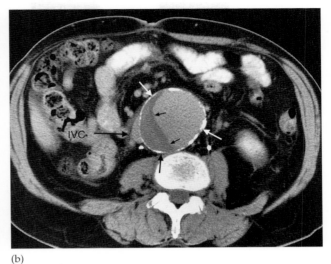

(b)

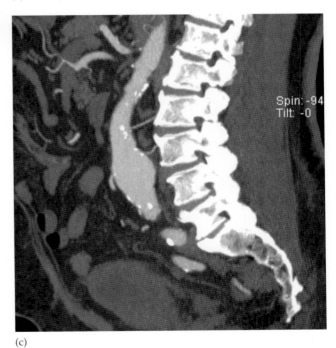

Fig. 8.20 Abdominal aortic aneurysm. (a) Ultrasound. Transverse scan showing a blood clot lining the wall (small white arrows) within the aneurysm (large black arrows). (b) CT scan with intravenous contrast enhancement. A 7 cm aneurysm (arrows) with a lower density blood clot (small black arrows) lining the wall. The wall shows patches of calcification. The inferior vena cava (IVC) is displaced by the aneurysm. (c) CT angiography of aorta. This sagittal reformat demonstrates a 3.5 cm fusiform aortic aneurysm (arrow).

(c)

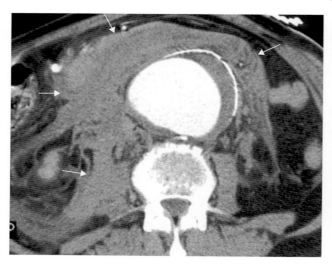

Fig. 8.21 CT scan of a leaking abdominal aortic aneurysm showing the aneurysm and the haemorrhage in the adjacent retroperitoneum (arrows).

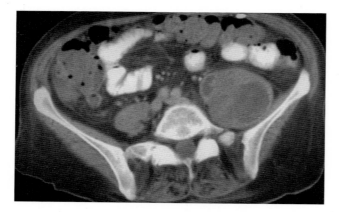

Fig. 8.22 CT scan of a large haematoma in the left iliopsoas muscle. Note the variable density, much of which is of lower density than the normal muscles.

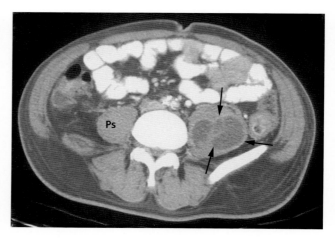

Fig. 8.23 Psoas abscess. CT scan showing left psoas abscess (arrows). Note the thick wall, which has a rim of enhancement, and low density fluid-like contents. Ps, normal right psoas muscle.

Retroperitoneal and psoas abscesses

Retroperitoneal and psoas abscesses are usually due to spread of infection from the appendix, colon, kidney, pancreas or spine. They are often found close to the organ of origin.

Retroperitoneal abscesses have many similar features to tumours and haematomas at both CT and ultrasound (Fig. 8.23). Usually, however, there is evidence of a fluid centre and there may be gas within the abscess. The wall of the abscess may enhance with contrast medium, a feature that is also seen with neoplasms.

9

Bones

Imaging techniques

Plain bone radiographs

Even with the introduction of the newer imaging modalities the plain radiograph is a very important investigation in many types of bone disease. It is helpful to understand the anatomical terms used to describe a normal long bone. These are shown in Fig. 9.1.

The radiological responses of bone to pathological process are limited; thus, similar x-ray signs occur in widely different conditions. It should be noted that it takes time for the various signs to develop; for example, in adults, it takes several weeks for a periosteal reaction to be visible after trauma and, in a child with osteomyelitis, the clinical features are present from 7 to 10 days before the first sign is visible on the radiograph. In general, the signs take longer to develop in adults than they do in children.

The signs of bone disease are:
• *Decrease in bone density*, which may be focal or generalized. Focal reduction in density is usually referred to as a 'lytic area' or an area of 'bone destruction'. When generalized, decrease in bone density is best referred to as 'osteo-

penia' until a specific diagnosis such as osteomalacia or osteoporosis can be made.
• *Increase in bone density (sclerosis)*, which may also be focal or generalized.
• *Periosteal reaction.* The periosteum is not normally visible on a radiograph. The term 'periosteal reaction' refers to excess bone produced by the periosteum, which occurs in response to such conditions as neoplasm, inflammation or trauma. Several patterns of periosteal reaction are seen (Fig. 9.2), but they do not correlate with specific diagnoses. At the edge of a very active periosteal reaction there may be a cuff of new bone known as a Codman's triangle (Fig. 9.2d). Although often seen in highly malignant primary bone tumours, e.g. osteosarcoma, a Codman's triangle is also found in other aggressive conditions.
• *Cortical thickening* also involves the laying down of new bone by the periosteum (Fig. 9.3), but here the process is very slow. The result is that the new bone, although it may be thick and irregular, shows the same homogeneous density as does the normal cortex. There are no separate lines or spicules of calcification as seen in a periosteal reaction. The causes are many, including chronic osteomyelitis, healed trauma, response to chronic stress or benign neoplasm. The feature common to all these conditions is that the process is either very slowly progressive or has healed.
• *Alteration in trabecular pattern* is a complex response usually involving a reduction in the number of trabeculae with an alteration in the remaining trabeculae, e.g. in osteo-

Diagnostic Imaging, 6th Edition. By Peter Armstrong, Martin Wastie and Andrea Rockall. Published 2009 by Blackwell Publishing. ISBN: 978-1-4051-7039.

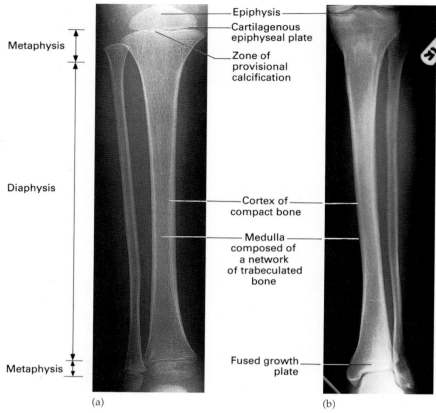

Metaphysis

Diaphysis

Metaphysis

Epiphysis
Cartilagenous epiphyseal plate
Zone of provisional calcification

Cortex of compact bone
Medulla composed of a network of trabeculated bone

Fused growth plate

(a)   (b)

Fig. 9.1 Normal long bones in (a) child and (b) adult. Increase in length takes place at the cartilagenous epiphyseal plate. In the growing child, calcification of cartilage occurs at the interface between the radiolucent growing cartilage and the bone to give the zone of provisional calcification, which is seen as a dense white line forming the ends of the shaft and surrounding the bony epiphyses. This calcified cartilage becomes converted to bone. (If there is temporary cessation of growth then the zone of provisional calcification may persist as a thin white line, known as a 'growth line', extending across the shaft of the bone.) As the child grows older the epiphyseal plate becomes thinner until, eventually, there is bony fusion of the epiphysis with the shaft.

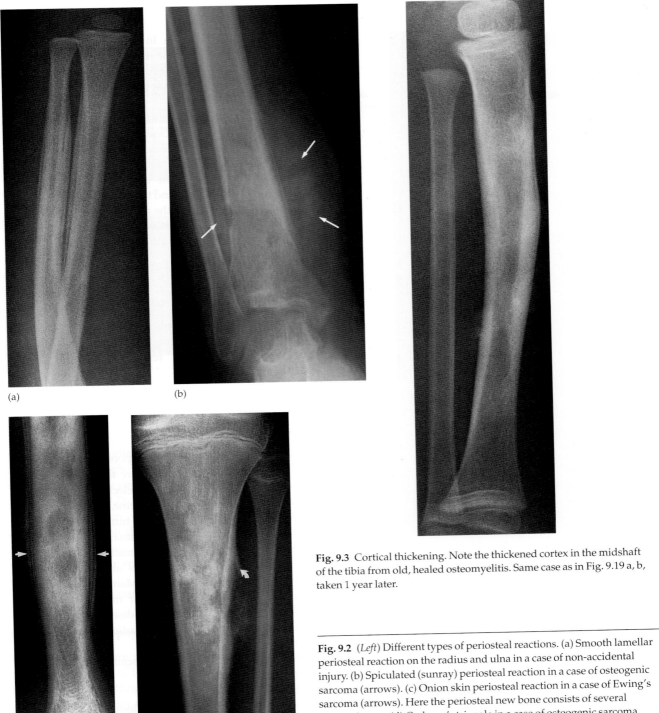

(a)

(b)

(c)

(d)

Fig. 9.3 Cortical thickening. Note the thickened cortex in the midshaft of the tibia from old, healed osteomyelitis. Same case as in Fig. 9.19 a, b, taken 1 year later.

Fig. 9.2 (*Left*) Different types of periosteal reactions. (a) Smooth lamellar periosteal reaction on the radius and ulna in a case of non-accidental injury. (b) Spiculated (sunray) periosteal reaction in a case of osteogenic sarcoma (arrows). (c) Onion skin periosteal reaction in a case of Ewing's sarcoma (arrows). Here the periosteal new bone consists of several distinct layers. (d) Codman's triangle in a case of osteogenic sarcoma. At the edge of the lesion the periosteal new bone is lifted up to form a cuff (arrow).

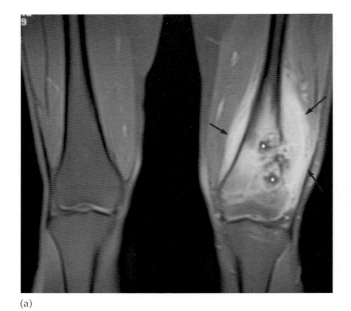

(a)

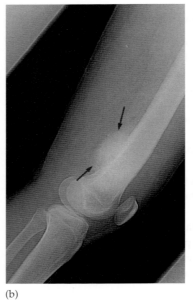

(b)

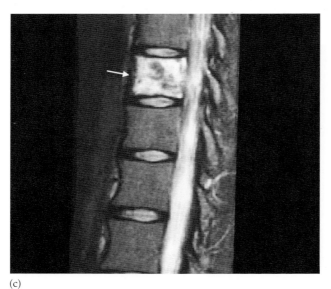

(c)

Fig. 9.9 Magnetic resonance imaging of bone tumours.
(a) T1-weighted post contrast scan of osteosarcoma in the lower
shaft and metaphysis of the left femur. The extent of tumour
(arrows) within the bone and the soft tissue extension are both very
well shown. The low signal in the medulla (*) is due to the calcified
osteogenic component of the tumour. The true extent of the tumour
cannot be assessed from the plain film (b), although the plain film
provides a more specific diagnosis, because the bone formation
within the soft tissue extension (arrows) is obvious.
(c) T2-weighted scan of lymphoma in the T10 vertebral body
(arrow). The very high signal of the neoplastic tissue is evident
even though there is no deformity of shape of the vertebral body.

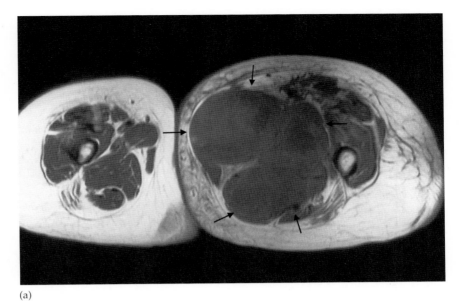

(a)

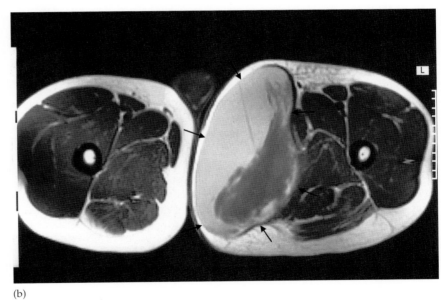

(b)

Fig. 9.10 Magnetic resonance imaging of soft tissue masses. (a) Soft tissue sarcoma producing an obvious soft tissue mass (arrows) in the medial compartment of the left thigh. (b) Large haematoma (arrows) in the medial compartment of the left thigh showing mixed signal, including the characteristic high signal of recent haemorrhage on T1-weighted sequence. (Both scans are T1-weighted.)

BONE DISEASES

When considering the diagnosis and differential diagnosis of bone diseases, it is convenient to divide disorders into those that:

- cause solitary lytic or sclerotic lesions
- produce multiple focal lesions, i.e. several discrete lytic or sclerotic lesions in one or more bones
- cause generalized lesions where all the bones show diffuse increase or decrease in bone density
- alter the trabecular pattern or change its shape.

Solitary lesions (fractures are dealt with separately in Chapter 12)

Solitary areas of lysis, sclerosis or a combination of the two, are usually one of the following:

- bone tumours
  - (a) malignant (primary or secondary)
  - (b) benign
- osteomyelitis
- bone cysts, fibrous dysplasia or other non-neoplastic defects of bone
- conditions of uncertain nature such as Langerhans histiocytosis and osteoid osteoma.

Primary malignant bone tumours and osteomyelitis are usually accompanied by periosteal reaction. Pathological fractures may be seen through benign and malignant bone tumours and through bone cysts.

The radiological diagnosis of a localized bone lesion can be a problem. Some conditions are readily diagnosed but, in others, even establishing which broad category of disease is present can be difficult. The initial radiological decision is usually to try and decide whether the lesion is benign, i.e. stable or very slow growing, or whether it is aggressive, i.e. a malignant tumour or an infection. It is also important to know the age of the patient, as certain lesions tend to occur in a specific age range.

The features to look for on plain radiographs and CT when trying to decide the nature of a localized bone lesion are:

1 *Zone of transition.* The edge of any lytic or sclerotic lesion should be examined carefully to see whether it is well demarcated or whether there is a wide zone of transition between the normal and the abnormal bone. There are

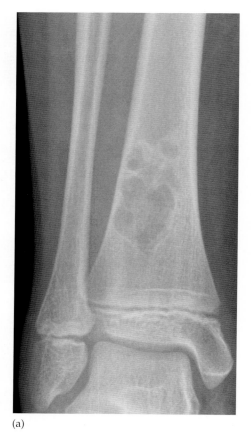

(a)

Fig. 9.11 The localized lesion. (a) A well-defined sclerotic edge indicating a benign lesion – a fibrous cortical defect. (b) Bone island. There is a small, well-defined area of compact bone in the neck of the femur (arrow). This common finding is without significance. (c) An ill-defined edge – in this case a metastasis; this type of bone destruction is known as permeative. (d) A well-defined edge – a metastasis in the shaft of the femur. (e) Destruction of the cortex indicating an aggressive lesion – another metastasis. *(f–h on p. 298)* (f) Expansion of the cortex – fibrous dysplasia. (g) Periosteal reaction (arrow) – osteomyelitis. (h) Containing calcium (arrow) – a cartilage tumour, in this case a chondrosarcoma.

two extremes: a lesion with a well-defined sclerotic edge is almost certainly benign, e.g. a fibrous cortical defect (Fig. 9.11a) or a bone island (Fig. 9.11b), whereas a lytic area with an ill-defined edge is likely to be aggressive. Aggressive lesions are fast-acting ones and include both tumour and infection (Fig. 9.11c). In the middle of this spectrum lies

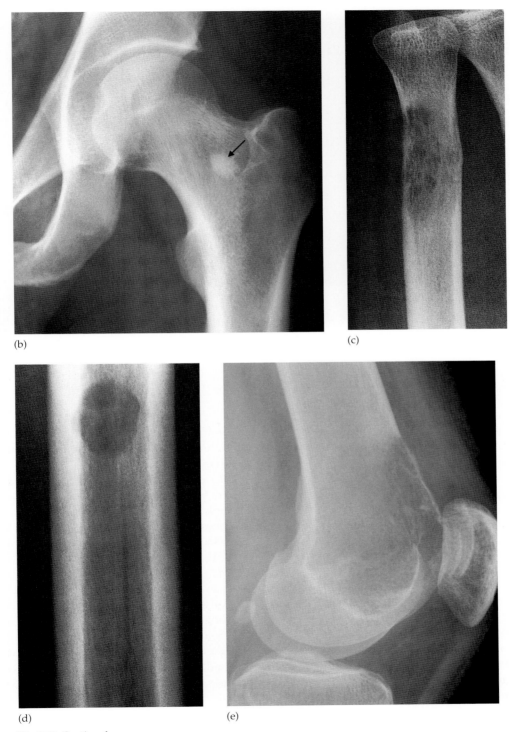

(b)

(c)

(d)

(e)

Fig. 9.11 *Continued*

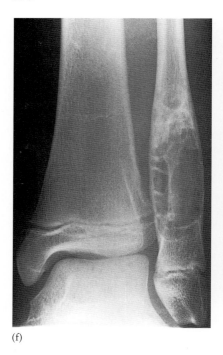

(f)

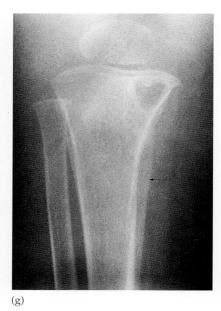

(g)

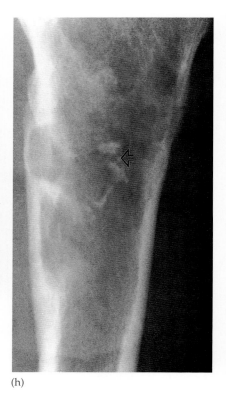

(h)

Fig. 9.11 *Continued*

the lytic area with no sclerotic rim, which may be a benign or malignant lesion. Metastases and myeloma (Fig. 9.11d) are a frequent cause of this pattern.

2 *The adjacent cortex.* Any destruction of the adjacent cortex indicates an aggressive lesion such as a malignant tumour or osteomyelitis (Fig. 9.11e).

3 *Expansion.* Bone expansion with an intact well-formed cortex usually indicates a slow-growing lesion such as an enchondroma or fibrous dysplasia (Fig. 9.11f).

4 *Periosteal reaction.* The presence of an active periosteal reaction in the absence of trauma usually indicates an aggressive lesion (Fig. 9.11g). The causes of localized periosteal reactions adjacent to a lytic or sclerotic lesion are:

- osteomyelitis
- malignant bone tumour, particularly Ewing's sarcoma and osteosarcoma
- occasionally metastasis, particularly neuroblastoma
- Langerhans histiocytosis.

A periosteal reaction is also a feature of trauma to a bone, but trauma while it causes fracture does not cause focal bone destruction.

5 *Calcific densities within the lesion.* Calcification within an area of bone destruction occurs in specific conditions; for example, patchy calcification of a popcorn type usually indicates a cartilage tumour (Fig. 9.11h), whereas diffuse ill-defined calcification suggests osteoid formation and indicates an osteosarcoma.

6 *Soft tissue swelling.* The presence of a soft tissue mass suggests an aggressive lesion; the better defined it is, the more likely it is that the lesion is a neoplasm. Ill-defined soft tissue swelling adjacent to a focal destructive lesion suggests infection. Sometimes a tumour arising primarily in the soft tissues may destroy bone by pressure erosion or direct invasion.

7 *Site.* The site of a lesion is important as certain lesions tend to occur at certain sites; for example, osteomyelitis characteristically occurs in the metaphyseal areas, particularly of the knee and lower tibia, whereas giant cell tumours are subarticular in position.

Bone tumours

The precise diagnosis of a bone tumour can be notoriously difficult both for the radiologist and the pathologist. Accurate histological diagnosis is essential for all malignant lesions and it is important to realize that separate portions of a tumour may show different histological appearances. In general, plain film radiography is the best imaging technique for making a diagnosis, whereas MRI or CT often show the full extent of a tumour to advantage and show the effects on surrounding structures and the relationship to the neurovascular bundle. The main role for radionuclide bone scanning is to diagnose metastatic bone disease. Metastatic malignant tumours are by far the commonest bone neoplasm, outnumbering many times primary malignant tumours. They are discussed on p. 306.

Primary malignant tumours

On plain films, primary malignant tumours usually have poorly defined margins, often with a wide zone of transition between the normal and abnormal bone. The lesion may destroy the cortex of the bone. A periosteal reaction is often present and a soft tissue mass may be seen.

Radionuclide bone scans show substantially increased activity in the lesion.

MRI is the most accurate technique for showing the local extent of the tumour with the additional advantage that images may be produced in the coronal and sagittal planes. Extension into both the medullary cavity and the soft tissues can be accurately defined, as can the relationship to important nerves and blood vessels. MRI provides this information better than CT.

Osteosarcoma (osteogenic sarcoma) (Fig. 9.9) occurs mainly in the 5–20-year-old age group, but is also seen in the elderly following malignant change in Paget's disease. The tumour often arises in a metaphysis, most commonly around the knee. There is usually bone destruction with new bone formation, and typically a florid spiculated periosteal reaction is present, the so-called sunray appearance (see Fig. 9.2b). The tumour may elevate the periosteum to form a Codman's triangle (see Fig. 9.2d, p. 289).

Chondrosarcoma occurs mainly in the 30–50-year-old age group, most commonly in the pelvic bones, scapulae, humeri and femora. A chondrosarcoma produces a lytic expanding lesion containing flecks of calcium, a sign that indicates its origin from cartilage cells. It can be difficult to distinguish from its benign counterpart, the enchondroma, but a chondrosarcoma is usually less well defined in at least one portion of its outline and it may show a periosteal reaction (Fig. 9.11h). Pelvic chondrosarcomas often have large extraosseus components best seen with CT or MRI (Fig. 9.12). A chondrosarcoma may arise from malignant degeneration of a benign cartilagenous tumour.

Fibrosarcoma and malignant fibrous histiocytoma are rare bone tumours with similar histological and radiological features. They most often present in young and middle-aged adults, usually around the knee. The feature on plain radiographs is an ill-defined area of lysis with periosteal reaction. Frequently the cortex is breached. There are no imaging features that distinguish these tumours from metastases or lymphoma.

Ewing's sarcoma is a highly malignant tumour, commonest in children, arising in the shaft of long bones. It produces ill-defined bone destruction with periosteal reaction that is typically 'onion skin' in type (see Fig. 9.2c, p. 289).

Giant cell tumour has features of both malignant and benign tumours. It is locally invasive but rarely metastasizes. It occurs most commonly around the knee and at the wrist after the epiphyses have fused. It is an expanding destructive lesion, which is subarticular in position (Fig. 9.13). The margin is fairly well defined but the cortex is thin and may in places be completely destroyed.

Primary lymphoma of bone is rare; most osseous malignant lymphoma is associated with generalized lymph node disease. When solitary primary lymphomas are encountered they may produce sclerotic bone lesions or they may cause destruction of bone, indistinguishable on imaging grounds from fibrosarcoma/malignant fibrous histiocytoma.

Benign tumours and tumour-like conditions

Included under this heading are benign tumours such as enchondroma, certain benign conditions similar to tumours, such as fibrous dysplasia, and some abnormalities which are difficult to classify, such as osteoid osteoma and Langerhans histiocytosis. Some of these lesions are discussed

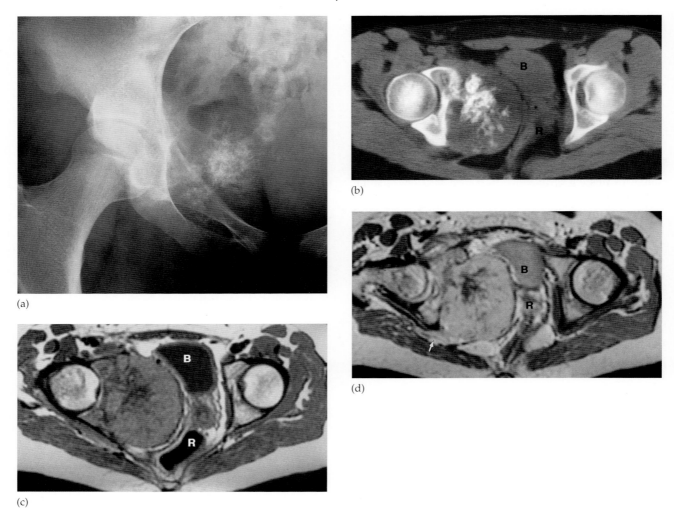

Fig. 9.12 Chondrosarcoma. (a) Plain film shows a large mass containing calcification arising from the pubic ramus. (b) CT shows the large mass containing calcium. There is also displacement of the bladder (B) and rectum (R). (c) Axial MRI scan at the same level. Note that the calcification gives no signal. (d) MRI scan at a lower level showing the tumour extending into the gluteal muscles (arrow).

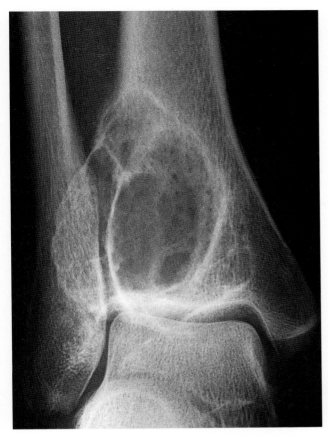

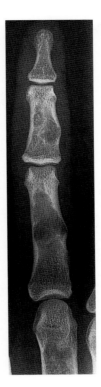

Fig. 9.14 Enchondromas in the metacarpal, proximal and middle phalanges showing lytic areas that expand but do not breach the cortex.

Fig. 9.13 Giant cell tumour. Eccentric expanding lytic lesion which has thinned the cortex crossed by strands of bone. The subarticular position is characteristic of this tumour.

below. In general, benign lesions have an edge which is well demarcated from the normal bone by a sclerotic rim. They cause expansion but rarely breach the cortex. There is no soft tissue mass and a periosteal reaction is unusual unless there has been a fracture through the lesion.

Radionuclide scans in benign tumours usually show little or no increase in activity, provided no fracture has occurred. CT and MRI scanning are infrequently needed in the evaluation of benign tumours.

Enchondromas are seen as lytic expanding lesions most commonly in the bones of the hand (Fig. 9.14). They often contain a few flecks of calcium and frequently present as a pathological fracture.

Fibrous cortical defects (non-ossifying fibromas) are common chance findings in children and young adults. They produce well-defined lucent areas in the cortex of long bones (Fig. 9.11a, p. 296).

Fibrous dysplasia may affect one or several bones. It occurs most commonly in the long bones and ribs as a lucent area with a well-defined edge and may expand the bone (Fig. 9.11f, p. 298). There may be a sclerotic rim around the lesion.

A *simple bone cyst* has a wall of fibrous tissue and is filled with fluid. It occurs in children and young adults, most commonly in the humerus and femur. Bone cysts form a lucency across the width of the shaft of the bone, with a well-defined edge. The cortex may be thin and the bone expanded (Fig. 9.15). Often, the first clinical feature is a pathological fracture.

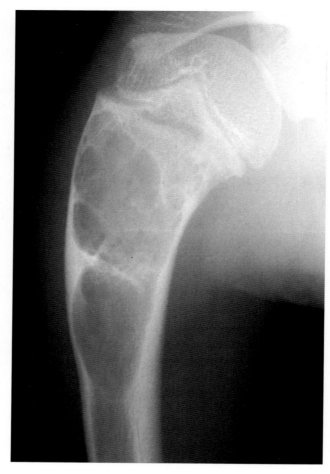

Fig. 9.15 Bone cyst. There is an expanding lesion crossed by strands of bone in the upper end of the humerus in a child. The lesion extends to, but does not cross, the epiphyseal plate.

Aneurysmal bone cysts are not true neoplasms, but they probably form secondarily to an underlying primary tumour. Mostly they are seen in children and young adults in the spine, long bones or pelvis. These lesions are purely lytic and cause massive expansion of the cortex, hence the name 'aneurysmal'. They may grow quickly and appear very aggressive but are, nevertheless, benign lesions. Computed tomography and MRI may show the blood pools within the cyst. The major differential diagnosis is from giant-cell tumour.

An *osteoid osteoma* is a painful condition found most commonly in the femur and tibia in young adults. It has a characteristic radiological appearance: a small lucency, sometimes with central specks of calcification, known as a nidus, surrounded by dense sclerotic rim. A periosteal reaction may also be present (Fig. 9.16). Computed tomography shows these features to advantage and osteoid osteomas can also be shown by MRI. An important imaging investigation is radionuclide bone scanning, which shows marked focal increased activity. Radionuclide bone scanning is par-

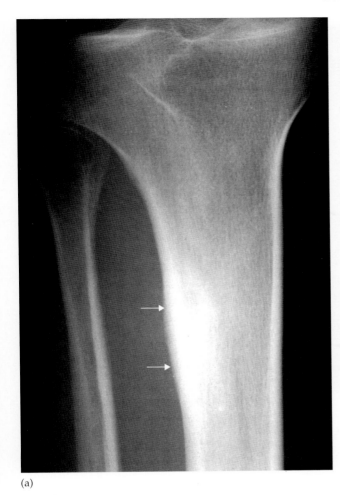

(a)

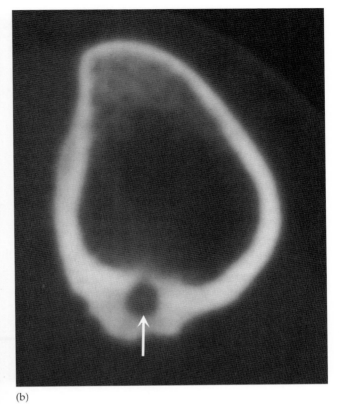

(b)

Fig. 9.16 Osteoid osteoma. (a) Plain film showing an area of sclerosis at the upper end of the tibia (arrows). (b) CT scan shows the sclerosis with a central lucency known as a nidus (arrow).

ticularly useful when the osteoid osteoma is difficult to see on plain film (see Fig. 9.6, p. 291) and is helpful in locating the tumour during surgery by using a small probe which detects gamma rays.

An *osteoma* is a benign tumour consisting of dense bone (Fig. 9.17). They may occur in the paranasal sinuses.

Eosinophil granuloma is the mildest and most frequent form of Langerhans histiocytosis (previously referred to as histiocytosis X). It occurs in children and young adults and produces lytic lesions which may be single or multiple, most frequently in the skull, pelvis, femur and ribs. Extensive

lesions may be seen giving rise to the so-called geographic skull (see Fig. 13.3, p. 400). Long bone lesions show bone destruction which may be ill defined having the features of an aggressive lesion, or well defined and may have a sclerotic rim. A periosteal reaction is sometimes seen.

Osteomyelitis

Osteomyelitis is most often caused by *Staphylococcus aureus* and usually affects infants and children. The initial radiographs are normal as bone changes are not visible until

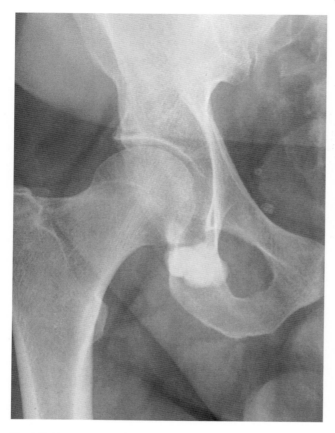

Fig 9.17 Osteoma. A well-defined area of dense cortical bone is present below the right acetabulum.

pool) images reflecting hyperaemia and on the delayed bone phase images. Ultrasound can demonstrate subperiosteal collections of pus well before bone changes are evident on plain film. Magnetic resonance imaging is the imaging investigation of choice and shows evidence of bone oedema and pus accumulation in the bone and soft tissues (Fig. 9.20).

In chronic osteomyelitis, the bone becomes thickened and sclerotic with loss of differentiation between the cortex and the medulla. Within the bone there may be sequestra and areas of bone destruction. This type of lesion is known as a Brodie's abscess (see Fig. 9.19d, p. 305). Computed tomography can be used in selected cases to show sequestra and sinus tracks. Magnetic resonance imaging may be useful in assessing activity by identifying medullary inflammation.

Tuberculous osteomyelitis is a particular problem in African and Asian populations and is being seen with increased frequency in patients with AIDS. The spine is the most frequent site of infection, followed by the large joints, but any bone may be affected. The disease is relatively indolent and produces large areas of bone destruction which, unlike pyogenic osteomyelitis, may be relatively asymptomatic in the early stages.

Distinction of neoplasm from osteomyelitis

It is not always possible using imaging tests to distinguish osteomyelitis from a bone tumour and biopsy is then needed. The clinical history is clearly important. With malignant bone tumours, the radiographs are usually abnormal when the patient first presents, whereas with osteomyelitis the initial films are often normal. But if early films are not available, difficulties may arise in distinguishing acute osteomyelitis from a highly malignant tumour such as Ewing's sarcoma or osteosarcoma. Chronic osteomyelitis may simulate a benign bone tumour on imaging examinations, but the presence of fever, and sometimes of discharging sinuses, usually helps to diagnose an infective lesion. Computed tomography and magnetic resonance imaging are more informative because they show the lesion better, but even with these imaging modalities there can be considerable difficulty deciding between infection and neoplasm.

The ^{99m}Tc bone scan is positive in both osteomyelitis and malignant tumours and cannot be used in differentiation.

10–14 days after the onset of the infection, but the ^{99m}Tc radionuclide bone scan and MRI show changes much earlier in the course of the disease within a day or two (Fig. 9.18).

Typically, acute osteomyelitis affects the metaphysis of a long bone, usually the femur or tibia. The earliest signs on plain radiographs are soft tissue swelling and bone destruction in the metaphysis, with a periosteal reaction that eventually may become very extensive and surround the bone to form an involucrum (Fig. 9.19b). A part of the original bone may die and form a separate dense fragment known as a sequestrum (Fig. 9.19c). A radionuclide bone scan will show increased activity both on the early (blood

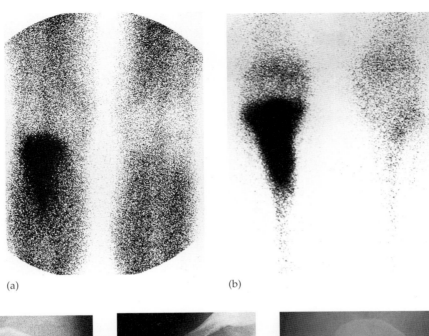

Fig. 9.18 Osteomyelitis. Radionuclide scans of knees. (a) The blood pool scan taken 1 minute after injection of radionuclide shows increased uptake in the upper part of the leg due to hyperaemia. (b) The delayed scan taken 3 hours later shows substantially increased uptake in the bone itself.

(a)

(b)

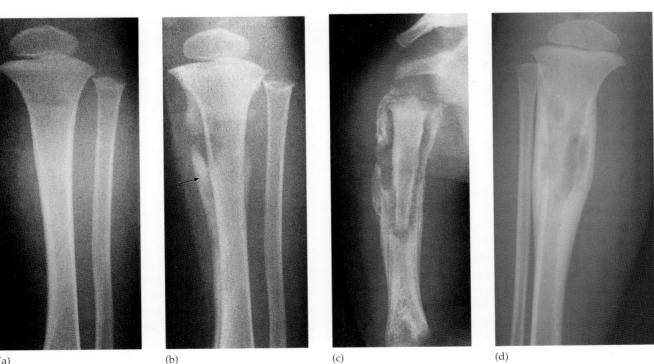

(a) (b) (c) (d)

Fig. 9.19 Osteomyelitis. (a) Initial films reveal no abnormality. (b) Films taken 3 weeks later show some destruction of the upper end of the tibia and an extensive periosteal reaction along the tibia, particularly the medial side (arrow). (c) Late acute osteomyelitis in another young child. The upper part of the humerus has separated to form a sequestrum. It is surrounded by an extensive periosteal reaction to form an involucrum. (d) Chronic osteomyelitis (Brodie's abscess) showing a lucency in the tibia surrounded by substantial sclerosis.

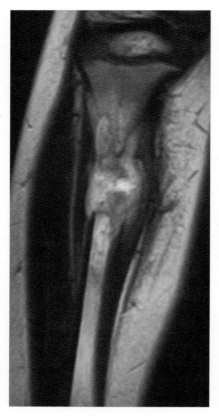

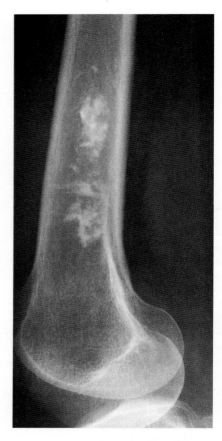

Fig. 9.20 Osteomyelitis. T2-weighted magnetic resonance imaging scan showing high signal in the medulla of the tibia extending into the cortex and soft tissues (same patient as Fig. 9.19d).

Fig. 9.21 Bone infarct. There is calcification in the medulla of the lower end of the femur.

Bone infarction

Bone infarction occurs most often in the intra-articular portions of the bones and is therefore described in the chapter on joint disease (p. 333). However, infarcts can occur in the shaft of a bone in several diseases including caisson disease, sickle cell disease or following radiation therapy. Sometimes, they are found incidentally in older people with no known cause. In the acute phase no abnormality is visible, other than a very occasional periosteal reaction. Once healed, they appear as irregular calcification in the medulla of a long bone (Fig. 9.21).

Multiple focal lesions

Metastases

Metastases are by far the commonest malignant bone tumour, outnumbering many times primary tumours. Metastases may be sclerotic, lytic or a mixture of lysis and sclerosis. Those bones containing red marrow are the ones most frequently affected, namely the spine, skull, ribs, pelvis, humeri and femora.

Many tumours metastasize to bone but lytic metastases in adults most commonly arise from a carcinoma of the breast and bronchus, less commonly from carcinoma of the thyroid,

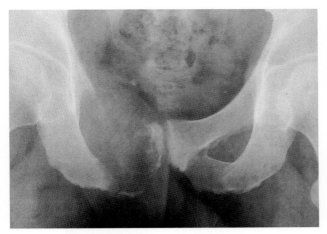

Fig. 9.22 Metastasis from a carcinoma of the kidney causing a large area of bone destruction with an ill-defined edge in the right superior and inferior pubic rami.

kidney or colon and in children from neuroblastoma or leukaemia. Lytic metastases give rise to well-defined or ill-defined areas of bone destruction without a sclerotic rim. The lesions vary from small holes to large areas of bone destruction (Fig. 9.22). In the long bones, metastases usually arise in the medulla and as they grow they enlarge and destroy the cortex. Metastases and myeloma are virtually the only causes of multiple obvious lytic lesions in bone.

Sclerotic metastases appear as ill-defined areas of increased density of varying size with ill-defined margins. In men, they are most commonly due to metastases from carcinoma of the prostate (Fig. 9.23), and in women from carcinoma of the breast. Metastases with bone expansion occur in primary tumours of the kidney and thyroid.

Mixed lytic and sclerotic metastases are not uncommon. They are often seen with carcinoma of the breast (Fig. 9.24).

A periosteal reaction is uncommon with metastases, except in neuroblastoma (Fig. 9.25).

A radionuclide bone scan is much more sensitive for detecting metastases than plain films. Not only are more lesions detected, but it is also an easier examination for the patient than a radiographic skeletal survey, which involves taking numerous films. Approximately 30% of metastases seen on a bone scan will not be visible on plain films. Increased radionuclide uptake in a patient with a known primary tumour but normal bone radiographs suggests

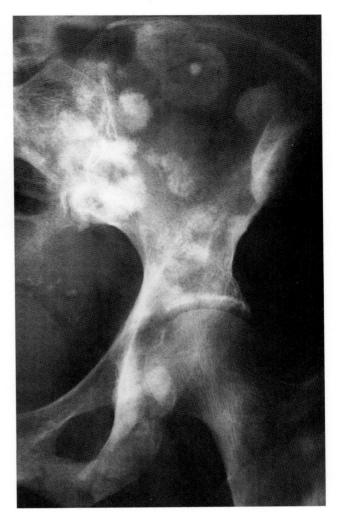

Fig. 9.23 Sclerotic metastases showing scattered areas of increased density.

metastases. If numerous areas of increased activity are seen in a patient with a known primary carcinoma, then the diagnosis of metastases is virtually certain (Fig. 9.26). If only one or a few areas of increased activity are present, radiographs will be needed to exclude the possibility of a benign condition such as degenerative change or fracture being responsible for the increased uptake of the radionuclide. If the bone scan is normal, it is most unlikely that radiographs will show metastases.

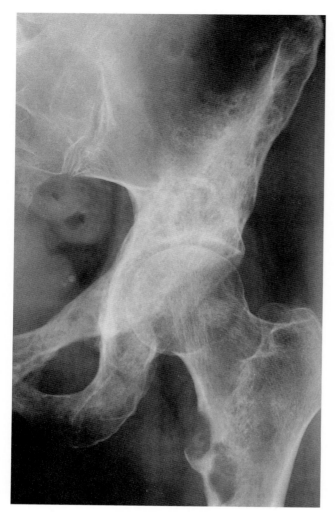

Fig. 9.24 Multiple metastases from carcinoma of the breast showing both lytic and sclerotic areas.

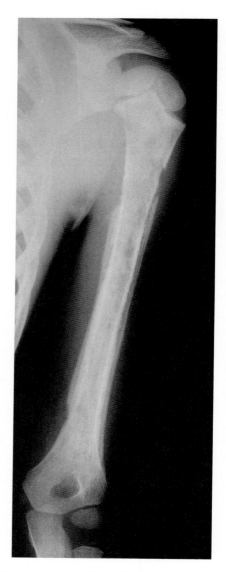

Fig. 9.25 Neuroblastoma. In this child's humerus there are several lytic areas and a florid periosteal reaction.

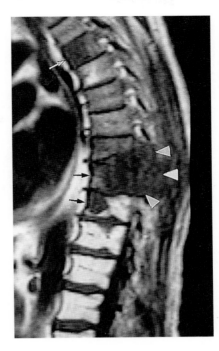

Fig. 9.27 Metastases from carcinoma of the prostate. Sagittal MRI scan showing low signal intensity in several vertebral bodies (arrows). Note the metastases also involve the posterior elements of two adjacent vertebrae (arrow heads).

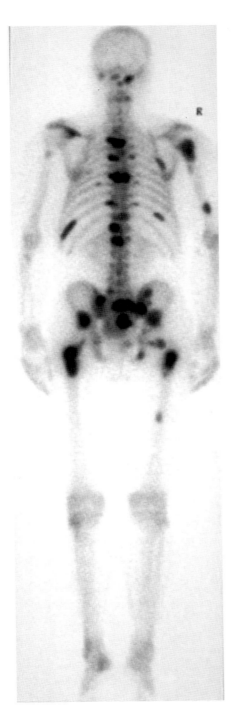

Fig. 9.26 Metastases. Radionuclide bone scan showing numerous discrete areas of increased uptake in the bones in a patient with carcinoma of the prostate.

Magnetic resonance imaging is better than radionuclide scanning for the detection of metastases and shows more metastases, but it is more difficult to survey the whole skeleton with MRI but with modern scanners the whole of the spine can readily be imaged. MRI has an important role to play when the bone scan is normal or equivocal in the face of strong clinical suspicion of metastases. MRI is used if there is a possibility of metastases causing spinal cord compression because it will show both the bone metastases and its effect on the spinal cord (Fig. 9.27). CT is less sensitive than MRI for detecting metastases. However, CT can readily demonstrate lytic and sclerotic metastases and images should be reviewed on bone windows on all staging scans (Fig. 9.28).

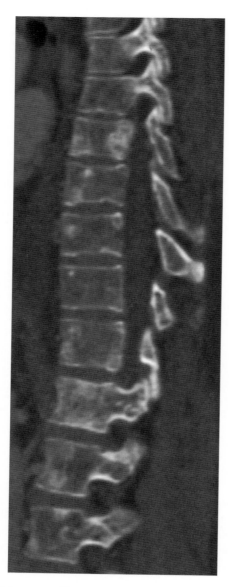

Fig. 9.28 Metastases. CT scan sagittal reconstruction in a staging scan for a patient with carcinoma of the breast showing multiple mixed, but mainly sclerotic, metastases in the thoracic and lumbar spine.

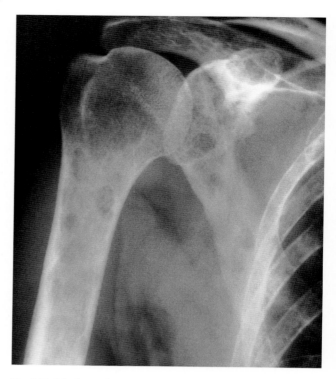

Fig. 9.29 Myeloma deposits causing multiple well-defined lytic lesions.

Multiple myeloma

Although myeloma deposits may be found in any bone, they are most frequently seen in bones with active haemopoiesis. The bone lesions may resemble lytic metastases in every way (Fig. 9.29), but are often better defined and may cause expansion of the bone. Diffuse marrow involvement may give rise to generalized loss of bone density, producing a picture similar to that of osteoporosis.

Most myeloma deposits show increased activity on radionuclide bone scans. In some instances, however, even large areas of bone destruction, which are clearly visible on plain radiographs, show no abnormality on the scan. Nevertheless, it is rare for all the lesions in a particular patient to be invisible, so bone scanning is still used for survey purposes, with radiographic skeletal surveys held in reserve. The role of MRI for detecting metastases applies also to multiple myeloma.

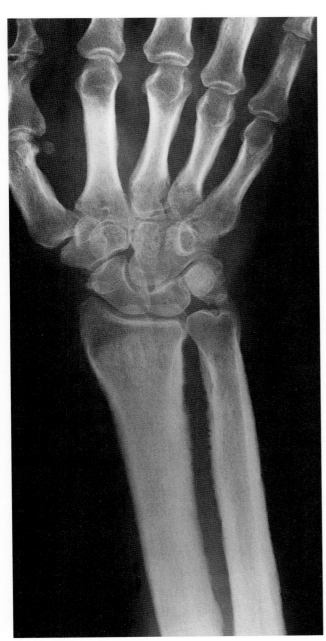

Fig. 9.30 Hypertrophic pulmonary osteoarthropathy. There is a periosteal reaction which is present bilaterally along the shafts of the radius and ulna and the metacarpals. In this case, it was associated with a bronchial carcinoma.

Lymphoma and leukaemia

Malignant lymphoma involving bone may give rise to lesions closely resembling metastases on all imaging modalities (Fig. 9.9c, p. 294).

Bone involvement in acute leukaemia in children is not uncommon. Leukaemic deposits produce ill-defined permeative bone destruction, mostly in the metaphyseal regions. Bone lesions are very rare in adult leukaemias.

Multiple periosteal reactions

Multiple periosteal reactions are seen in conjunction with other signs in:
- non-accidental injury
- widespread bone infection, e.g. congenital syphilis, neonates with infected intravenous catheters
- venous stasis and ulceration of the legs, where low-grade periosteal reaction and cortical thickening of the tibia and fibula may be encountered
- hypertrophic pulmonary osteoarthropathy. In this condition, there is widespread periosteal reaction around the bones of the forearms and lower legs which, when severe, extends to involve the hands and feet (Fig. 9.30). Finger clubbing is invariably present. Hypertrophic pulmonary osteoarthropathy is seen in a number of conditions, mostly intrathoracic, of which carcinoma of the bronchus is by far the commonest
- scurvy.

Generalized decrease in bone density (osteopenia)

The radiographic density of bone is dependent on the amount of calcium present in the bones. Calcium content may be reduced due to a disorder of calcium metabolism, as in osteomalacia or hyperparathyroidism, or to a reduction in protein matrix, as in osteoporosis. The radiological diagnosis of decreased bone density is often difficult, especially as the appearances of the bones are markedly affected by radiographic exposure factors.

The main causes of generalized decrease in bone density are:
- osteoporosis
- osteomalacia

- hyperparathyroidism
- multiple myeloma, which may cause generalized loss of bone density, with or without focal bone destruction.

Each of these conditions may have other radiological features that enable the diagnosis to be made, but when they are lacking, as they frequently are in osteoporosis and osteomalacia, it becomes very difficult to distinguish between them radiologically.

Osteoporosis

Osteoporosis is the consequence of a deficiency of protein matrix (osteoid). The remaining bone is normally mineralized and appears normal histologically, but because the matrix is reduced in quantity there is necessarily a reduction in calcium content. Osteoporosis predisposes to fractures, particularly of the vertebral bodies and hips.

The more frequent causes of osteoporosis are:
- idiopathic, often subdivided according to age of onset, e.g. juvenile, postmenopausal, senile. Postmenopausal and senile osteoporosis are the commonest forms: up to 50% of women over 60 years of age have osteoporosis
- Cushing's disease and steroid therapy
- disuse.

A radiological diagnosis of osteoporosis is only made after other diseases have been excluded. Bone destruction, which could indicate metastatic carcinoma or myeloma, and evidence of hyperparathyroidism and osteomalacia should be sought, because these conditions can closely resemble osteoporosis.

The changes of osteoporosis are best seen in the spine (Fig. 9.31). Although there is an overall decrease in bone density, the cortex stands out clearly as if pencilled in. An important feature is collapse of the vertebral bodies, representing compression fractures, which result in the vertebral bodies appearing wedged or biconcave. Several vertebrae may be involved and the disc spaces often appear widened.

The long bones have thin cortices. Many of the trabeculae are resorbed but those that remain stand out clearly.

Disuse osteoporosis can be caused by localized pain or immobilization of a fracture (Fig. 9.32). Besides a reduction in density and thinning of the cortex, the bone may sometimes have a spotty appearance (Fig. 9.32c).

Reflex sympathetic dystrophy syndrome (Sudeck's atrophy) is a disorder of the sympathetic nervous system comprising

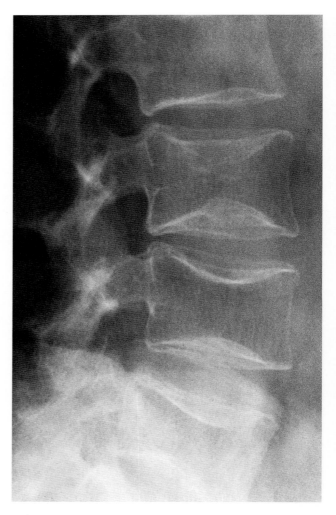

Fig. 9.31 Senile osteoporosis. There is decreased bone density but the edge of the vertebral bodies are well demarcated. Note the partial collapse of several of the vertebral bodies and the widening of the disc spaces.

severe osteoporosis and oedema of the soft tissues following a fracture. The degree of osteoporosis is disproportionate to the trauma or the degree of disuse.

Screening for osteoporosis

Because osteoporosis is such a prevalent problem and, once established, is difficult to treat, attempts have been made to

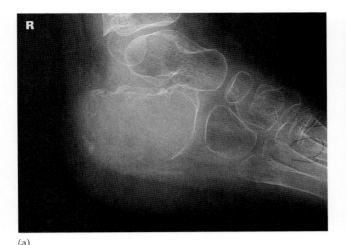

(a)

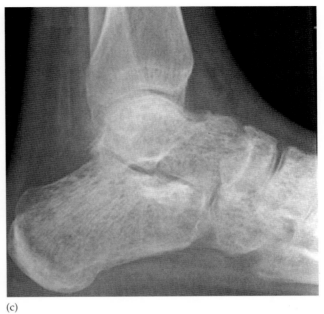

(c)

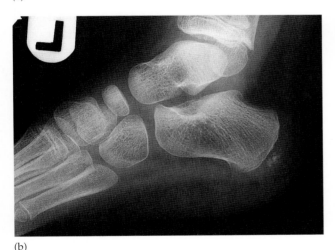

(b)

Fig. 9.32 (a) Disuse osteoporosis due to osteomyelitis of the right calcaneum. The calcaneum is partly destroyed by infection. The remaining bones of the right foot show a marked reduction in bone density with well-defined cortex. Compare these bones with those in the normal left foot (b). (c) In this patient with paraplegia the osteoporosis has a spotty appearance.

develop screening tests for the at-risk population in order to institute preventive treatment, e.g. hormone replacement therapy. Bone mass is usually measured by dual energy x-ray absorption, often abbreviated to DEXA. Bone mineral density is expressed as a T score, which is the number of standard deviations above or below the mean for a young healthy adult population. Osteoporosis is defined as a T score ≤ -2.5. Although bone density can be accurately and reproducibly measured, bone mineral density is a poor predictor of an individual's fracture risk and it has not been possible to use bone densitometry to select patients for preventive therapy on a population-wide basis.

Rickets and osteomalacia

In these conditions there is poor mineralization of osteoid. If this occurs before epiphyseal closure, the condition is known as rickets – in adults the condition is known as osteomalacia.

The main causes of rickets and osteomalacia are:
• Dietary deficiency of vitamin D, or lack of exposure to sunlight, resulting in decreased production of endogenous vitamin D.
• Malabsorption, resulting in impaired absorption of calcium or vitamin D.

• Renal disease, where rickets develops despite normal amounts of vitamin D in the diet, hence the term 'vitamin D-resistant rickets':

  tubular defects: hypophosphataemia, Fanconi syndrome and renal tubular acidosis

  chronic renal failure: impaired ability to activate vitamin D.

Regardless of the cause of the osteomalacia or rickets, the bone changes are similar. When it is due to chronic renal failure, the changes of hyperparathyroidism may also be present.

In *rickets* the changes are maximal where bone growth is occurring, so they are best seen at the knees, wrists and

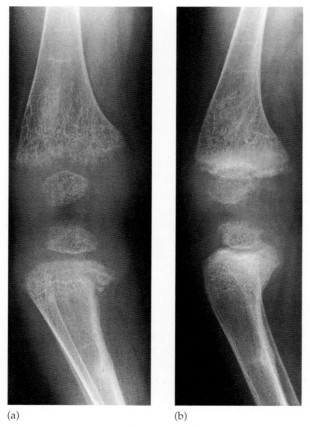

(a)   (b)

Fig. 9.33 (a) Rickets. Dietary rickets showing widening and irregular mineralization of the metaphyses which have a frayed appearance. There is reduced bone density and bowing of the limbs. (b) After commencement of vitamin D treatment, mineralization of the metaphyses has occurred.

ankles. The zone of provisional calcification is deficient and the metaphyses are irregularly mineralized, widened and cupped (Fig. 9.33). This results in an increased distance between the visible epiphysis and the calcified portion of the metaphysis. The generalized decrease in bone density, however, may not be very obvious. Deformities of the bones occur because the undermineralized bone is soft. Greenstick fractures are common.

In *osteomalacia* the characteristic features are loss of bone density, thinning of the trabeculae and the cortex, and Looser's zones (pseudofractures) (Fig. 9.34a). Looser's zones are short lucent bands running through the cortex at right-angles, usually going only part way across the bone thought to be insufficiency fractures. They may have a sclerotic margin making them more obvious. They are commonest in the scapulae, medial aspects of the femoral necks and in the pubic rami.

Bone deformity, consequent upon bone softening, is an important feature. In the spine, the vertebral bodies are biconcave (Fig. 9.34b), the femora may be bowed and in severe cases the side walls of the pelvis may bend inwards, giving the so-called triradiate pelvis.

Hyperparathyroidism

Excess parathyroid hormone secretion mobilizes calcium from the bones, resulting in a decrease in bone density.

Hyperparathyroidism may be primary, from hyperplasia or a tumour of the parathyroid glands, or secondary to chronic renal failure (see next section on Renal osteodystrophy).

Many patients with primary hyperparathyroidism present with renal stones and only a small minority have bone changes radiologically.

The signs of hyperparathyroidism in the bones are:
• A generalized loss of bone density, with loss of the differentiation between cortex and medulla. The trabecular pattern may have a fine lacework appearance. With advanced disease there may be marked deformity of the skeleton.
• The hallmark of hyperparathyroidism is subperiosteal bone resorption (Fig. 9.35a), which occurs particularly in the hands on the radial side of the middle phalanges and at the tips of the terminal phalanges. There may also be resorption of the outer ends of the clavicles.

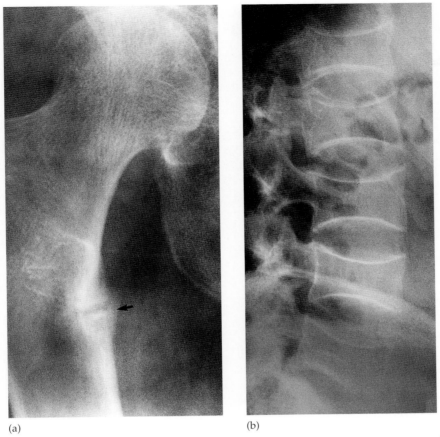

(a)   (b)

Fig. 9.34 Osteomalacia. (a) Looser's zone showing the horizontal lucent band with sclerotic margins running through the cortex of the medial side of the upper femur (arrow). (b) There is decreased bone density and partial collapse of all the vertebral bodies to approximately the same extent.

• Soft tissue calcification, vascular calcification and chondrocalcinosis sometimes occur.

• Brown tumours are occasionally present. These are lytic lesions, which may be single or multiple. They are of varying size and may expand the bone. They occur most commonly in the mandible and pelvis but any bone may be involved (Fig. 9.35b).

The bone changes in primary and secondary hyperparathyroidism are similar except that 'brown tumours' are much rarer and vascular calcification is commoner in secondary hyperparathyroidism.

Renal osteodystrophy

Three distinct bone lesions can occur, often together, in patients with chronic renal failure:

• osteomalacia in adults; rickets in children
• hyperparathyroidism
• sclerosis, an infrequent feature. It may be seen in the spine as bands across the upper and lower ends of the vertebral bodies, giving the so-called rugger jersey spine (Fig. 9.36) or at the metaphyses of the long bones.

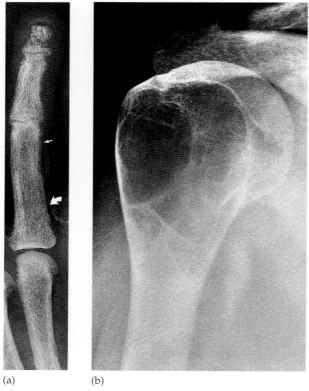

(a)   (b)

Fig. 9.35 Hyperparathyroidism. (a) Note the characteristic features of subperiosteal bone resorption (straight arrow), resorption of the tip of the terminal phalanx and the altered bone architecture. Arterial calcification is also present (curved arrow). (b) Brown tumour. There is a lytic area in the upper end of the humerus with a well-defined edge.

Generalized increase in bone density

Several conditions can cause a generalized increase in bone density, including:

• *Sclerotic metastases* are by far the commonest cause, particularly from prostatic or breast carcinoma. These may affect the skeleton diffusely (Fig. 9.37).

• *Osteopetrosis* (*marble bone disease*). In this congenital disorder of bone formation the bones are densely sclerotic (Fig. 9.38). The bones are brittle and may fracture readily, but if fractured they heal easily.

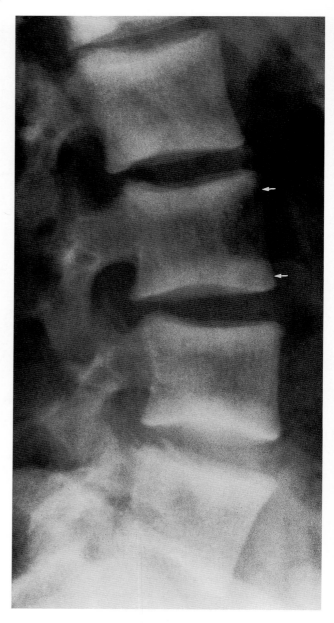

Fig. 9.36 Rugger jersey spine (renal osteodystrophy). There are sclerotic bands running across the upper and lower ends of the vertebral bodies of the lumbar spine (arrows).

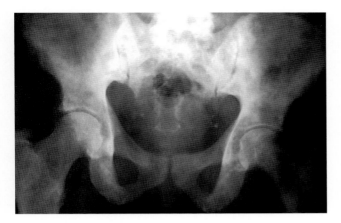

Fig. 9.37 Metastases from carcinoma of the prostate causing a widespread increase in bone density.

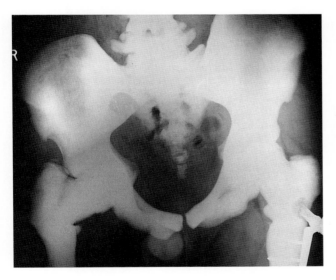

Fig. 9.38 Osteopetrosis. There is a marked generalized increased bone density affecting all bones. There are multiple healed fractures, with a pin and plate in the left femur.

• *Myelosclerosis* is a form of myelofibrosis in which, in addition to the replacement of bone marrow by fibrous tissue, the process extends to lay down extratrabecular bone, usually in a rather patchy fashion (Fig. 9.39). The spleen is invariably enlarged because it becomes the site of haemopoiesis. It may reach a very large size and forms an important sign on abdominal radiographs.

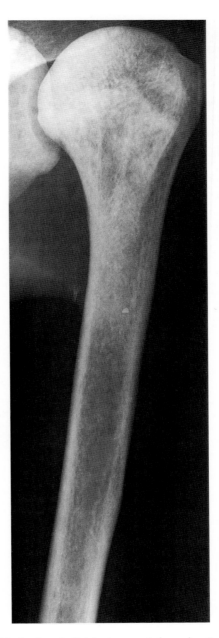

Fig. 9.39 Myelosclerosis. Patchy increase in bone density in the humerus is seen. In this condition the bone marrow becomes replaced with bone.

Alteration of trabecular pattern and change in shape

Paget's disease

The incidence of Paget's disease varies greatly from country to country, being common in the UK but rare in the USA and Asia. It is usually a chance finding in an elderly patient. One or more bones may be affected, the usual sites being the pelvis, spine, skull and long bones. Bone softening causes bowing and deformity of the bones and pathological fractures may also occur (see Fig. 12.54, p. 396).

Although there is a rare lytic form of Paget's disease, e.g. osteoporosis circumscripta of the skull, the cardinal features are thickening of the trabeculae and of the cortex, leading to loss of corticomedullary differentiation and increased bone density, together with enlargement of the affected bone (Fig. 9.40).

In the skull there are many circumscribed areas of sclerosis scattered in the skull vault, giving a mottled appearance which has been likened to cotton wool. An increased thickness of the calvarium is a particularly obvious feature.

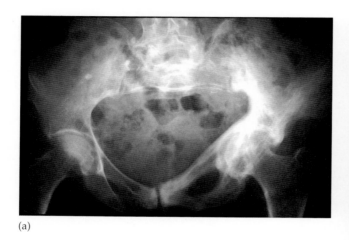

(a)

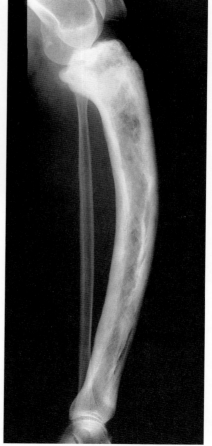

(b)

Fig. 9.40 (a) Paget's disease showing typical sclerosis with coarse trabeculae in the left side of the pelvis. Note that the width of the affected bones is increased. The pelvis is deformed consequent upon the bone softening. (b) Similar signs in the tibia of another patient. Note the bowing of the bone from softening.

These changes of sclerosis, cortical thickening, coarse trabeculae and, most particularly, increase in the size of the bone, distinguish Paget's disease from metastases due to prostatic or breast carcinoma, which are also common in the elderly.

Malignant degeneration, with development of an osteosarcoma in abnormal bone, is an occasional occurrence (Fig. 9.41).

There is greatly increased uptake of radionuclide at bone scanning in bones involved by Paget's disease (see Fig. 1.9, p. 9), which can be useful to define the extent of disease and response to treatment. Perhaps more importantly, it should be realized that Paget's disease may mimic tumours on radionuclide bone scans as well as on plain radiographs.

Haemolytic anaemia

There are several types of haemolytic anaemia, but radiological changes are seen in two main types: thalassaemia and sickle cell disease. Both show changes of marrow hyperplasia, but sickle cell anaemia may also show evidence of bone infarction and infection.

Marrow hyperplasia

Overactivity and expansion of the bone marrow causes thinning of the cortex and resorption of some of the trabeculae so that those that remain are thickened and stand out more clearly. In the skull, there is widening of the diploë and there may be perpendicular striations giving an appearance known as 'hair-on-end' (Fig. 9.42a). The ribs may enlarge and the phalanges may become rectangular (Fig. 9.42b).

Infarction and infection

Infarction at bone ends causes flattening and sclerosis of the humeral and femoral heads.

Areas of bone destruction with periosteal new bone formation, or just a periosteal reaction, may be seen in the shafts of the bones. These signs are due to bone infarction. It is not possible to determine from the radiographs whether or not these infarcts are infected.

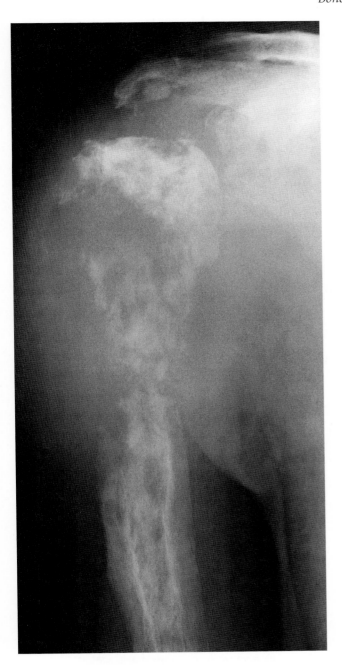

Fig. 9.41 Sarcoma in Paget's disease. There is extensive bone destruction in the humeral head and shaft. Evidence of the underlying Paget's disease can be seen.

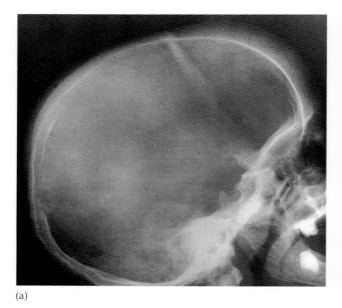

(a)

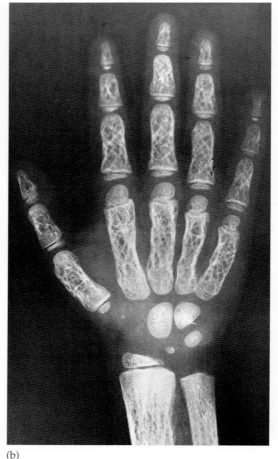

Fig. 9.42 Haemolytic anaemia – thalassaemia. (a) Skull showing thickened diploë. (b) Hand. Due to marrow expansion the bones are expanded and those trabeculae that remain are very thickened.

(b)

Sarcoidosis

Sarcoidosis occasionally involves the bones. The phalanges of the hands and feet are virtually the only bones affected. The signs are either small cysts with a well-defined edge or areas of bone destruction showing a lace-like pattern (Fig. 9.43). If the bones are involved, there is invariably evidence of sarcoidosis in the chest and sarcoid skin lesions are usually present.

Radiation-induced disease of bone

Radiotherapy may damage bones in the radiation field. Early change may be limited to osteoporosis. In severe cases the bone thins and shows patchy increased density with small lytic areas – an appearance known as osteonecrosis. Pathological fracture is a serious complication. The commonest sites are in the ribs following radiotherapy for breast cancer and in the pelvis or femora following treatment for cervical carcinoma.

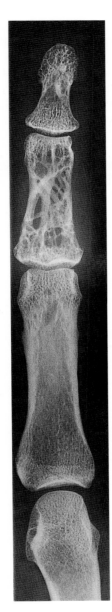

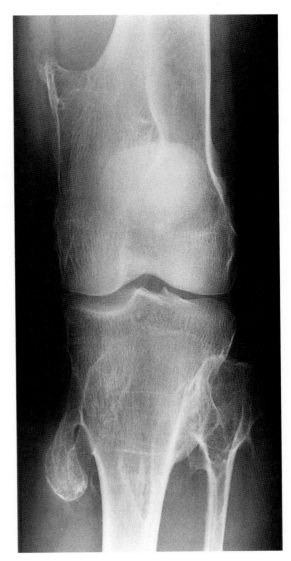

Fig. 9.44 Diaphyseal aclasia. Several bony projections (exostoses) are seen arising around the knee, directed away from the joint. The opposite knee was similarly affected.

Fig. 9.43 Sarcoidosis, showing the characteristic lace-like trabecular pattern in the middle phalanx.

Occasionally, radiation may induce sarcomatous change, usually an osteosarcoma which occurs several years after the radiation therapy.

Changes in bone shape

Bone dysplasias

Bone dysplasias are congenital disorders resulting in abnormalities in the size and shape of the bones. There are a large number of different dysplasias; many of them are hereditary and all of them are rare. Only diaphyseal aclasia will be mentioned here. Osteopetrosis has been described on p. 316.

Diaphyseal aclasia is a congenital disorder resulting in abnormalities of the size and shape of the bones. In diaphyseal aclasia (multiple exostoses), there are multiple bony projections known as osteochondromas or exostoses. They have a cartilagenous cap which may contain calcification. When osteochondromas occur on the long bones they are near the metaphyses and are directed away from the joint (Fig. 9.44).

Occasionally, a chondrosarcoma may develop in the cartilage cap. This should be suspected if there is either rapid growth, an ill-defined edge to the bone, or extensive calcification extending into the soft tissues.

10

Joints

Imaging techniques

The *plain film* examination remains important for imaging joint disease (Fig. 10.1), but magnetic resonance imaging (MRI) is being used with increasing frequency. MRI is particularly useful for:
- meniscal and ligamentous tears in the knee
- rotator cuff tears of the shoulder
- avascular necrosis of the hip
- septic arthritis.

Arthrography involves injecting contrast medium into the joint space directly and then performing an MR scan. Magnetic resonance arthrography has a role in the shoulder and wrist.

Plain film signs of joint disease

Synovial joints have articular surfaces covered by hyaline cartilage. Both articular and intra-articular cartilage (such as the menisci in the knee) are of the same radiodensity on plain films as the soft tissues, and, therefore, are not visualized as such; only the space between the adjacent articular cortices can be appreciated, which is referred to as the 'joint space' (Fig. 10.1). The synovium, synovial fluid and capsule also have the same radiodensity as the surrounding soft tissues and, unless outlined by a plane of fat, cannot be identified as discrete structures. The articular cortex forms a thin, well-defined line which merges smoothly with the remainder of the cortex of the bone.

Diagnostic Imaging, 6th Edition. By Peter Armstrong, Martin Wastie and Andrea Rockall. Published 2009 by Blackwell Publishing. ISBN: 978-1-4051-7039.

Signs indicating the presence of an arthritis

Joint space narrowing

Joint space narrowing is due to destruction of articular cartilage. It occurs in practically all forms of joint disease, except avascular necrosis.

Soft tissue swelling

Swelling of the soft tissues around a joint may be seen in any arthritis accompanied by a joint effusion and whenever periarticular inflammation is present. It is, therefore, a feature of inflammatory, and particularly infective, arthritis. Discrete soft tissue swelling around the joints can be seen in gout due to gouty tophi.

Osteoporosis

Osteoporosis of the bones adjacent to joints occurs in many painful conditions. Underuse of the bones seems to be an important mechanism, but is not the only factor. Osteoporosis is particularly severe in rheumatoid and tuberculous arthritis.

Signs that point to the cause of an arthritis

Articular erosions

An erosion is an area of destruction of the articular cortex and the adjacent trabecular bone (Fig. 10.2), usually accompanied by destruction of the articular cartilage. Erosions are

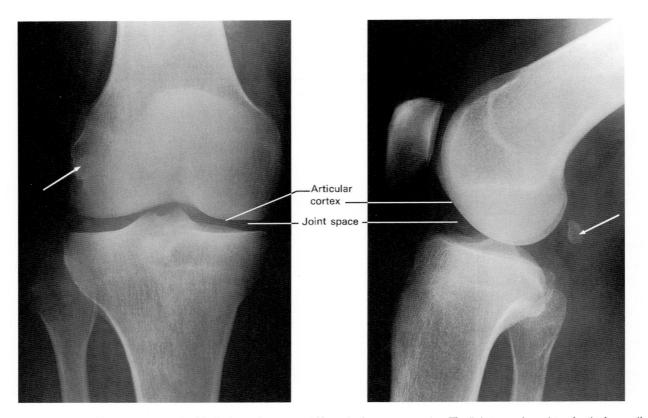

Fig. 10.1 Normal knee joint. Note the fabella (arrow), a sesamoid bone in the gastrocnemius. The 'joint space' consists of articular cartilage and synovial fluid.

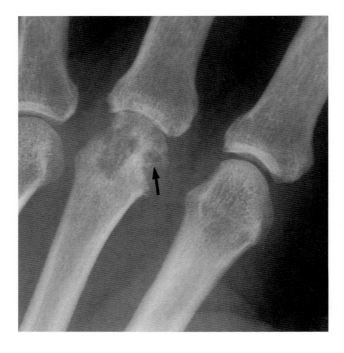

Fig. 10.2 Erosions. Areas of bone destruction are seen affecting the articular cortex of the metacarpophalangeal joint. A typical erosion is arrowed. The joint space is also narrowed.

easily recognized when seen in profile, but when viewed *en face* the appearances can be confused with a cyst. Oblique views designed to show erosions in profile are often taken.

There are several causes of erosions:

1 Inflammatory overgrowth of the synovium (pannus) which occurs in:

- rheumatoid arthritis, which is by far the commonest cause of an erosive arthropathy
- juvenile rheumatoid arthritis (Still's disease)
- psoriasis
- Reiter's disease
- ankylosing spondylitis
- tuberculosis.

2 Response to the deposition of urate crystals in gout.

3 Destruction caused by infection:

- pyogenic arthritis
- tuberculosis.

4 Synovial overgrowth caused by repeated haemorrhage in haemophilia and related bleeding disorders.

5 Neoplastic overgrowth of synovium, e.g. synovial sarcoma.

Osteophytes, subchondral sclerosis and cysts

Osteophytes, subchondral sclerosis and cysts are all features of osteoarthritis. A characteristic increase in the density of subchondral bone is seen in avascular necrosis (see p. 333).

Alteration in the shape of the joint

Several conditions lead to characteristic alterations in the shape or relationship of the bone ends, e.g. slipped epiphysis, developmental dysplasia of the hip, osteochondritis dissecans and avascular necrosis in its later stages.

Diagnosis of arthritis

When considering an arthritis it is important to have the following information:

1 *Is more than one joint involved?* Certain diseases typically involve several joints, e.g. rheumatoid arthritis, while others rarely do, e.g. infections and synovial tumours.

2 *Which joints are involved?* Many arthropathies have a predilection for certain joints and spare others:

- Rheumatoid arthritis virtually always involves the hands and feet, principally the metacarpo- and metatarsophalangeal joints, the proximal interphalangeal joints and the wrist joints. Psoriatic arthritis usually affects the terminal interphalangeal joints.
- Gout characteristically involves the metatarsophalangeal joint of the big toe.
- When osteoarthritis is seen in the hands it almost always involves the terminal interphalangeal joints and often affects the carpometacarpal joint of the thumb. In the feet, it is almost always the first metatarsophalangeal joint that is affected. In the large joints, osteoarthritis is common in the hips and knees but relatively rare in the ankle, shoulders and elbows unless there is some underlying deformity or disease.
- The distribution of neuropathic arthritis depends on the neurological deficit; for example, diabetes affects the ankles and feet, whereas syringomyelia affects the shoulders, elbows and hands.

3 *Is a known disease present?* Sometimes an arthritis is part of a known disease, e.g. haemophilia or diabetes.

Rheumatoid arthritis

Rheumatoid arthritis is a polyarthritis caused by inflammatory overgrowth of synovium known as pannus.

The earliest change is periarticular soft tissue swelling and osteoporosis. This osteoporosis is believed to be due to a combination of disuse and synovial hyperaemia. Destruction of the articular cartilage by pannus leads to joint space narrowing. Further destruction leads to small bony erosions which occur, initially, at the joint margins (Fig. 10.3). These erosions are often seen first around the metatarso- or metacarpophalangeal joints, proximal interphalangeal joints and on the styloid process of the ulna. Later, extensive erosions may disrupt the joint surfaces. Ulnar deviation is usually present at this stage. With very severe destruction, the condition is referred to as arthritis mutilans (Fig. 10.4).

Similar changes are seen in the large joints (Fig. 10.5). In such cases, osteoarthritis may be superimposed on the rheumatoid arthritis and may dominate the picture.

With severe disease, there may be subluxation at the atlantoaxial joint (Fig. 10.6) due to laxity of the transverse ligament which holds the odontoid peg against the

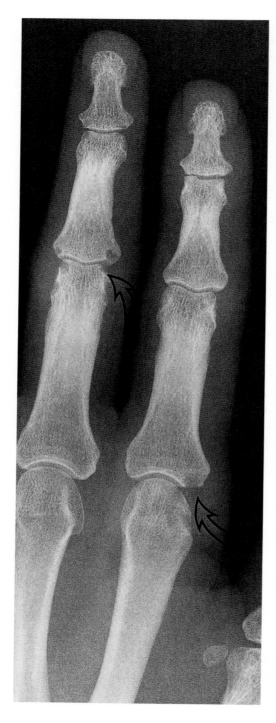

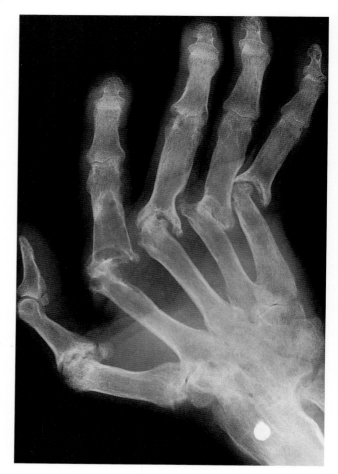

Fig. 10.4 Advanced rheumatoid arthritis (arthritis mutilans). There is extensive destruction of the articular cortex of the metacarpophalangeal joints with ulnar deviation of the fingers. Fusion of the carpal bones and wrist joint has occurred.

Fig. 10.3 (*Left*) Early rheumatoid arthritis. Small erosions are present in the articular cortex (arrows) and there is soft tissue swelling around the proximal interphalangeal joints.

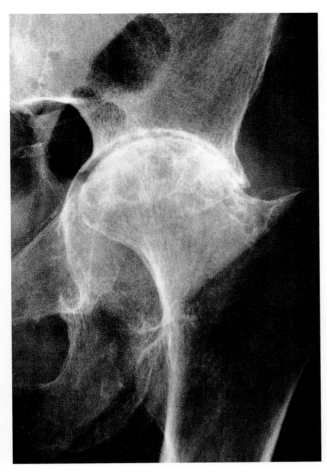

Fig. 10.5 Rheumatoid arthritis. Uniform loss of joint space is seen in this hip joint. Sclerosis is also present due to associated osteoarthritis.

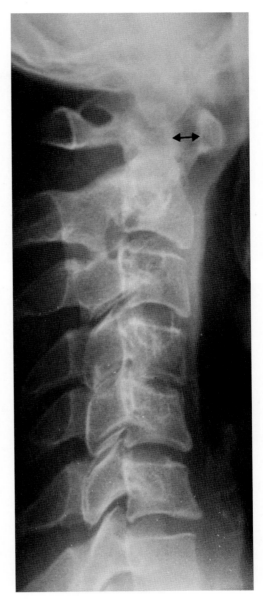

Fig. 10.6 Rheumatoid arthritis – atlantoaxial subluxation. C1 is displaced anteriorly upon C2. The distance between the arch of the atlas and the odontoid peg (arrow) is increased from the normal value (2 mm) to 8 mm. (This is the same patient whose hand is illustrated in Fig. 10.4.)

anterior arch of the atlas. Atlantoaxial subluxation may only be demonstrable in a film taken with the neck flexed. Even though it is frequently asymptomatic, there is always the possibility of neurological symptoms from compression of the spinal cord by the odontoid process and it is important to be aware of its existence if the patient is to have a general anaesthetic. Atlantoaxial instability can be well demonstrated with MRI.

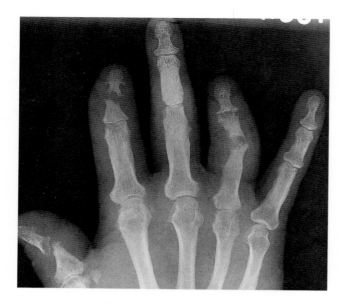

Fig. 10.7 Psoriatic arthropathy. There are extensive erosive changes affecting the interphalangeal joints but sparing the metacarpophalangeal joints.

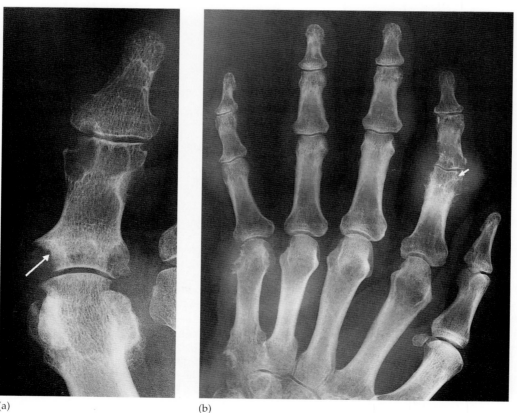

(a)

(b)

Fig. 10.8 Gout. (a) Erosion: there is a typical well-defined erosion with an overhanging edge (arrow) at the metatarsophalangeal joint of the big toe. (b) Tophi: these are the large soft tissue swellings. A good example is seen around the proximal interphalangeal joint of the index finger. Several erosions are present (one of these is arrowed).

Role of radiology in rheumatoid arthritis

Radiographs assist in the diagnosis of doubtful cases. To this end, the detection of erosions is extremely helpful. A widespread erosive arthropathy is almost diagnostic of rheumatoid arthritis. Radiographs are also useful in assessing the extent of the disease and in observing the response to treatment.

Other erosive arthropathies

A number of other arthropathies, such as juvenile rheumatoid arthritis and the HLA-B27 spondyloarthropathies, which include psoriasis and Reiter's disease, produce articular erosions.

Juvenile rheumatoid arthritis (Still's disease; juvenile chronic polyarthritis) shows many features similar to rheumatoid arthritis but erosions are less prominent. The knee, ankle and wrist are the joints most commonly affected. Hyperaemia from joint inflammation causes epiphyseal enlargement and premature fusion.

In *psoriasis*, there is an erosive arthropathy with predominant involvement of the terminal interphalangeal joints (Fig. 10.7).

Gout

In gout, the deposition of urate crystals in the joint and in the adjacent bone gives rise to an arthritis which most commonly affects the metatarsophalangeal joint of the big toe.

The earliest change is soft tissue swelling. At a later stage, erosions occur that, unlike rheumatoid arthritis, may be at a distance from the articular cortex. These erosions have a well-defined, often sclerotic, edge and frequently have overhanging edges (Fig. 10.8a). They are due to urate deposits in the bone. These deposits may be very large, causing extensive bony destruction. There is usually no osteoporosis.

Localized soft tissue lumps caused by collections of sodium urate, known as tophi, may occur in the periarticular tissues (Fig. 10.8b). These swellings can be large and occasionally show calcification.

Joint infection

Joint infection is most often due to pyogenic bacterial infection or tuberculosis. Usually only one joint is affected.

Synovial biopsy or examination of the joint fluid is necessary in order to identify the infecting organism.

Pyogenic arthritis

In pyogenic arthritis, which is usually due to *Staphylococcus aureus*, there is rapid destruction of the articular cartilage followed by destruction of the subchondral bone and a soft tissue swelling around the joint may be visible (Fig. 10.9). A pyogenic arthritis may occasionally be due to spread of osteomyelitis from the metaphysis into the adjacent joint. A joint effusion is the earliest finding which can readily be detected with ultrasound, which can also be used to guide aspiration of the fluid. If the diagnosis is still in doubt then MRI is often performed.

Tuberculous arthritis

An early pathological change is the formation of pannus, which explains why tuberculous arthritis may be radiologically indistinguishable from rheumatoid arthritis. The hip and knee are the most commonly affected peripheral joints. The features to look for are joint space narrowing and erosions, which may lead to extensive destruction of the articular cortex. A very important sign is a striking osteoporosis, which may be seen before any destructive changes are visible (Fig. 10.10).

At a late stage there may be gross disorganization of the joint with calcified debris near the joint.

Haemophilia and bleeding disorders

In haemophilia and Christmas disease, repeated haemorrhages into the joints result in soft tissue swelling, erosions and cysts in the subchondral bone. The epiphyses may enlarge and fuse prematurely (Fig. 10.11).

Osteoarthritis

Osteoarthritis is the commonest form of arthritis. It is due to degenerative changes resulting from wear and tear of the articular cartilage. The hip and the knee are frequently involved but, despite being a weight-bearing joint, the ankle is infrequently affected. The wrist, joints of the hand and the metatarsophalangeal joint of the big toe are also frequently involved.

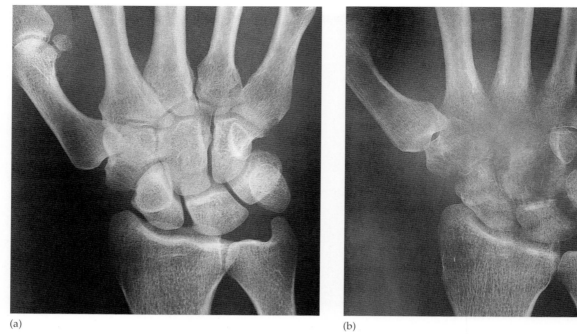

(a)

(b)

Fig. 10.9 Pyogenic arthritis. (a) Initial film of the wrist was normal. (b) Film taken 3 weeks later shows destruction of the carpal bones and bases of the metacarpals.

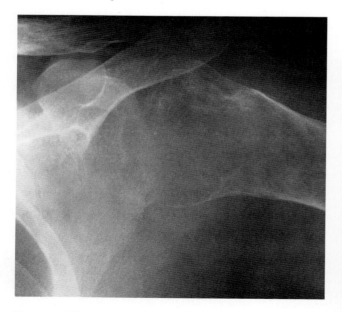

Fig. 10.10 Tuberculous arthritis of the shoulder. Note the striking osteoporosis and erosion of the humeral head.

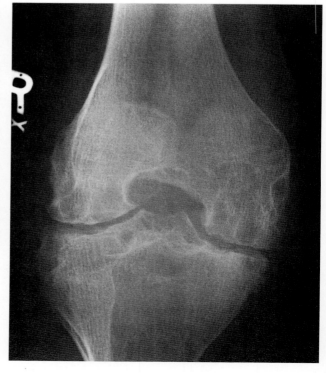

Fig. 10.11 Haemophilia. Subchondral cysts have formed caused by repeated haemorrhages into the joint. Note the soft tissue swelling around the joint and the deep intercondylar notch – a characteristic feature of haemophilia.

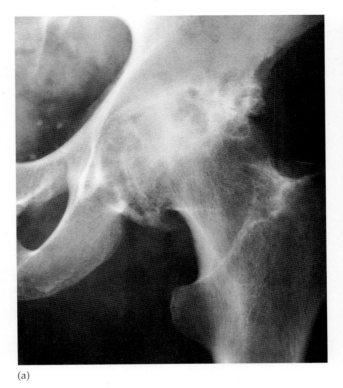
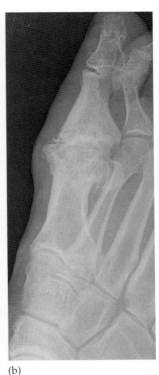

Fig. 10.12 Advanced osteoarthritis. (a) Note the narrowed superior part of the joint space of the hip, subchondral sclerosis and cyst formation and osteophytes. (b) Similar changes are seen in the metatarsophalangeal joint of the big toe, which is known as hallux rigidus.

(a)

(b)

In osteoarthritis, a number of features can usually be seen (Fig. 10.12):

• *Joint space narrowing.* The loss of joint space is maximal in the weight-bearing portion of the joint; for example, in the hip it is often maximal in the superior part of the joint, whereas in the knee it is the medial compartment that usually narrows the most. Even when the joint space is very narrow it is usually possible to trace out the articular cortex.

• *Osteophytes* are bony spurs, often quite large, which occur at the articular margins.

• *Subchondral sclerosis* usually occurs on both sides of the joint; it is often worse on one side.

• *Subchondral cysts* may be seen beneath the articular cortex often in association with subchondral sclerosis. Normally, the cysts are easily distinguished from an erosion as they are beneath the intact cortex and have a sclerotic rim but, occasionally, if there is crumbling of the joint surfaces, the differentiation becomes difficult.

• *Loose bodies* are discrete pieces of calcified cartilage or bone lying free within the joint, most frequently seen in the knee. It is important not to call the fabella, a sesamoid bone in the gastrocnemius, a loose body in the knee joint (see Fig. 10.1, p. 324).

Osteoarthritis and rheumatoid arthritis are the two types of arthritis most commonly encountered. They show many distinguishing features which are listed in Table 10.1.

Neuropathic joint

Changes are seen in the feet of diabetics with peripheral neuropathy. The predominant feature is resorption of the bone ends and calcification of the arteries in the feet is often present. There may also be bone destruction due to infection (Fig. 10.13). Diagnosing osteomyelitis in the bones of the feet in diabetic patients can be difficult because bone destruction can be due to neuropathy or infection, or to a combination of the two.

Table 10.1 Comparison of osteoarthritis and rheumatoid arthritis.

Osteoarthritis	Rheumatoid arthritis
Joint space narrowing maximal at weight-bearing site	Joint space narrowing uniform
Erosions do not occur but crumbling of the joint surfaces may mimic erosions	Erosions a characteristic feature
Subchondral sclerosis and cysts may be seen	Not a feature but erosions *en face* may mimic cysts
Sclerosis is a prominent feature	Sclerosis not a feature unless there is secondary osteoarthritis
No osteoporosis	Osteoporosis often present

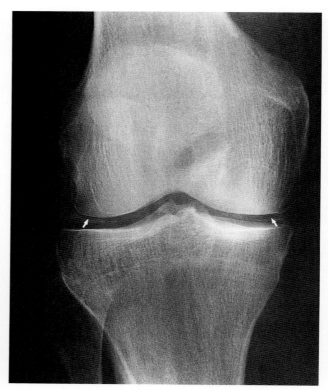

Fig. 10.14 Chondrocalcinosis. Calcification seen in the menisci in the knee (arrows).

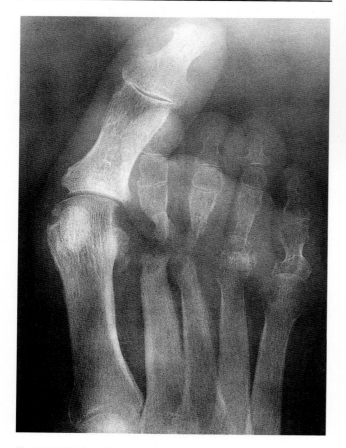

Fig. 10.13 Diabetic foot. There is resorption of the heads of the second and third metatarsals and bases of the proximal phalanges causing disorganization of the metatarsophalangeal joints. The patient had a peripheral neuropathy with an anaesthetic foot.

Calcium pyrophosphate dihydrate (CPPD) crystal deposition disease

In this condition there is deposition of CPPD crystals in the joint manifested by chondrocalcinosis, which is a descriptive term for calcification occurring in articular cartilage. In the knee, which is the most frequently affected joint, calcification may occur in the fibrocartilage of the menisci (Fig. 10.14) as well as the articular cartilage. Calcium pyrophosphate deposition disease may give rise to an arthritis clinically simulating gout, hence the alternative name 'pseudogout'. A severe arthritis resembling degenerative disease may follow. Chondrocalcinosis is, however, often an incidental asymptomatic finding.

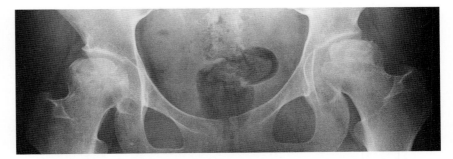

Fig. 10.15 Avascular necrosis. There is fragmentation with some sclerosis of both femoral heads.

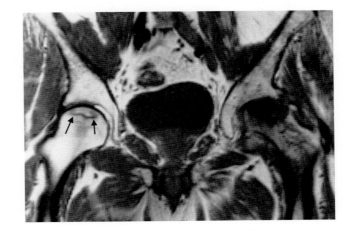

Fig. 10.16 Avascular necrosis of both femoral heads. Coronal MRI scan. The changes on the left are very severe and advanced. The changes in the right hip are relatively early and show a rim of low signal demarcating the ischaemic area (arrows).

Synovial sarcoma (synovioma)

This tumour appears as a soft tissue mass adjacent to a joint. Bone destruction on one or both sides of the joint occurs at a later stage. The soft tissue mass may contain visible calcification. The diagnosis is most readily made by MRI, which can demonstrate the full extent of the soft tissue mass.

Avascular (aseptic) necrosis

Avascular necrosis, also known as osteonecrosis, is where there is death of bone due to interruption of the blood supply. It occurs most commonly in the intra-articular portions of bones and is associated with numerous underlying conditions including:
- steroid therapy
- collagen vascular diseases
- radiation therapy
- sickle cell anaemia
- exposure to high pressure environments, e.g. tunnel workers and deep-sea divers (caisson disease)
- fractures.

The plain radiographic features of avascular necrosis are increased density of the subchondral bone with irregularity of the articular contour or even fragmentation of the bone (Fig. 10.15). A characteristic crescentic lucent line may be seen just beneath the articular cortex. The cartilage space is preserved until secondary degenerative changes supervene. Magnetic resonance imaging has now become the imaging modality of choice for demonstrating avascular necrosis and may show changes at a time when the radiographs may be normal. The appearances at MRI depend on the stage of disease, but the typical site of involvement and signal pattern allows a specific diagnosis to be made (Fig. 10.16).

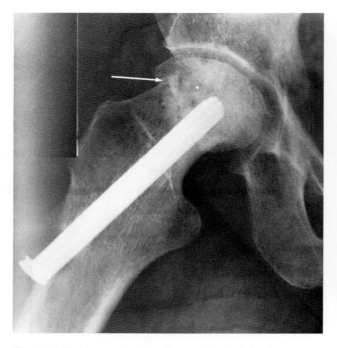

Fig. 10.17 Post-traumatic avascular necrosis. A pin has been inserted because of a subcapital fracture of the femoral neck (arrow), which occurred 10 months before this film was taken. Avascular necrosis has occurred in the head of the femur, which has become sclerotic.

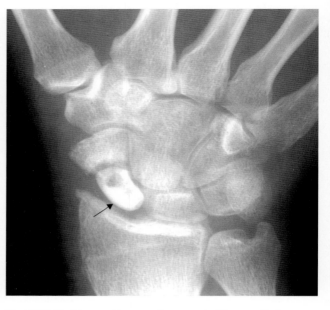

Fig. 10.18 Post-traumatic avascular necrosis. The ununited scaphoid fracture shows a sclerotic proximal pole (arrow) due to avascular necrosis of this part of the bone.

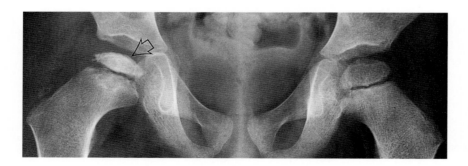

Fig. 10.19 Perthe's disease. The right femoral epiphysis (arrow) in this child is sclerotic and flattened. Compare it with the normal left side.

After a *fracture* the blood supply may become interrupted and avascular necrosis may then supervene, particularly in subcapital fractures of the femoral neck (Fig. 10.17) and fractures through the waist of the scaphoid. The femoral head and proximal pole of the scaphoid become fragmented and dense due to the ischaemia (Fig. 10.18).

Osteochondritis

There is also a group of conditions, some of which are called osteochondritis, in which no associated cause for avascular necrosis can be found. The osteochondrites are now regarded as being due to impaired blood supply associated with repeated trauma.

Perthe's disease, an avascular necrosis of the femoral head in children, is the most important example. The earliest plain radiographic change is increase in density and flattening of the femoral epiphysis which later may progress to collapse and fragmentation (Fig. 10.19). The epiphysis may widen and, in consequence, the femoral neck enlarges and may contain small cysts. The joint space is widened but the acetabulum is not affected. With healing, the femoral head reforms but may remain permanently flattened and, therefore, be responsible for osteoarthritis in later life.

Other forms of avascular necrosis are: *Freiberg's disease*, which affects the metatarsal heads; *Kohler's disease*, which affects the navicular bone of the foot; *Osgood–Schlatter's disease* of the tibial tuberosity and *Kienböck's disease* of lunate bone in the wrist.

Osteochondritis dissecans is thought to be a localized form of avascular necrosis. A small fragment of bone becomes separated from the articular surface of a joint leaving a defect, and the bony fragment can often be detected lying free within the joint. It occurs most frequently in the knee and ankle. The diagnosis can be established with plain film radiography (Fig. 10.20). Computed tomography and MRI are excellent imaging methods to diagnose small lesions or osteochondritis dissecans in portions of the articular bone that are difficult to see in standard plain film projections.

Slipped femoral epiphysis

Slipped femoral epiphysis occurs between the ages of 9 and 17 years, and may present with pain in the hip or pain referred to the knee. The epiphysis slips posteriorly from its normal position: this is best appreciated on a lateral film of the hip (Fig. 10.21). With a greater degree of slip, the condition can be recognized on the frontal view as a downward displacement of the epiphysis.

The films of the hip must be very carefully evaluated if the diagnosis is suspected clinically, because the diagnosis is easy to miss in the early stage at a time when further slip can be prevented surgically.

Developmental dysplasia of the hip (DDH)

Ultrasound has now replaced x-rays for detecting dislocation or subluxation of the hip in the infant in whom clinical examination is suspicious but not diagnostic. Ultrasound allows visualization of cartilagenous structures which are not seen on x-ray films, so the relationship of the cartilagenous femoral head and acetabulum can be determined.

Later in life, the condition is easier to diagnose on plain radiographs, but fortunately such cases are now rare, as the condition is usually treated in the neonatal period, the diagnosis having been made clinically. The features to look for are lateral and upper displacement of the head of the femur (Fig. 10.22). Increased slope to the acetabular roof is sometimes present.

Osteitis condensans ilii

Osteitis condensans ilii occurs almost exclusively in women who have borne children. The condition is thought to be a stress phenomenon associated with childbearing and is usually asymptomatic. There is a zone of sclerosis on the iliac side of the sacroiliac joints, but the sacroiliac joints themselves are normal (Fig. 10.23).

Scleroderma

Scleroderma may cause calcification and atrophy of soft tissues of the hands with loss of the tips of the terminal phalanges (Fig. 10.24).

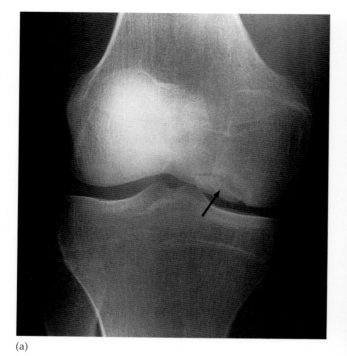

(a)

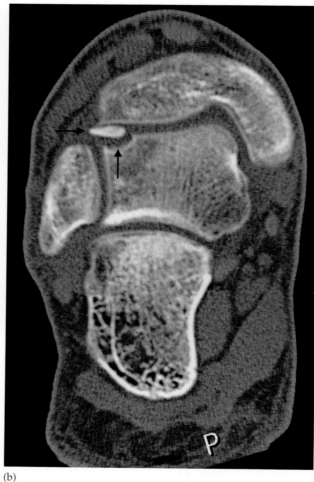

(b)

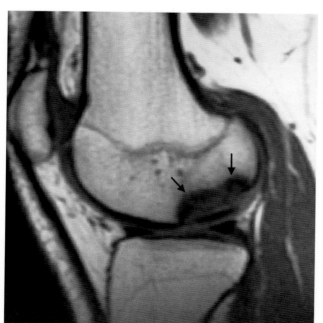

(c)

Fig. 10.20 Osteochondritis dissecans. (a) A fragment (arrow) has become separated from the articular cortex of the medial femoral condyle. (b) Coronal CT scan through an ankle showing small osteochondritis dissecans fragment (horizontal arrow) separated from the rest of the talus with a well-corticated defect in the underlying bone (vertical arrow). (c) MRI scan of the knee showing an osteochondritis defect (arrows) of the medial femoral condyle.

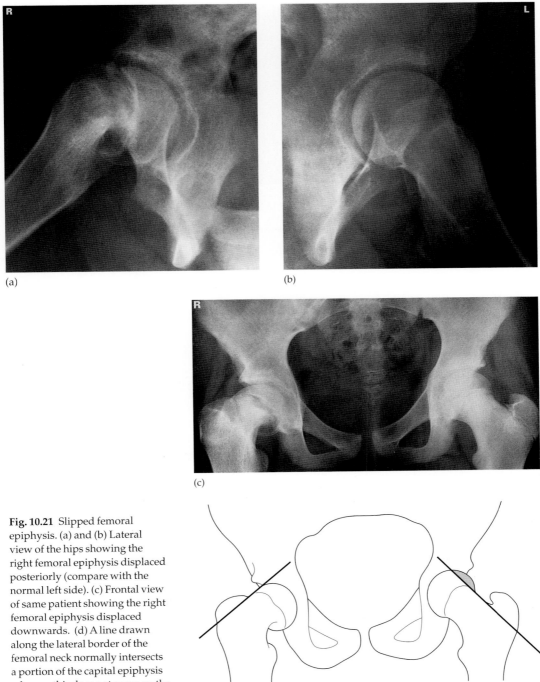

(a)

(b)

(c)

Fig. 10.21 Slipped femoral epiphysis. (a) and (b) Lateral view of the hips showing the right femoral epiphysis displaced posteriorly (compare with the normal left side). (c) Frontal view of same patient showing the right femoral epiphysis displaced downwards. (d) A line drawn along the lateral border of the femoral neck normally intersects a portion of the capital epiphysis whereas this does not occur on the side with slip.

(d) Slipped capital epiphysis   Normal

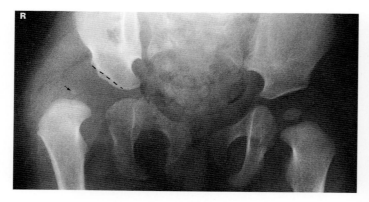

Fig. 10.22 Developmental dysplasia of right hip. The right femoral epiphysis (arrow) is smaller than on the normal left side and it does not lie within the acetabulum. Note the sloping roof of the right acetabulum (dotted lines).

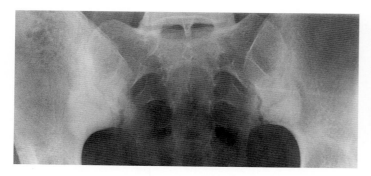

Fig. 10.23 Osteitis condensans ilii. Anteroposterior view. Sclerosis is seen in both iliac bones just adjacent to the sacroiliac joints. The joints themselves, however, are normal. The patient was a young woman who had borne children.

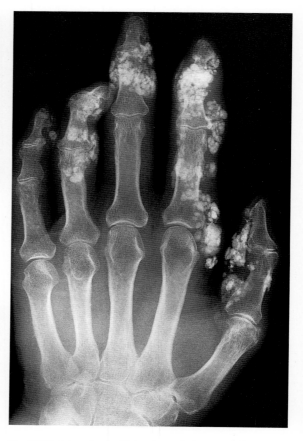

Fig. 10.24 Scleroderma. Extensive soft tissue calcification is present as well as atrophy of soft tissues at the ends of the fingers.

Internal derangements of the knee

Most knee injuries produce soft tissue damage, notably meniscal or ligamentous tears, either alone or in conjunction with bony fracture. Plain film examination can only demonstrate the state of the bones and show an effusion. Magnetic resonance imaging is the best imaging modality for detecting internal derangement, with many investigators believing that MRI is more accurate than arthroscopy.

Menisci

The menisci, which are composed of fibrocartilage, are well demonstrated on MRI as they have a different signal intensity from the hyaline cartilage covering the adjacent femoral condyles and tibial plateau. The normal menisci are of uniform low signal on all sequences and have the appearance on sagittal images described as a bow tie. A meniscal tear (Fig. 10.25) can be recognized as a break in the meniscus disrupting the articular surface allowing synovial fluid, which has a higher signal intensity, to enter the substance of the meniscus. Meniscal signal not disrupting the articular surface is caused by intrasubstance degeneration as a result of wear and tear due to ageing.

Some surgeons proceed directly to arthroscopy in patients with clear-cut clinical features of internal derangement, reserving MRI for those patients with suspicious but not definite clinical signs or symptoms, although many surgeons prefer to have a preliminary MRI. Magnetic resonance imaging can show bone bruises and other pathology adjacent to, but not within, the joint, entities that cannot be diagnosed at arthroscopy. Magnetic resonance imaging can also, on occasion, show meniscal tears not seen at arthroscopy.

Cruciate ligaments

The anterior cruciate ligament is seen as a low signal linear structure in the intercondylar notch. A torn ligament may just not be visible or a disruption of the ligament can be identified (Fig. 10.26). Partial tears may be seen as high signal within the ligament. Demonstration of the posterior cruciate ligament is not so important as these are rarely repaired even if torn.

Collateral ligaments

The medical and lateral collateral ligaments are of low signal on all sequences, and damage to the ligaments can be recognized by high signal in or around the ligaments.

Shoulder rotator cuff degeneration/tear

The rotator cuff of the shoulder consists of the supraspinatus, infraspinatus, teres minor and subcapularis muscles together with their tendons and they provide dynamic stability of the gleno humeral joint allowing the shoulder to perform a wide range of movements. Of the four muscles, the supraspinatus is the one that most commonly causes significant clinical problems. Tears of the supraspinatus tendon are thought to be due to impingement between the acromium and greater tuberosity of the humerus, and can lead to acute or chronic symptoms. Magnetic resonance imaging and/or ultrasound can be useful in selected patients when corrective surgery is being considered. On MRI, the normal low signal of the supraspinatus tendon is interrupted by the higher signal of fluid, and in complete tears it may be possible to see the retracted ends of the torn tendon–muscle junction (Fig. 10.27).

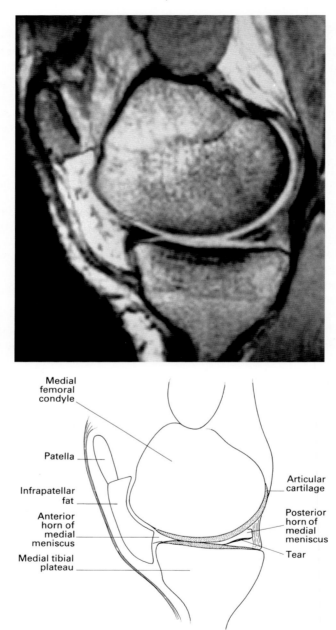

Fig. 10.25 Tear of medial meniscus. Sagittal MRI through the medial part of the knee joint showing a tear in the posterior horn of the medial meniscus. The anterior horn appears normal.

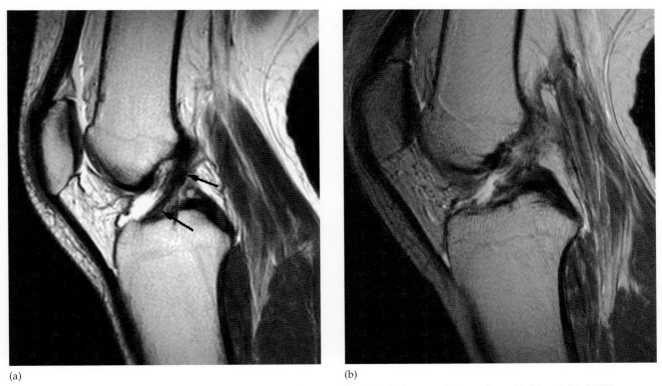

(a)

(b)

Fig. 10.26 (a) Normal anterior cruciate ligament is shown as a low signal band in the intercondylar notch on this T1-weighted MRI (arrows). (b) With a tear the ligament is disrupted.

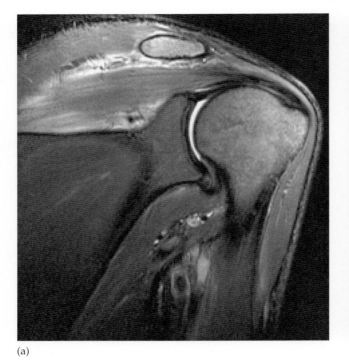

(a)

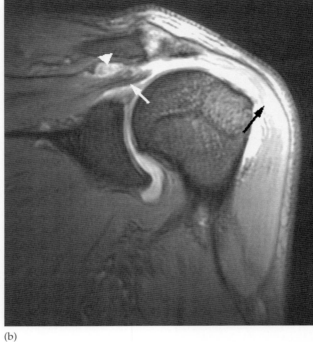

(b)

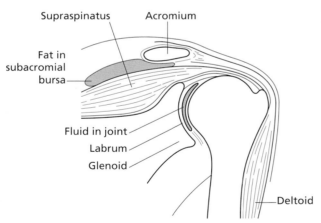

Fig. 10.27 (a) Normal shoulder MRI showing the supraspinatus tendon inserting into the greater tuberosity of the humerus (diagram).(b) Supraspinatus tendon tear. MRI showing complete disruption of the supraspinatus tendon (white arrow) with fluid in the subacromial bursa (arrow head) and oedema of the adjacent deltoid muscle (black arrow).

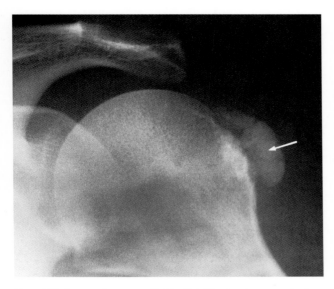

Fig. 10.28 Supraspinatus tendinitis. Calcification is present in the supraspinatus tendon (arrow).

Tears of the supraspinatus tendon may be associated with tears or detachment of the glenoid labrum, which is a fibrocartilaginous ring surrounding the glenoid of the scapula.

Calcific tendonitis

Calcification occurs in the periarticular regions and is most commonly seen in the shoulder in the supraspinatus tendon as amorphous calcification adjacent to the greater tuberosity of the humerus (Fig. 10.28).

11

Spine

Spinal imaging has been revolutionized by the introduction of magnetic resonance imaging (MRI). Plain films have a role in spinal disorders, especially in spinal trauma, though the value of plain films in back pain is questionable. The spinal cord and spinal nerves are invisible on plain films but MRI is able to visualize not only the vertebrae and the intervertebral discs but also the spinal canal and contents as well. Magnetic resonance imaging is the preferred examination for degenerative, inflammatory and malignant conditions of the spine.

The detailed structure of the vertebrae differs in the cervical, thoracic and lumbar regions, but the general structure is similar. The appearance of a normal vertebra is illustrated in Fig. 11.1. In the lateral projection, the vertebral bodies are approximately rectangular in shape. There may be shallow indentations on the upper and lower surfaces due to protrusion of disc material into the vertebral end plates. These indentations are known as Schmorl's nodes and are of no clinical significance (Fig. 11.2).

The appearances of normal vertebrae at MRI are illustrated in Fig. 11.3. On a T1-weighted MRI scan, fat appears as high signal while cerebrospinal fluid (CSF) and the intervertebral discs are of low signal. On a T2-weighted scan, normal discs and CSF are of high signal. It should be appreciated that bone produces no signal at MRI; the signal responsible for showing the spine on an MR image comes from the bone marrow, thecal contents and discs. Normal bone marrow has a different MRI signal to most soft tissues and, in particular, has a different signal to tumour and infection.

Other imaging methods for examining the spine are *radionuclide bone scans*, which are particularly useful for the detection of bony metastases, and *computed tomography (CT)*, which has an important role in spinal trauma. *Myelography*, which entailed injecting contrast into the subarachnoid space by lumbar puncture, has now been replaced by MRI.

Signs of abnormality

The abnormalities detected on plain radiographs often permit a diagnosis to be made, though other imaging may be performed for confirmation.

Disc space narrowing (Fig. 11.4)

The intervertebral discs are radiolucent on plain radiographs as they are composed of fibrous tissue and cartilage. Normally, the disc spaces are the same height at all levels in the cervical and thoracic spine. In the lumbar spine, the disc spaces increase slightly in height going down the spine, except for the disc space at the lumbosacral junction, which is usually narrower than the one above it. Magnetic resonance imaging shows the internal structure of the disc, and any loss of disc height together with alteration of the normal signal characteristics can be readily appreciated. Disc space narrowing occurs with degenerative disease and with disc space infection.

Collapse of vertebral bodies

A collapsed vertebral body is one which has lost height. Loss of height is most easily appreciated on plain lateral radiographs of the spine, though it is, of course, well demonstrated on sagittal sections with MRI and CT. If any collapse is present, it is essential to look at the adjacent disc to see if it is narrowed and to check if part of any pedicle

Diagnostic Imaging, 6th Edition. By Peter Armstrong, Martin Wastie and Andrea Rockall. Published 2009 by Blackwell Publishing. ISBN: 978-1-4051-7039.

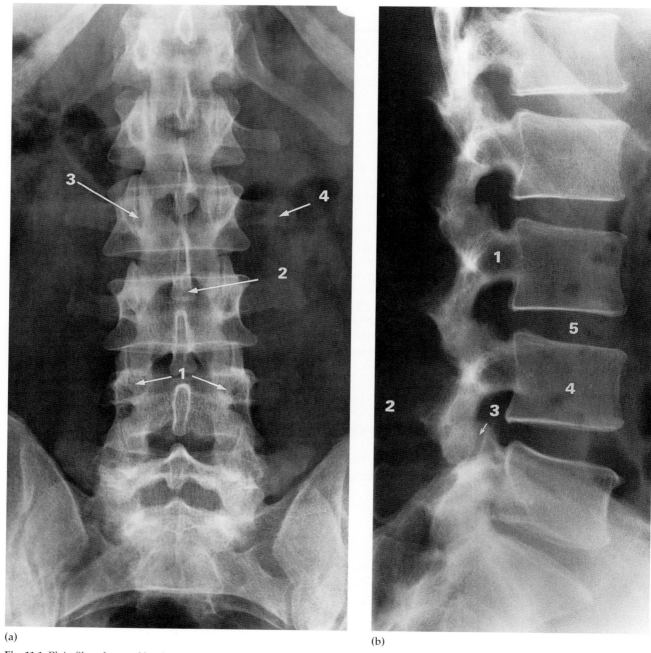

(a)   (b)

Fig. 11.1 Plain film of normal lumbar spine. (a) Frontal. **1**, pedicles; **2**, spinous process; **3**, facet joint; **4**, transverse process. (b) Lateral. **1**, pedicles; **2**, spinous process; **3**, facet joint; **4**, vertebral body; **5**, disc space. Note how the height of the disc spaces increases from L1 to L5 with the exception of the L5–S1 disc space which is normally narrower than the one above.

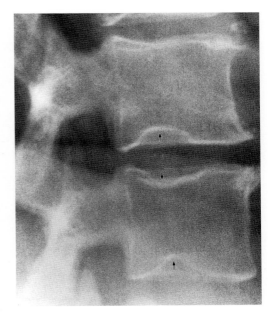

Fig. 11.2 Schmorl's nodes. These are indentations into the end plates of the vertebral bodies (arrows) and are without significance.

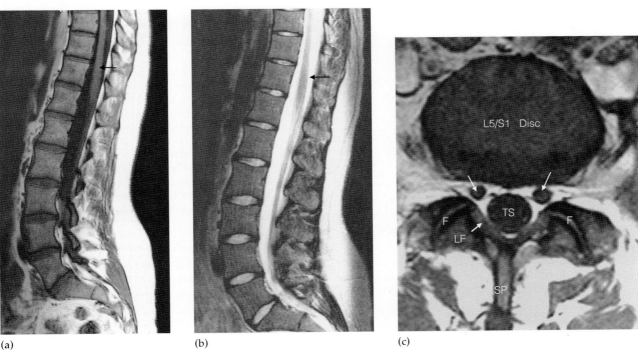

(a)   (b)   (c)

Fig. 11.3 MRI of normal lumbar spine. (a) T1-weighted scan. The discs and spinal cord (arrow) are of intermediate signal. (b) T2-weighted scan. The discs and cerebrospinal fluid appear as high signal. The spinal cord is arrowed. (c) Axial T1-weighted scan through the L5/S1 disc space. Note the high signal fat surrounding the S1 nerve roots (arrows). F, facet joints; LF, ligamentum flavum; SP, spinous process; TS, thecal sac.

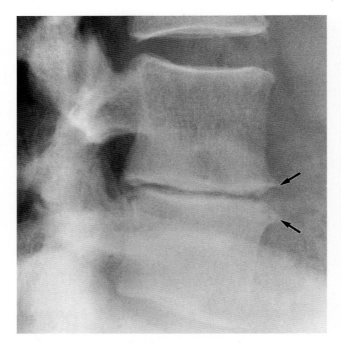

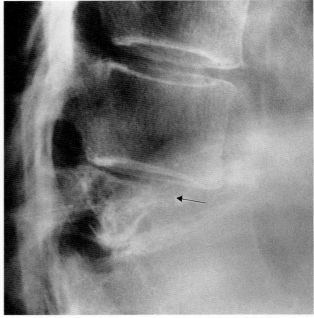

(a)

Fig. 11.4 Disc space narrowing caused by disc degenerative changes between L3 and L4. Note the osteophytes (arrows) and sclerosis of the adjoining surfaces of the vertebral bodies.

Fig. 11.5 Collapsed vertebra. (a) Metastasis (arrow) causing complete collapse of the vertebral body. The adjacent vertebral discs are unaffected. (b–e *facing page.*) (b) Osteomyelitis. The disc space is narrowed and there is destruction of the surfaces of the adjacent vertebral bodies (arrows). (c) Traumatic collapse. Note the concave superior surface of the collapsed vertebral body. Some fragments have been extruded anteriorly (arrow). (d) Osteoporotic collapse. There is decreased bone density with a collapse of a vertebral body due to a compression fracture. (e) Collapse due to eosinophil granuloma. In this child the vertebral body is so collapsed that it resembles a thin disc (arrow).

is destroyed. The commoner causes of vertebral collapse are listed below together with a synopsis of the signs of importance in differential diagnosis:

• *Metastases and myeloma.* Bone destruction, or replacement of normal marrow signal by tumour in the case of MRI, may be visible. The pedicles are a good place to look for evidence of bone destruction on plain film examination. The disc spaces are usually normal (Fig. 11.5a).

• *Infection.* The adjacent disc space is nearly always narrow or obliterated. There may be bone destruction next to the affected disc but the pedicles are usually intact (Fig. 11.5b). Magnetic resonance imaging will show altered signal within the affected vertebral body and disc.

• *Osteoporosis and osteomalacia.* There is generalized reduction in bone density leading to compression fractures. The disc spaces are normal or even slightly increased in height and the pedicles are intact. Marrow signal at MRI is normal.

• *Trauma.* A compression fracture is commonly due to forward flexion of the spine, causing the vertebral body

to become wedge-shaped. The superior surface is usually concave (Fig. 11.5c,d). The discs are normal but may be impacted into the fractured bone – a feature well shown on sagittal MRI and CT. Associated fractures may be seen in the pedicles or neural arch, but otherwise the bone and discs are normal.

• *Eosinophil granuloma.* Complete collapse of one or more vertebral bodies may occur in children or young adults with Langerhans histiocytosis (eosinophil granuloma). The vertebral body is flattened and sometimes referred to as a 'vertebra plana' (Fig. 11.5e). The adjacent discs are normal and the pedicles are usually preserved.

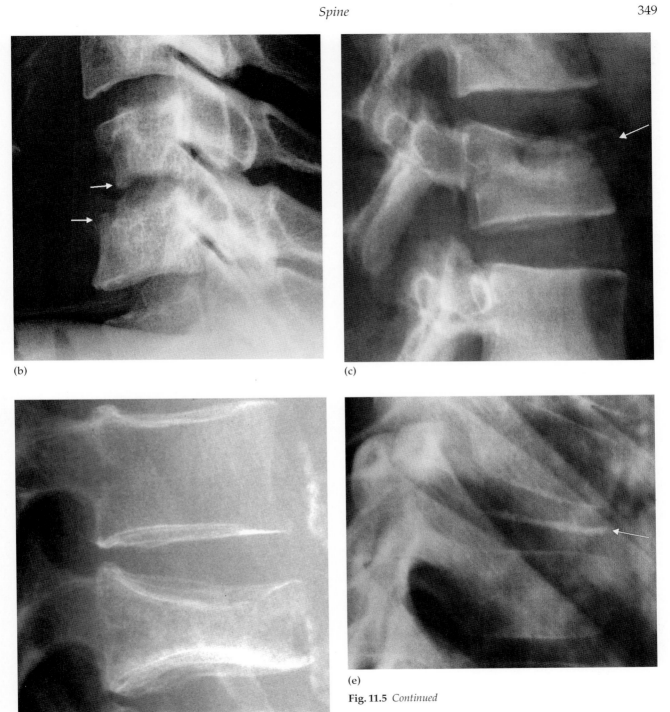

(b)

(c)

(d)

(e)

Fig. 11.5 *Continued*

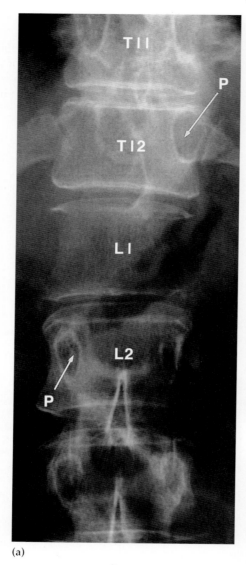

(a)

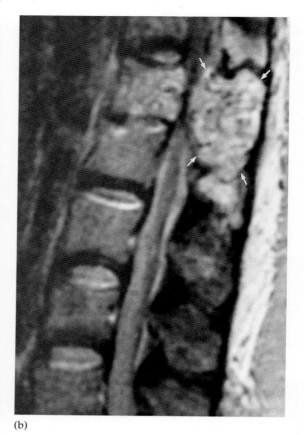

(b)

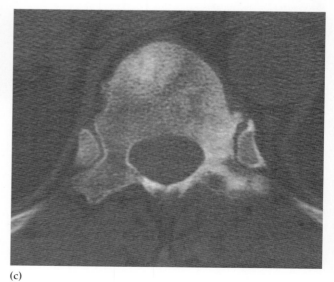

(c)

Fig. 11.6 Destruction of the pedicles due to metastatic renal cell carcinoma. (a) The pedicles of L1 have both been destroyed, as has the right pedicle of T12. Arrows point to representative normal pedicles (P). (b) MRI scan in the same patient showing extensive tumour in the vertebral body and a posterior mass of tumour (arrows) which is compressing the dural sac. (c) CT scan in a patient with prostatic metastases showing sclerosis of the left pedicle of a lower thoracic vertebra together with sclerosis in the vertebral body and transverse process.

Pedicles

On plain films the pedicles are best assessed in the frontal view, except in the cervical spine where oblique views are necessary. They are very well demonstrated on CT scans. Destruction or sclerosis of one or more of the pedicles (Fig. 11.6) is a fairly reliable sign of spinal metastases.

Flattening and widening of the distance between the pedicles occurs with tumours arising within the spinal canal, e.g. neurofibroma or meningioma. Although neurofibromas may be completely intradural, some have a dumb-bell shape with a portion lying outside the spinal canal.

Dense vertebrae

Sclerosis, which is demonstrated on plain films or CT, may affect just one vertebra or may be part of a generalized process involving many bones. Common causes are:

• *Metastases*, particularly from primary tumours of the prostate or breast (Fig. 11.7).

• *Malignant lymphoma.*

• *Paget's disease*, which may be difficult to distinguish from neoplastic disease. (An important diagnostic feature is increase in the size of the vertebra. A coarse trabecular pattern typical of Paget's disease is usually but not invariably present; Fig. 11.8.)

• *Haemangioma*, which gives rise to characteristic vertical striations in a vertebra that is normal in size (Fig. 11.9).

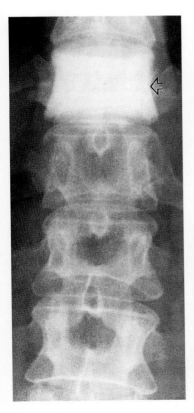

Fig. 11.7 Dense vertebra (arrow) due to metastases from carcinoma of the breast.

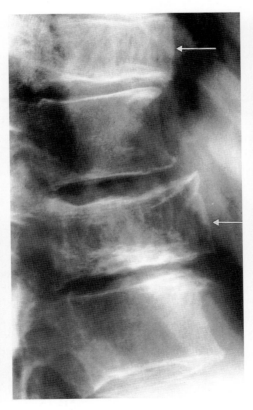

Fig. 11.8 Paget's disease. Note the increased density and coarse trabeculae in the vertebral bodies (arrows). They are also wider than the normal ones.

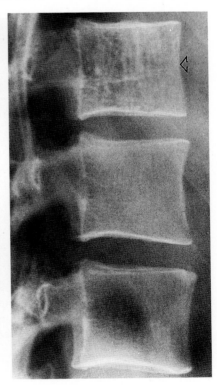

Fig. 11.9 Haemangioma. Vertical striations are present in this normal-sized vertebra (arrow).

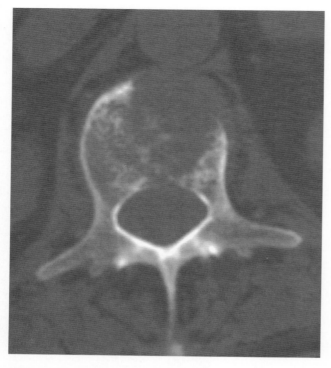

Fig. 11.10 Metastasis causing a large lytic area in the body of a lumbar vertebra.

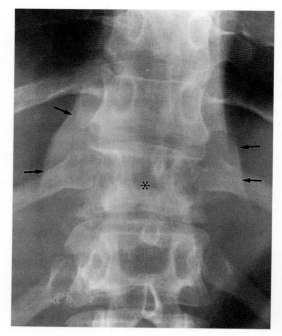

Fig. 11.11 Fusiform paravertebral shadow (arrows) around a thoracic vertebra partially destroyed by Hodgkin's disease (*).

Lysis within a vertebra

As with sclerosis, lysis, which is demonstrated on plain films or CT, may be part of a widespread process or be confined to one vertebra. The common causes are:

• *Metastases*, particularly from primary tumours of the lungs, breasts or kidneys (Fig. 11.10).
• *Multiple myeloma/plasmacytoma.*
• *Malignant lymphoma* occasionally gives rise to a lytic lesion.
• *Infection*. Here the lysis usually involves one body or two adjacent bodies and the adjacent disc space is almost invariably narrowed (see below).

Paravertebral shadow

A paravertebral soft tissue shadow may first draw attention to an abnormality in the spine. The easiest place to recognize such swelling on plain radiographs is in the thoracic region, where the soft tissue density adjacent to the spine assumes a characteristic fusiform shape (Fig. 11.11). Swellings in the lumbar region have to be very large if they are to displace the psoas outline and be recognizable on plain films. Anterior swelling in the cervical region can be recognized by the forward displacement of the pharyngeal air shadow. Paravertebral soft tissue swelling is readily recognized at all levels with CT and MRI scanning.

Paravertebral soft tissue swelling occurs with infection, with malignant neoplasms and with haematomas following trauma. Specific diagnostic signs are often present in such cases in the adjacent bones.

Metastases/myeloma/lymphoma

As with the remainder of the skeleton, the important signs of metastases and lymphoma on plain films or CT are areas of lysis or sclerosis, or a mixture of the two (Fig. 11.12). Multiple myeloma, which almost always gives rise to lytic lesions in the vertebral bodies, is frequently indistinguishable from lytic metastases. A point of difference is that metastases often involve the pedicles as well as the vertebral bodies.

Collapse of one or more vertebral bodies may occur with metastases and is a particular feature of myeloma. The collapse may mask the areas of bone destruction in the vertebral body. True destruction of the disc space does not occur with metastases or myeloma.

Radionuclide bone imaging may reveal increased activity around neoplastic tumour deposits, because of increased bone turnover, but myeloma lesions may or may not give rise to focal areas of increased activity.

Magnetic resonance imaging is the most accurate test for demonstrating metastases, lymphoma and myeloma, and with modern scanners large areas of the body can be scanned quite quickly (Fig. 11.13). Tumour tissue has significantly different signal characteristics (low signal on T1-weighted images, high signal on T2-weighted images) than normal bone marrow (Fig. 11.14), and thus the tumour deposits stand out clearly from the adjacent marrow. The normal bone does not generate any signal and, therefore, does not impair the visibility of the tumour. Magnetic resonance imaging has the advantage that it can additionally detect any spinal cord or nerve root compression (see Figs 11.6 and 11.32, pp. 350 and 368).

Infection

The hallmark of infection is destruction of the intervertebral disc and adjacent vertebral bodies. Early in the course of the disease, there is narrowing of the disc space with erosion of the adjoining surface of the vertebral body. Later, bone destruction may lead to collapse of the vertebral body, resulting in a sharp angulation known as a gibbus (Fig. 11.15a). A paravertebral abscess is usually present.

Computed tomography shows the bone destruction and paravertebral soft tissue swelling to advantage and disc space narrowing can be shown with sagittal reconstructions. MRI is the preferred investigation as it can, with one examination, demonstrate disc space narrowing, altered signal in the adjacent vertebral body, adjacent soft tissue swelling and any spinal cord or nerve root compression (Fig. 11.15b). Needle biopsy/aspiration of the infected disc or adjacent vertebral body under plain film or CT control is a very useful technique to confirm the diagnosis and identify the responsible organism. It should be remembered, however, that positive cultures are rare once antibiotics have been commenced.

The common infecting organisms are *Mycobacterium tuberculosis* and *Staphylococcus aureus*. Though there are some differences in the signs produced by these two infections, there is considerable overlap. The lesion in tuberculosis is usually purely lytic, whereas some sclerosis is often seen in pyogenic infection. Paravertebral abscesses tend to be larger in tuberculosis.

Bony fusion of the vertebral bodies across the obliterated disc spaces occurs with healing. Eventually, tuberculous paravertebral abscesses may calcify.

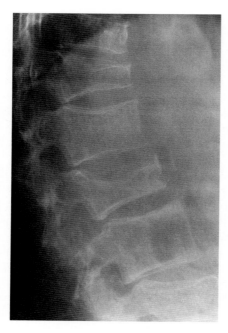

Fig. 11.12 Metastases. Lateral view of the upper lumbar spine. Note the abnormal bony architecture and varying degrees of collapse of several of the vertebral bodies.

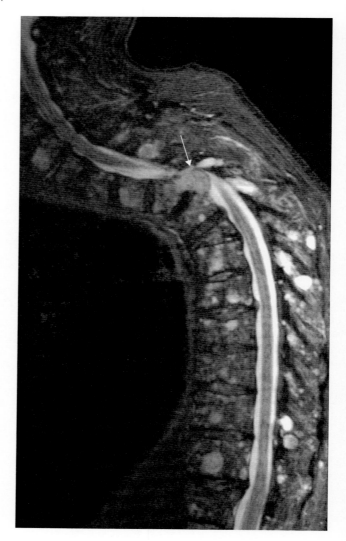

Fig. 11.13 Myeloma. MRI scan of the cervical and thoracic spine showing many deposits as high signal areas in the spine. The scan readily demonstrates a kyphus due to bone destruction and myeloma extending into the spinal canal causing spinal cord compression (arrow).

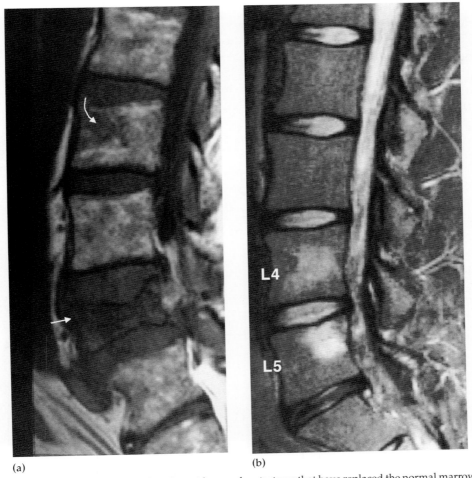

Fig. 11.14 (a) Metastases. T1-weighted MRI scan showing widespread metastases that have replaced the normal marrow signal and appear as low signal areas: a particularly large metastasis is seen in L2 (curved arrow). L4 is collapsed (straight arrow). (b) Lymphoma. T2-weighted scan showing high signal areas in L4 and L5.

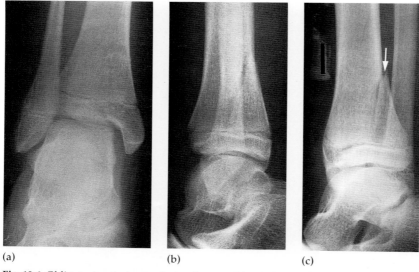

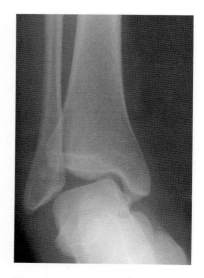

(a)   (b)   (c)

Fig. 12.6 Oblique view to demonstrate a fracture. (a) and (b) Anteroposterior and lateral views in this child's ankle do not show an obvious fracture. (c) Oblique view clearly demonstrates the fracture (arrow).

Fig. 12.7 Stress view to demonstrate ligamentous rupture. Inversion stress on ankle opens up lateral joint indicating rupture of lateral ligaments.

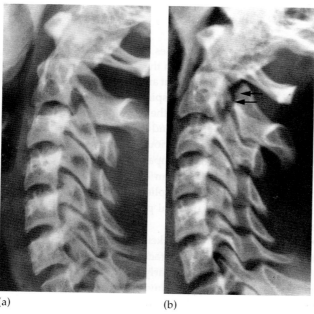

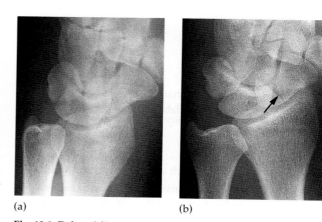

(a)   (b)

Fig. 12.9 Delayed films to demonstrate a fracture. (a) Films taken immediately after injury do not show a fracture. (b) Films taken 2 weeks after injury show a fracture through the scaphoid (arrow).

(a)   (b)

Fig. 12.8 Flexion and extension views to demonstrate a fracture. (a) Extension view of cervical spine does not reveal a fracture. (b) Flexion view clearly shows the fracture of the arch of C2 (arrows).

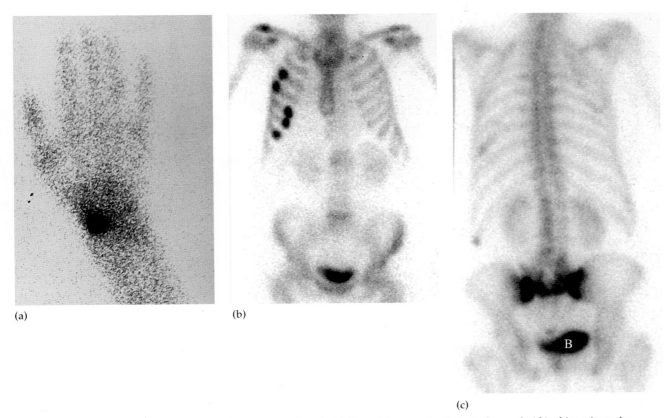

(a)

(b)

(c)

Fig. 12.10 Radionuclide bone scans in trauma. (a) Fracture of scaphoid. There is increased activity in the scaphoid in this patient who suffered continuing pain after trauma to the wrist. In spite of normal x-rays, the bone scan indicates there is a fracture which was not visible on the radiographs. (b) Fractures in five of the ribs on the right. The distribution of increased uptake is diagnostic of injury. (c) Insufficiency fracture. There is increased uptake in the sacrum in this elderly lady who had a normal pelvic x-ray. B, isotope in the bladder.

Radionuclide bone scanning in bone trauma (Fig. 12.10)

Fractures may not be visible on plain films, and, in these instances, radionuclide bone scanning is particularly helpful. The bone scans show increased activity at injured sites within 2–3 days. Increased activity persists for as long as the fractures are healing, often lasting several months. Multiple fractures occasionally give a picture resembling metastases, but usually the distribution suggests injury.

Computed tomography in bone trauma

The major advantages of computed tomography (CT) over plain films are:
• Better assessment of fractures in bones of complex shape, such as the spine and pelvis (Fig. 12.11) which can be aided by three-dimensional reconstruction of the CT image. Reconstructions to any desired plane (Fig. 12.12) or three-dimensional images (Fig. 12.13) are easily obtained on

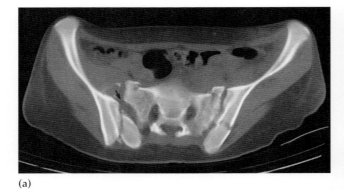

(a)

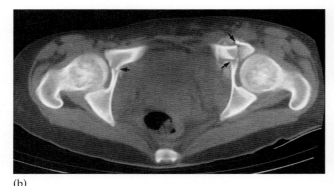

(b)

Fig. 12.11 Fracture of the pelvis. (a) A section through the sacrum shows fractures of the sacrum and iliac bones. There is separation of the right sacroiliac joint (arrow). (b) A lower section shows fractures through the acetabula (arrows). The fractures and their displacement were much better demonstrated with CT than with radiographs of the pelvis.

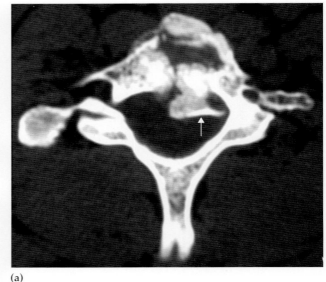

(a)

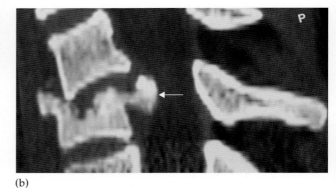

(b)

Fig. 12.12 CT scanning in a spinal fracture. (a) A comminuted fracture of C7 with displacement of a large bone fragment (arrow) into the spinal canal. (b) Sagittal reconstruction also shows the fractured vertebra and displaced fragment (arrow).

modern equipment. In the spine, fractures of the pedicles, laminae and articular facets as well as fragments displaced into the spinal canal are particularly well seen (Fig. 12.12). In fractures of the pelvis, especially those around the hip joints, CT shows the relationship of the fractures to the joint as well as loose fragments within the joint (Fig. 12.11). Computed tomography is invariably performed in acetabular fractures and fracture dislocations of the hip. It is also very helpful in tibial plateau fractures and fractures of the ankle, calcaneum and midfoot.

• Better assessment of the extent of soft tissue damage and haematomas and of internal visceral injuries.
• In general, less manipulation of the patient is required, so that the examination of the severely injured individual is more comfortable and often safer. The examination is quick, an important factor in patients with serious internal injuries.

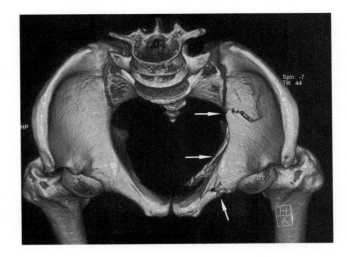

Fig. 12.13 Multiple fractures through the left innominate bone shown by three-dimensional CT. The two horizontal arrows point to a complex fracture with a displaced fragment. The oblique arrow points to another fracture in the superior pubic ramus. A further view of this scan is shown in Fig. 1.4, p. 4).

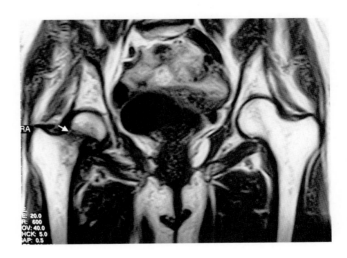

Fig. 12.14 Coronal MRI showing a fracture of the right femoral neck (arrow) which was not visible on x-rays of the hip.

Magnetic resonance imaging in bone trauma

Even though cortical bone does not produce a magnetic resonance signal, a fracture can be seen as a dark line across the bright signal of the fat in the marrow on a T1-weighted scan (Fig. 12.14). Altered signal is seen within the bone, representing haemorrhage and/or oedema. Sometimes a bone bruise may be visible on magnetic resonance imaging (MRI) even though there is no discernible fracture (Fig. 12.15) on a conventional radiograph. Magnetic resonance imaging is also very useful for demonstrating injury to soft tissues such as muscle, tendons and ligaments and is particularly useful in knee injuries (Fig. 12.16). Magnetic resonance imaging is the best examination for sports injury and repetitive strain injuries.

Magnetic resonance imaging is the best method for demonstrating scaphoid fractures and its use has been advocated as the initial investigation.

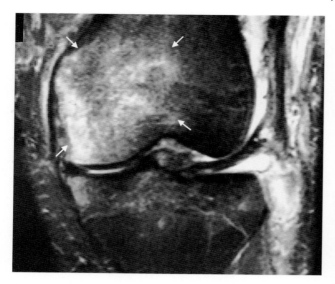

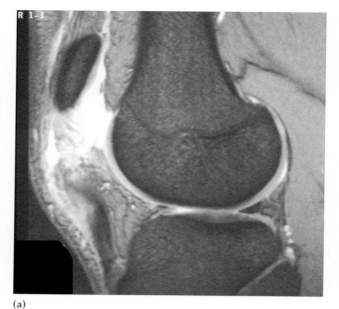

(a)

Fig. 12.15 Bone bruise. MRI in a patient who suffered severe soft tissue damage to the lateral side of his knee. The high signal in the medial femoral condyle (arrows) is due to a bone bruise. The plain films of the knee showed no bony injury.

Fig. 12.16 Rupture of patella tendon. (a) MRI showing diffuse high signal in region of the patella tendon. (b) Normal knee for comparison. The arrows point to the patella tendon.

(b)

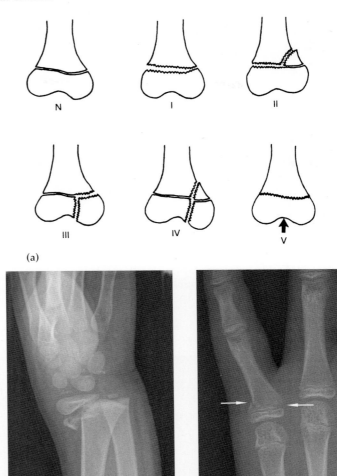

Fig. 12.17 (a) Salter–Harris classification (N, normal):
- Type I – epiphyseal separation by a fracture through the growth plate
- Type II is the commonest – a fragment of the metaphysis accompanies the displaced epiphysis
- Type III – a fracture through the epiphysis and growth plate
- Type IV – a fracture occurs through the epiphysis, growth plate and metaphysis
- Type V – is a crush injury of the growth plate and usually no changes are seen on the radiograph.

(a)

Fig. 12.17 (b, c) Two examples of Salter–Harris type II fractures. Note that in both examples the fracture runs through the metaphysis as well as through the epiphyseal plate.

(b)

(c)

Salter–Harris classification

Specific injuries

Numerous types of fractures and dislocations may be encountered and it is not practical to describe and illustrate them all in this book. The following section is an atlas illustrating a selection of the more common and important injuries.

Fractures of an epiphysis, growth plate or metaphysis of the long bones often occur in children and may lead to subsequent growth deformities because of damage to a growth plate. Five types are recognized in the Salter–Harris classification (Fig. 12.17a). Types I and II usually have favourable outcomes. Types III, IV and V require more complex treatment.

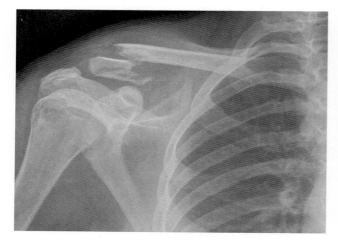

Fig. 12.18 Fracture of clavicle. This common fracture usually occurs in the outer half of the clavicle. Upward displacement of the medial fragment is frequently seen, as in this example.

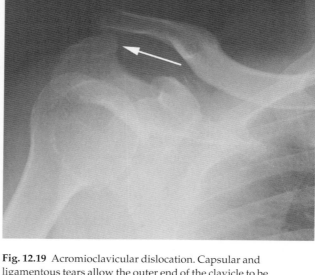

Fig. 12.19 Acromioclavicular dislocation. Capsular and ligamentous tears allow the outer end of the clavicle to be displaced upward relative to the medial aspect of the acromion process (arrow).

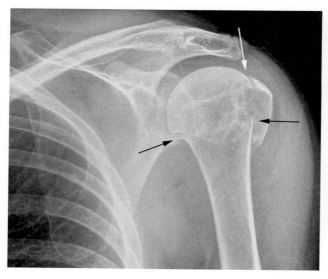

Fig. 12.20 Fracture of the neck of humerus (black arrows) is a common fracture in the elderly and may be overlooked clinically if the fracture is impacted. The greater tuberosity is also fractured (white arrow) in this example.

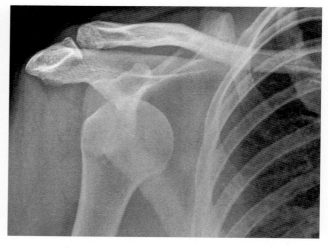

Fig. 12.21 Anterior dislocation of shoulder. The head of the humerus is displaced inferior and anterior to the glenoid fossa to lie beneath the coracoid process.

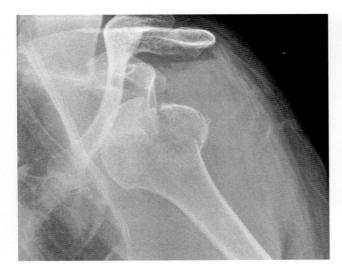

Fig. 12.22 Anterior dislocation of the shoulder may be associated with a fracture of the greater tuberosity.

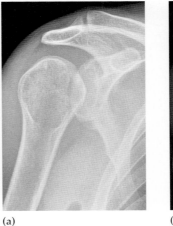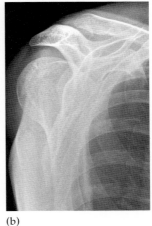

(a)   (b)

Fig. 12.23 Posterior dislocation of the shoulder is often a consequence of an electric shock or epileptic seizure. (a) The dislocation may be difficult to see on the frontal view. Note the internal rotation of the humerus and lack of congruity of the humeral head with the glenoid. (b) Lateral view shows the humeral head behind the posterior rim of the glenoid fossa beneath the spine of the scapula.

Fig. 12.24 Elbow effusion with fracture of radial head. (a) The anterior and posterior fat pads (arrows) are displaced away from the humerus which almost invariably means a fracture is present. (b) Oblique view in this patient shows the fracture of the radial head (arrow) which was only demonstrated on the oblique view.

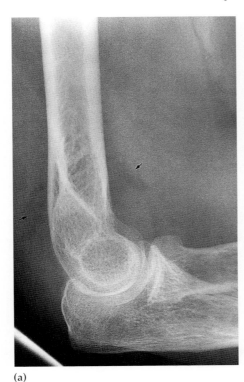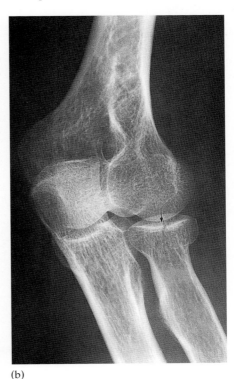

(a)   (b)

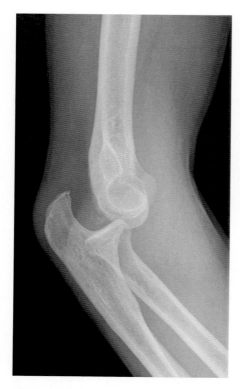

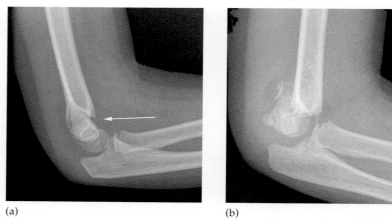

(a)   (b)

Fig. 12.26 Supracondylar fracture. Two examples (a) with minor displacement (b) with severe displacement. These fractures occur in children and are potentially dangerous because of possible injury to the brachial artery and nerve damage.

Fig. 12.25 Dislocation of the elbow. The common form is backward and lateral displacement of the radius and ulna.

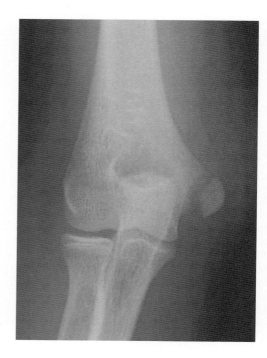

Fig. 12.27 Epicondylar fracture: medial epicondyle separation. Fractures of the epicondyles occur in children before the epiphyses fuse fully.

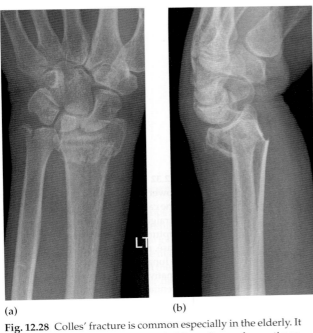

(a)   (b)

Fig. 12.28 Colles' fracture is common especially in the elderly. It is a fracture through the lower end of the radius and sometimes the ulnar styloid is avulsed in addition, as in this example. (a) Anteroposterior view. (b) Lateral view showing posterior displacement and angulation giving rise to the 'dinner fork' deformity.

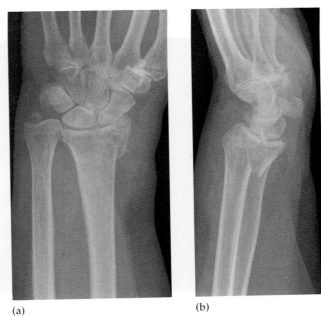

(a)   (b)

Fig. 12.29 Smith's fracture is a fracture of the lower radius with the reverse deformity to a Colles' fracture. It has anterior displacement and angulation. (a) Anteroposterior view. (b) Lateral view.

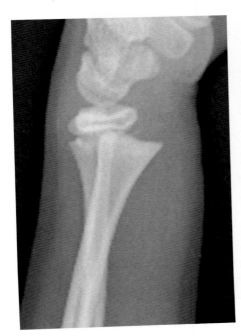

Fig. 12.30 Fracture through lower radial epiphysis resulting in separation of epiphysis (Salter–Harris I fracture).

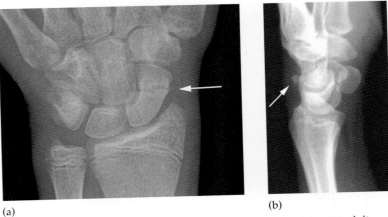

(a)   (b)

Fig. 12.31 Fractures of wrist bones. (a) Scaphoid fractures occur in young adults following a fall on the outstretched hand. They are serious injuries because if missed non-union or avascular necrosis may supervene. The fracture (arrow), as in this example, is usually across the waist of the scaphoid. (b) Triquetral fracture – a flake fracture detached from the posterior aspect of the triquetral is seen only on the lateral view.

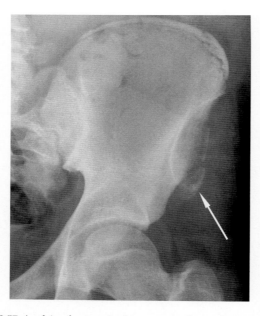

Fig. 12.57 Avulsion fracture. In this example, the avulsed anterior inferior iliac spine appears as a bone fragment adjacent to the ilium (arrow) and is caused by violent contraction of the rectus femoris muscle.

The fractures are caused by squeezing the baby and are thus usually seen in the axillary and posterior portions of the ribs.

• *Epiphyseal separation* is frequently associated with a metaphyseal fracture.

• *Metaphyseal sclerosis* is probably due to repeated injury and repair.

• *Periosteal reactions.* Haemorrhage under the periosteum occurs easily in children. The elevated periosteum lays down new bone, which may be so extensive that it envelops the shaft.

A CT scan or ultrasound of the head may be necessary to detect brain damage or subdural haemorrhage.

Avulsion fractures

Avulsion fractures occur in sports people and are found in recognized sites such as the inferior iliac spine from avulsion of the rectus femoris muscle or the ischium from avulsion of the adductor muscles (Fig. 12.57).

13

Skull and Brain

Computed tomography (CT) and magnetic resonance imaging (MRI) are the standard investigations for disorders of the brain and skull. Angiography is undertaken to demonstrate arterial stenoses, venous occlusions, aneurysms and arteriovenous malformations particularly prior to interventional procedures. Plain films of the skull are restricted to showing abnormalities of the skull bones. A lateral view of the skull is often included in a skeletal survey for myeloma. Skull radiographs, once the mainstay for investigating head injury, have now been replaced by CT except as part of a skeletal survey in suspected non-accidental injury.

Plain skull films

Normal

The bones of the normal vault have an inner and outer table of compact bone with spongy bone (diploë) between them; the sutures remain visible even when fused and should not be mistaken for fractures. Blood vessels cause impressions on the bones of the vault, resulting in linear or star-shaped translucencies (Fig. 13.1) and small lucencies are often seen in the inner table near the vertex caused by normal arachnoid granulations; they may be difficult to distinguish from small lytic lesions.

Bone lysis

Abnormal focal areas of bone lysis usually indicate metastasis or myeloma (Fig. 13.2). Large areas of bone destruction

Diagnostic Imaging, 6th Edition. By Peter Armstrong, Martin Wastie and Andrea Rockall. Published 2009 by Blackwell Publishing. ISBN: 978-1-4051-7039.

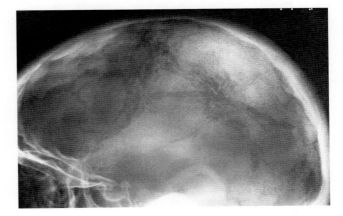

Fig. 13.1 Vascular markings. In this normal skull the vascular markings are very prominent. Note how they form a star-shaped translucency in the parietal region.

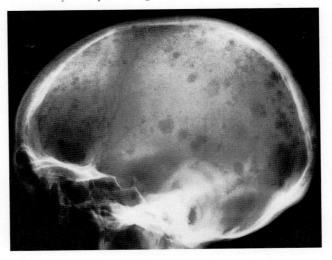

Fig. 13.2 Myeloma. Many well-defined lytic lesions of various sizes are seen in all areas of the skull vault.

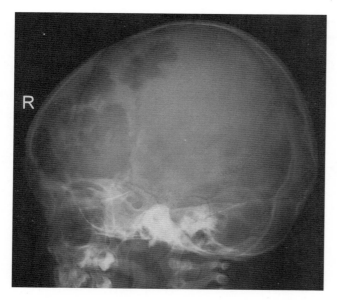

Fig. 13.3 Langerhans histiocytosis. In this child's skull vault there are large irregularly shaped lytic areas. This appearance is known as a geographical skull.

are seen in Langerhans histiocytosis (histiocytosis X), giving the appearance known as 'geographical skull' (Fig. 13.3), and in a form of Paget's disease known as osteoporosis circumscripta.

CT AND MRI

In most neurological disorders, plain films are either normal or the abnormalities are too non-specific for the diagnosis to be made. CT and MRI give vastly more information and one or other investigation is indicated in practically all patients with intracranial disease.

Computed tomography of the brain

A routine CT examination of the brain involves making 20–30 axial sections. The axial plane is the routine projection but computer reconstructions can be made from the axial sections, which then provide images in the coronal or sagittal planes (Fig. 13.4). The window settings are selected for the brain and are also altered to show the bones (Fig. 13.5).

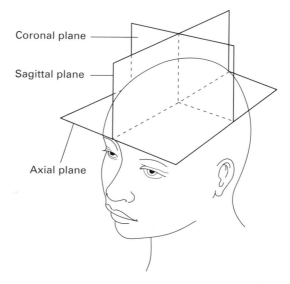

Fig. 13.4 Illustration of the axial, coronal and sagittal planes.

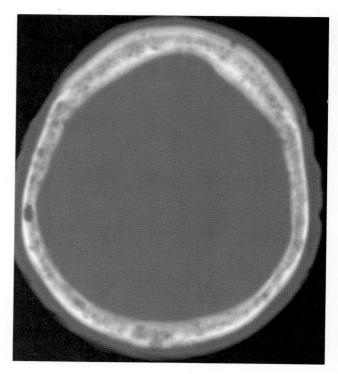

Fig. 13.5 Myeloma. Examination on bone windows shows multiple lytic lesions in the skull vault.

Contrast enhancement for CT

An intravenous injection of contrast medium is often given because an abnormality not seen on pre contrast scans may be rendered visible following contrast enhancement. Contrast enhancement is predominantly a consequence of breakdown of the blood–brain barrier allowing contrast to enter the lesion. Such breakdown occurs mainly with neoplasm, ischaemia and inflammation.

The use of contrast enhancement varies in different centres. It tends not to be used in patients who are known to have a very recent cerebral haemorrhage or infarct. Areas of calcification may be obscured on post contrast scans.

Normal head CT

A normal CT scan of the head is illustrated in Fig. 13.6. The cerebrospinal fluid (CSF) is seen as water density within the ventricular system and subarachnoid space, and is clearly different in density to the normal brain substance and it is possible to distinguish the white and grey matter of the brain. The larger arteries at the base of the brain as well as the venous sinuses can be recognized when opacified by contrast medium. The falx appears denser than the brain. Calcification may be seen in the pineal gland and choroid plexuses. The supratentorial regions are usually well shown, but details of the posterior fossa may be obscured by artefacts from the overlying temporal and occipital bones.

Abnormal head CT

When an abnormality is seen it is important to decide whether it has an intra-axial or extra-axial location. Intra-axial lesions involve the white and grey matter of the brain parenchyma, while extra-axial lesions involve the meninges, extracerebral spaces and skull vault.

The cardinal signs of an abnormality on a CT scan are:
- abnormal tissue density
- mass effect
- enlargement of the ventricles.

Abnormal tissue density

Abnormal tissue may be of higher or lower density than the normal surrounding brain. High density is seen with recent haemorrhage (see Fig. 13.21, p. 416), calcified lesions and areas of contrast enhancement (see Fig. 13.11, p. 407). Low density is usually due to neoplasms or infarcts, or to oedema, which commonly surrounds neoplasms, infarcts, haemorrhages and areas of inflammation. Oedema characteristically shows finger-like projections and does not enhance with intravenous contrast medium. As a rule, it is not possible to diagnose the nature of a mass based on attenuation values alone; an exception is lipoma which, because it contains fat, has a value of approximately minus 100 Hounsfield units.

Mass effect

The lateral ventricles should be examined to see if they are displaced or compressed. Shift of midline structures, such as the septum pellucidum (the thin membrane separating the lateral ventricles), the third ventricle, or the pineal, is a common finding with intracranial masses. Ventricular dilatation will occur if the mass obstructs the flow of CSF. Specific diagnoses are suggested by combining the clinical features with information about multiplicity, size, shape, position and density of the lesion, all of which are known with great accuracy from CT.

Enlargement of ventricles

There are two basic mechanisms which cause the cerebral ventricles to enlarge:
- Obstruction to the CSF pathway, either within the ventricular system (non-communicating hydrocephalus) or over the surface of the brain (communicating hydrocephalus) (Fig. 13.7).
- Secondary to atrophy of brain tissue (see Fig. 13.30, p. 422).

Computed tomography or MRI can provide an accurate picture of the size of the various ventricles, cerebral sulci and subarachnoid cisterns. With this information it may be possible to predict the nature of hydrocephalus.

CT angiography

Modern CT scanners can acquire slices very rapidly and the large volumes of high resolution data are ideal for three-dimensional imaging and can be subjected to

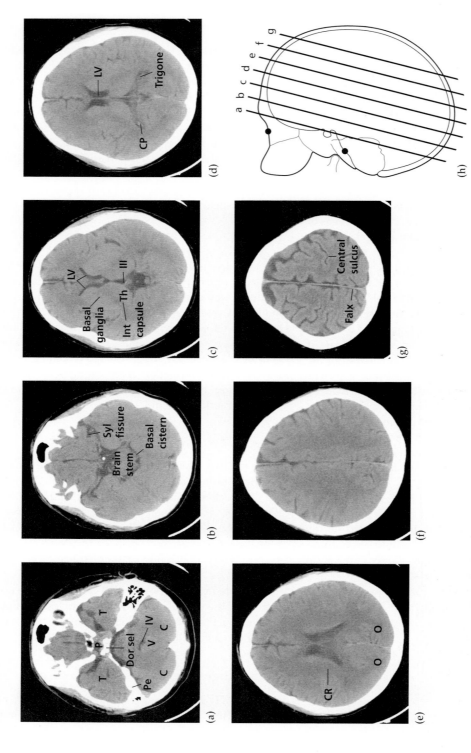

Fig. 13.6 Normal head CT. The images on the page opposite are representative sections from a post contrast series. Those on this page are the pre contrast images from the same patient. The levels at which the sections were taken are indicated in the diagram. aca, anterior cerebral artery; bas art, basilar artery; C, cerebellar hemisphere; Cav sinus, cavernous sinus; CP, choroid plexus; CR, corona radiata; Dor sel, dorsum sellae; F, frontal lobe; III, third ventricle; IV, fourth ventricle; Int capsule, internal capsule; int cer v, internal cerebral vein; LV, lateral ventricle; mca, middle cerebral artery; O, occipital lobe; P, pituitary gland; Par, parietal lobe; pca, posterior cerebral artery; Pe, petrous bone; str sinus, straight sinus; sup sag sinus, superior sagittal sinus; T, temporal lobe; Th, thalamus; Syl fissure, Sylvian fissure; V, vermis.

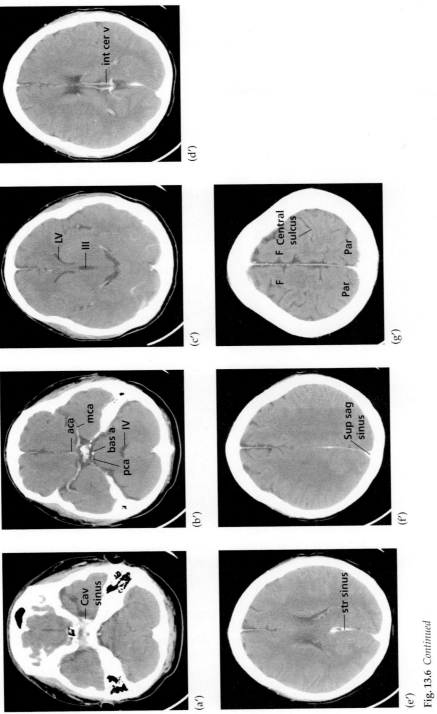

Fig. 13.6 *Continued*

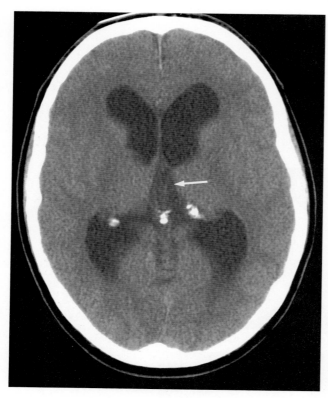

Fig. 13.7 Hydrocephalus. The lateral ventricles and third ventricle (arrow) are dilated but the fourth ventricle is normal in size. The hydrocephalus was due to stenosis of the aqueduct, which connects the third and fourth ventricles.

post-processing techniques. CT angiography has replaced conventional angiography for the diagnosis of arterial occlusions, aneurysms and arteriovenous malformations. The venous phase of the angiogram can give information on the venous sinuses of the brain. The data can be subjected to computer manipulation and an example of a three-dimensional surface-rendered reconstruction of an occipital arteriovenous malformation is shown in Plate 8.

Perfusion of selected portions of the brain can be assessed with CT angiography, which is valuable in the early diagnosis of stroke.

MRI of the brain

The routine techniques used for MRI vary from centre to centre. Axial, coronal and sagittal projections are all considered standard (Fig. 13.8) and two of these are usually chosen for a routine examination. This multiplanar capability is particularly useful for assessing the extent of pituitary tumours and for visualizing structures in the posterior fossa and craniovertebral junction. A variety of signal sequences are used to create the images: particularly T1-weighted and T2-weighted images.

It is possible to recognize flowing blood and, therefore, the larger arteries and veins stand out clearly without the need for contrast medium. The characteristics of grey and white matter are different, and both are clearly different from the CSF in the ventricular system and subarachnoid space. Therefore, the anatomy of the brain can be exquisitely displayed.

The disadvantages of MRI compared with CT are the inability to show calcification, lack of bone detail, the relative expense of the technique, and the difficulty of monitoring seriously ill patients whilst lying within the scanner.

Contrast enhancement for MRI

Although the natural differences in MRI signal intensity are great, contrast agents are often used to give additional information. Like the intravenous iodinated agents used for CT, the gadolinium compounds used for MRI enhancement are excluded from the normal brain substance by the blood–brain barrier (they do, however, accumulate in the pituitary gland). Breakdown of the blood–brain barrier by tumours, abscess and infarcts means that gadolinium will accumulate within these pathological processes. The tissues containing the gadolinium show very high signal intensity (i.e. they appear white) on T1-weighted images.

Magnetic resonance angiography

Magnetic resonance angiography (MRA) of the vascular system (Fig. 13.9) has now developed to such an extent that it can be used to show arterial and venous anatomy, as well as disorders such as occlusions, stenoses and aneurysms, and has replaced conventional arteriography.

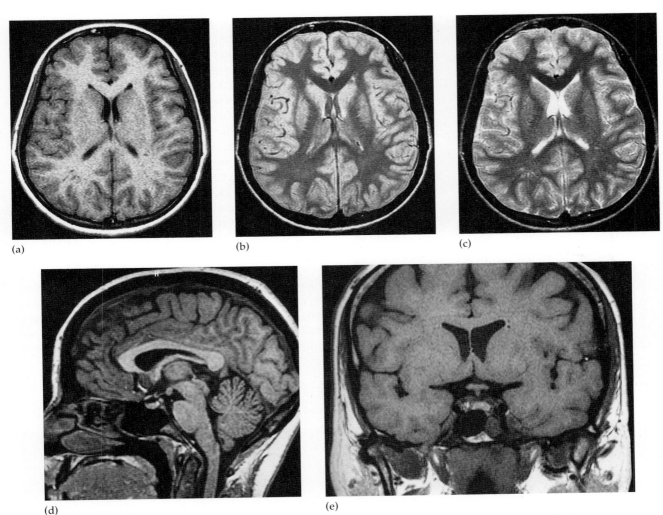

(a)　　　　　　　　　　(b)　　　　　　　　　　(c)

(d)　　　　　　　　　　(e)

Fig. 13.8 Normal brain MRI. The top row of images are axial sections at the level of the lateral ventricles. (a) T1-weighted image. (b) Proton density. (c) T2-weighted image. The bottom two images are (d) a midline sagittal section (T1-weighted) and (e) a coronal section through the level of the frontal horns (T1-weighted).

Abnormal MRI of the brain

The range of abnormalities that can be shown by MRI is very great. Fat, subacute and chronic haemorrhage, oedema, CSF and flowing blood all have characteristic signal intensities. Thus, it is more often possible to make a specific diagnosis of an intracranial disorder with MRI than with CT. Nevertheless, many mass lesions, such as the various cerebral neoplasms and infections, can be almost indistinguishable. A noteworthy feature of MRI is its ability to demonstrate plaques of demyelination in multiple sclerosis (see Fig. 13.29, p. 422) and abnormal blood vessels such as arteriovenous malformations (see Fig. 13.25, p. 418), so making it the imaging modality of choice for these conditions. MRI is the preferred investigation in encephalitis and both epilepsy and congenital malformations in children.

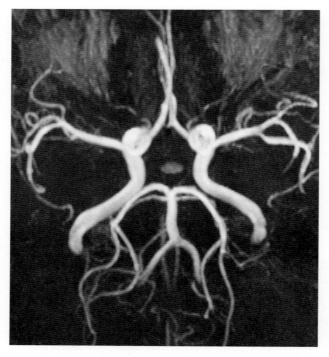

With the recent advent of fast scanning techniques, various sequences have been introduced. Perfusion imaging, using intravenous contrast, assesses arterial flow and tissue perfusion. Diffusion imaging depends on the random diffusion of water molecules in tissues which may be altered in pathological states, so generating a difference in contrast between an area of pathology and surrounding normal tissue. Diffusion and perfusion scans are proving very useful for the early diagnosis of stroke as they show very early changes. A mathematical computation of the diffusion weighted images is known as an apparent diffusion coefficient (ADC) map.

An advance in diffusion weighting has enabled the white matter to be imaged to demonstrate the location and orientation of the tracts: an investigation known as tractography which is helpful for surgical planning and for studying white matter pathways in disease.

Functional MRI depends on the contrast from blood oxygen levels. Neuronal activity alters the ratio of oxy- and deoxyhaemoglobin levels, which can be measured to produce a map of neuronal activation. The technique may be useful in understanding brain function particularly in psychiatric disorders.

Fig. 13.9 Magnetic resonance angiography (MRA). The arteries at the base of the brain, the circle of Willis, are very well shown by MRA without the use of any contrast agent.

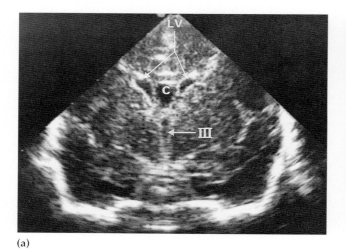

(a)

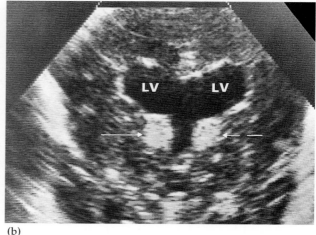

(b)

Fig. 13.10 Neurosonography. (a) Normal coronal section taken through the anterior fontanelle in a neonate. C, cavum septum pellucidum; III, third ventricle; LV, lateral ventricle. (b) Coronal section showing bilateral subependymal haemorrhages (arrows). The lateral ventricles are dilated.

Neurosonography (Fig. 13.10)

With ultrasound it is simple to scan the heads of neonates and young babies to obtain images of the ventricular system and the adjacent brain. Scanning is best done through an open fontanelle where there is no bone to impede the transmission of ultrasound. Little discomfort is caused to the baby and the procedure is readily carried out even on ill babies in intensive care units. Neurosonography has proved particularly useful in detecting intracerebral haemorrhage and the ventricular dilatation that may follow. It has also been used to demonstrate the presence and cause of other forms of hydrocephalus and congenital abnormalities of the brain.

Specific brain disorders

Brain tumours

Glioma

At CT (Fig. 13.11a), a glioma typically appears as a solitary, irregular mass surrounded by oedema. Compression or displacement of the ventricles can usually be demonstrated. The CT attenuation values of the tumour itself are usually low, but may be high or mixed. Gliomas may calcify; some, particularly the low grade tumours, may be very densely calcified. For accurate detection of gliomas both pre and post contrast scans should be performed. Most gliomas show

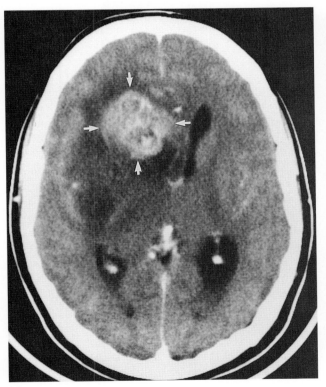

(a)

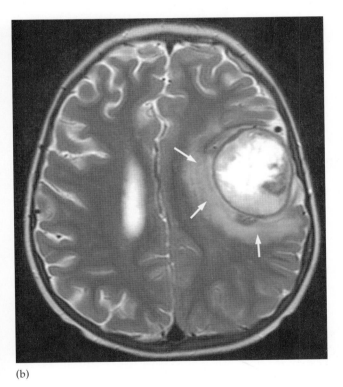

(b)

Fig. 13.11 Glioma. (a) CT scan, post i.v. contrast, showing round mass (arrows) with contrast enhancement and surrounding oedema. Note the compression and displacement of the adjacent lateral ventricles. (b) MRI scan (T2-weighted) in another patient, showing a large, high-intensity rounded lesion with displacement and compression of the adjacent ventricular system. The high-intensity tumour is surrounded by oedema (arrows).

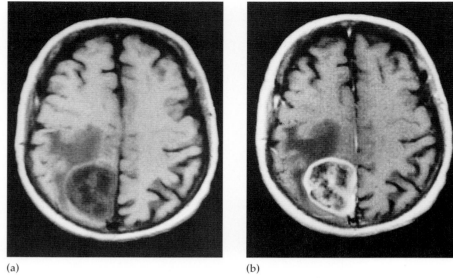

(a)   (b)

Fig. 13.12 Glioma. (a) Pre and (b) post contrast enhancement (with intravenous gadolinium) shows the obvious partial enhancement of the tumour. Note the adjacent low intensity white matter oedema.

partial enhancement with intravenous contrast medium; sometimes only the outer portion enhances, giving a so-called ring enhancement pattern.

AT MRI, the signs are basically the same as for CT. The essential features are a mass, often with adjacent oedema. The mass may show a variety of signal intensities. In general, the tumour is lower in signal intensity than the normal brain on the T1-weighted images and higher in signal intensity on the T2-weighted images (Fig. 13.11b). Calcification, though sometimes recognizable as absence of signal, is less evident than it is with CT. The enhancement pattern with gadolinium is similar to the pattern of contrast enhancement at CT (Fig. 13.12).

Brain metastases (Fig. 13.13)

Metastases in the brain may be of high or low density at CT. They usually show contrast enhancement and are often surrounded by substantial oedema. The MRI features are essentially similar. Metastases are typically multiple. A solitary metastasis is indistinguishable from a primary intracerebral brain tumour with either technique.

Meningioma

Meningiomas arise from the meninges of the vault, falx or tentorium in characteristic sites, the commonest being the parasagittal region over the cerebral convexities and the sphenoid ridges. On an unenhanced CT scan, a meningioma is slightly denser than the brain because of fine calcium in the lesion (Fig. 13.14a). Following intravenous contrast injection the tumour shows marked enhancement (Fig. 13.14b). Sclerosis and thickening of the adjacent bone may also be seen.

The multiplanar imaging capability of MRI makes it possible to predict the site of origin of the tumour with greater confidence than is usually possible with CT (Fig. 13.15). Once it can be ascertained that the tumour is extra-axial and compressing the brain from outside, the diagnosis of meningioma becomes highly likely.

Acoustic neuroma

Neurofibromas of the acoustic nerve arise in the internal auditory canal or immediately adjacent to the internal auditory meatus in the cerebellopontine angle. When large, they can be recognized at CT or MRI. When small, they may only be identifiable with MRI. Contrast enhancement improves their visibility with either technique (Fig. 13.16).

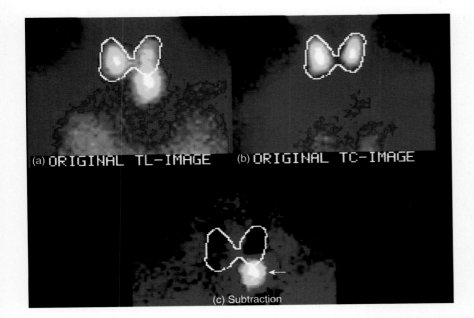

(a) ORIGINAL TL-IMAGE (b) ORIGINAL TC-IMAGE

(c) Subtraction

Plate 7 Parathyroid adenoma. (a) Thallium scan. Uptake occurs in the parathyroid adenoma and in the thyroid gland. (b) Pertechnetate scan. The pertechnetate is taken up by the thyroid gland and its outline has been drawn in. (c) Subtraction of the pertechnetate from the thallium scan reveals uptake in the parathyroid adenoma (arrow).

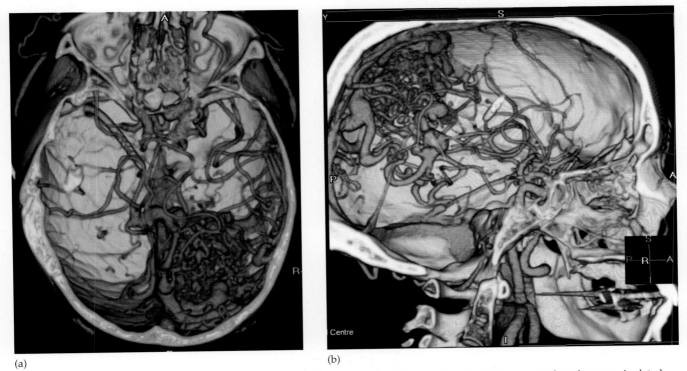

(a)

(b)

Plate 8 Occipital arteriovenous malformation. CT angiogram. (a) axial, (b) sagittal. The data from the CT angiogram have been manipulated to remove brain tissue and to highlight the vascular anatomy so that both the arterial supply and draining veins are demonstrated.

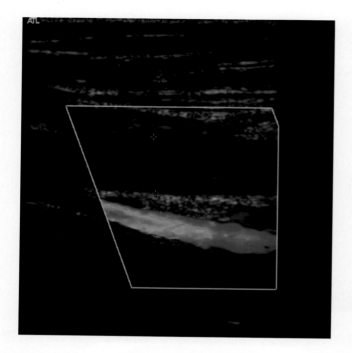

Plate 9 Colour duplex ultrasound. No flow is seen in the superficial femoral vein (between callipers) which also demonstrates increased echogenicity in the lumen diagnostic of deep vein thrombosis.

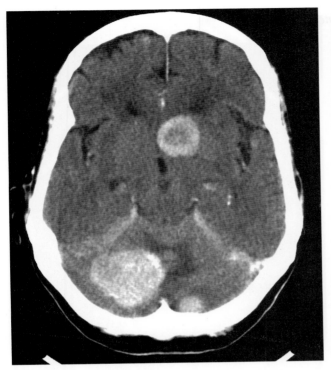

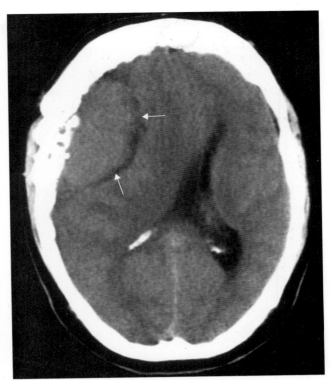

(a)

Fig. 13.13 Metastases. Enhanced CT scan showing several metastases as rounded areas of increased density.

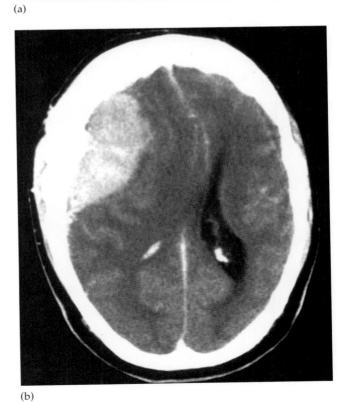

(b)

Fig. 13.14 Meningioma. (a) Pre contrast CT scan showing that the density of the meningioma (arrows) is slightly greater than the brain substance. (b) Enhanced scan showing marked contrast enhancement of the tumour. Note the thickening of the overlying bone.

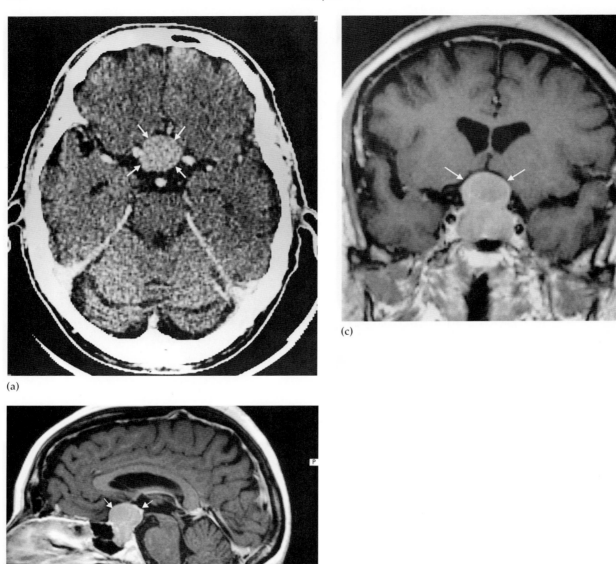

Fig. 13.17 Pituitary tumour. (a) Computed tomography scan after contrast shows a mass in the pituitary fossa which enhances vividly (arrows). (b) Sagittal MRI scan showing a tumour extending superiorly (arrows). (c) Coronal MRI, post contrast scan, in another patient showing a pituitary tumour (arrows).

Pituitary tumours

Pituitary tumours are divided into macroadenomas (>1 cm) and microadenomas (<1 cm). Large tumours may cause enlargement of the pituitary fossa.

Computed tomography can show a pituitary tumour (Fig. 13.17a), but MRI is now the investigation employed and is excellent for demonstrating the presence and extent of a pituitary tumour and can readily demonstrate its relationship to the optic chiasm and optic nerves which become compressed by upward extension of the tumour (Fig. 13.17b and c). The combined sagittal and coronal imaging planes are ideal, showing very small tumours, smaller than can be seen with CT. Gadolinium enhancement is particularly useful for finding microadenomas of the pituitary when the tumour is seen as a low intensity region compared with the normally enhancing pituitary gland (Fig. 13.18).

Stroke

Stroke is defined as a sudden focal neurological deterioration and is a common cause of hospital admission with a high morbidity. The important causes of stroke are:

- cerebral ischaemia and infarction
- cerebral haemorrhage
- subarachnoid haemorrhage.

Acute cerebral infarction and haemorrhage are often clinically similar, but it is important to distinguish between these two conditions as subsequent investigation and treatment differ. Infarction occurs much more commonly than haemorrhage. Patients with stroke should be imaged with CT as soon as possible to exclude a haemorrhage so that appropriate treatment can be instituted without delay. CT angiography may be helpful if patients are considered for thrombolysis. Diffusion-weighted MRI is more sensitive than unenhanced CT for acute stroke imaging.

Cerebral infarction

Following a thrombotic or embolic occlusion of a cerebral artery, an area of the brain may become ischaemic and undergo infarction. Changes of acute infarction are not usually recognized on CT before 6 hours when subtle signs of reduced parenchymal attenuation due to oedema may be

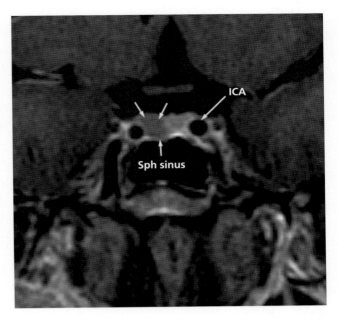

Fig. 13.18 Very small pituitary adenoma (microadenoma). Post-gadolinium contrast image showing the normal portion of the gland enhances whereas the adenoma (arrows) does not enhance. ICA, internal carotid artery; Sph sinus, sphenoid sinus.

seen. Over the next few days the infarct evolves into a low attenuation area conforming to the shape of a recognizable arterial distribution (Fig. 13.19). The infarct may gradually resolve, leaving an atrophic area and/or a persistent scar. Routine MRI scanning will detect abnormalities, which are most obvious as hyperintense areas on a T2-weighted scan, within 8 hours of the onset of symptoms. Enhancement with gadolinium shows changes sooner while special fast scanning techniques such as perfusion/diffusion scans show changes within minutes of the onset of symptoms. Diffusion-weighted imaging is the best method for the early detection of an infarct (Fig. 13.20). There is a brief period after the onset of symptoms when systemic thrombolysis is likely to be successful. Thrombolysis is most beneficial if given within 3 hours of the onset of symptoms. Because of its ability to make an early diagnosis of stroke, it is likely that MRI will come to play an increasingly important diagnostic role.

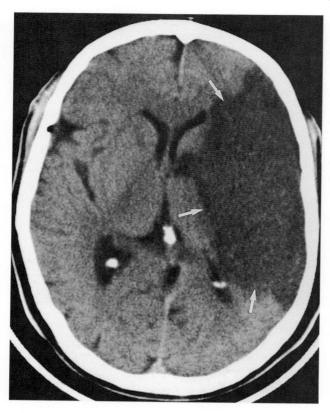

Fig. 13.19 Cerebral infarction. (a) Unenhanced CT scan showing a low density region of the left cerebral hemisphere conforming to the distribution of the middle cerebral artery (arrows).

taken. Endarterectomy or angioplasty has been shown to be beneficial in patients where there is a stenosis of more than 70% of the diameter of the artery.

Cerebral haemorrhage

Haemorrhage is demonstrable on CT immediately after the event as a region of high attenuation frequently causing mass effect. Depending on the site and amount of bleeding, blood may also be identified in the subarachnoid space and within the ventricles (Fig. 13.21). The initial high density of haemorrhage lessens over the following week or two leaving a low-density area indistinguishable from an infarct. Haemorrhage can be seen on MRI. In the subacute and chronic phases, MRI is the preferred investigation as haematoma develops a specific signal pattern owing to the breakdown products of haemoglobin which have a paramagnetic effect that profoundly alters the MR signal in a way which can be recognized on T1- and T2-weighted scans (Fig. 13.22).

Subarachnoid haemorrhage

Subarachnoid haemorrhage is usually due to a ruptured intracranial aneurysm or less commonly an arteriovenous malformation. CT is the best initial investigation to diagnose a subarachnoid haemorrhage and to demonstrate the site of bleeding.

A subarachnoid haemorrhage is recognized by high density blood in the cortical sulci, Sylvian fissures and basal cisterns. CT will also show any intracerebral haemorrhage or blood in the ventricles (Fig. 13.23). Diagnosing a subarachnoid haemorrhage on CT can obviate the need for lumbar puncture and CSF examination, but it should be realized that a normal CT examination does not exclude the diagnosis.

Only large aneurysms can be seen directly on contrast-enhanced CT. With multidetector CT, an unenhanced routine head CT is followed by CT angiography as a single investigation to diagnose subarachnoid haemorrhage, localize the bleeding and demonstrate the aneurysm. If multiple aneurysms are found, CT may indicate which aneurysm has bled.

Patients whose symptoms resolve within 24 hours are referred to as having a transient ischaemic attack (TIA). A common cause for a TIA is embolus from an atheromatous stenosis of the internal carotid artery. The presence of atheromatous plaque and degree of stenosis can be assessed with Doppler ultrasound of the neck. Ultrasound can also demonstrate a dissection of the carotid artery in the neck. The cerebral vessels may be imaged non-invasively with MR angiography (Fig. 13.20d and e). When non-invasive imaging is inconclusive and endarterectomy or angioplasty is being contemplated then arteriography is under-

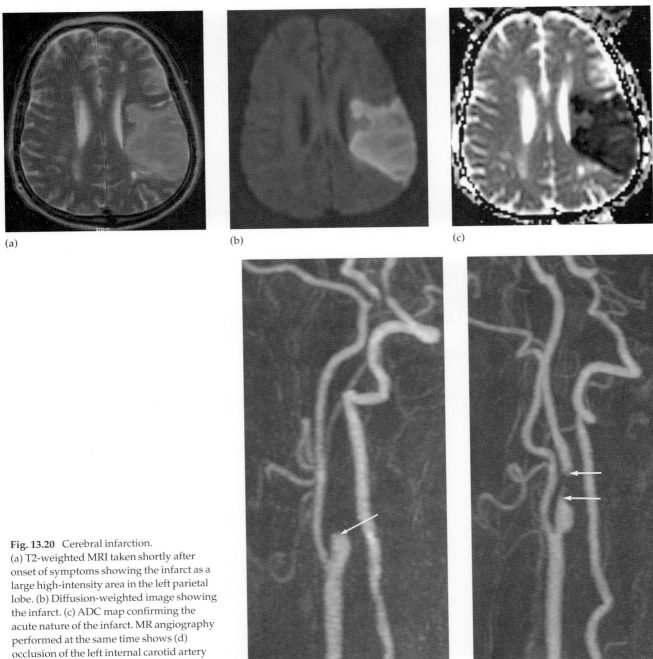

(a)

(b)

(c)

(d)

(e)

Fig. 13.20 Cerebral infarction.
(a) T2-weighted MRI taken shortly after onset of symptoms showing the infarct as a large high-intensity area in the left parietal lobe. (b) Diffusion-weighted image showing the infarct. (c) ADC map confirming the acute nature of the infarct. MR angiography performed at the same time shows (d) occlusion of the left internal carotid artery (arrow). (e) High-grade stenosis of the right internal carotid artery (arrows).

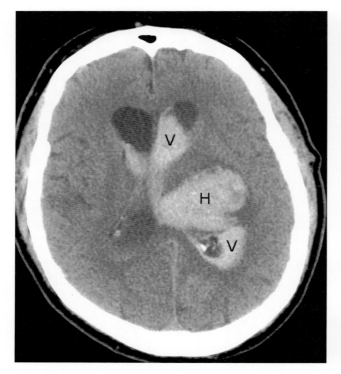

Fig. 13.21 Intracerebral haemorrhage. CT scan showing the haematoma as a high-density area (H) in the left basal ganglia. Blood has ruptured through into the ventricles (V). The patient was hypertensive.

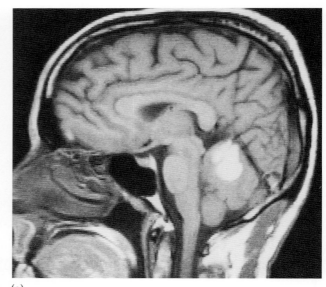

(a)

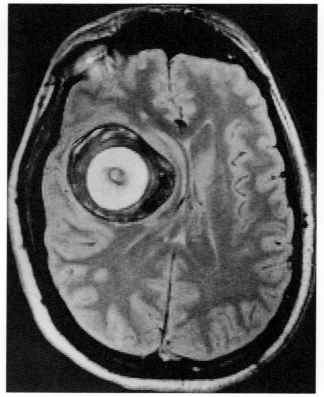

(b)

Fig. 13.22 Cerebral haemorrhage on MRI. (a) A 7-day-old haemorrhage into the superior portion of the cerebellum is clearly shown as a high signal intensity collection on a T1-weighted image. (b) A chronic haemorrhage in the right cerebral hemisphere shows the complex mixture of high and low signals typical of old haemorrhage.

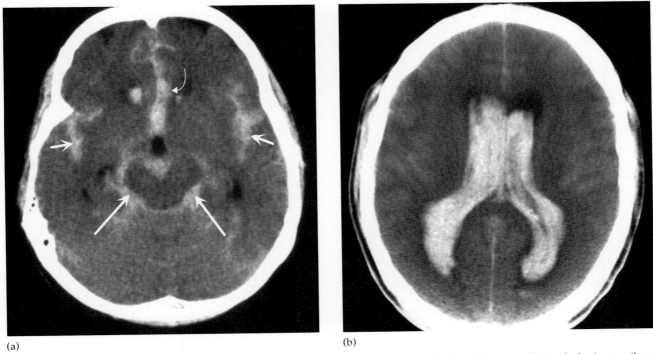

(a)   (b)

Fig. 13.23 Subarachnoid haemorrhage. (a) High-density subarachnoid blood can be seen in the basal cisterns outlining the brain stem (long arrows), the Sylvian tissues (short arrows) and adjacent to the falx (curved arrow). (b) In this patient the blood is mainly in the ventricles.

Aneurysms can nowadays be treated with interventional radiological microcatheter techniques by occluding the aneurysm with metal coils which invoke thrombosis of the lumen of the aneurysm (see Fig. 15.12, p. 446).

Arteriovenous malformation

Arteriovenous malformations may present with haemorrhage. CT can demonstrate the abnormal vessels in the region of the haemorrhage, particularly with contrast enhancement (Fig. 13.24). MRI is particularly suitable for demon-strating arteriovenous malformations, because the signal from fast-flowing blood even without intravenous contrast agent is so very different from that of stationary tissues (Fig. 13.25). It has become the best

method of investigation to confirm or exclude this particular diagnosis. MRI is better than CT in demonstrating subacute or chronic haemorrhage. As with aneurysms, angiography is then needed to define the vascular anatomy for those cases where surgery or percutaneous transvascular embolism is contemplated (Fig. 13.26, Plate 8).

Infection

In acute *meningitis* CT and MRI are usually normal. If meningitis is suspected clinically, antibiotic treatment should start immediately and not await the result of a scan. A lumbar puncture is frequently performed to obtain CSF to confirm the diagnosis. A CT scan prior to lumbar

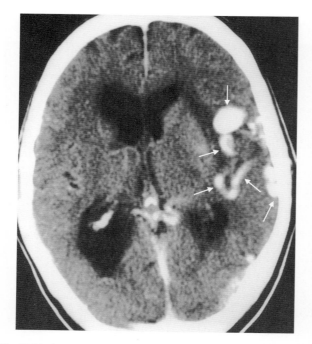

Fig. 13.24 Arteriovenous malformation. Enhanced CT scan showing the enlarged abnormal vessels (arrows).

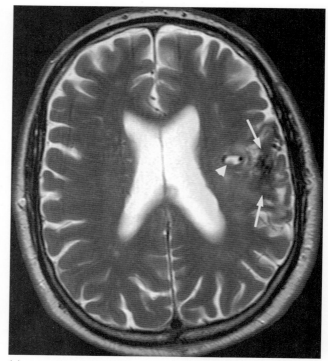

(a)

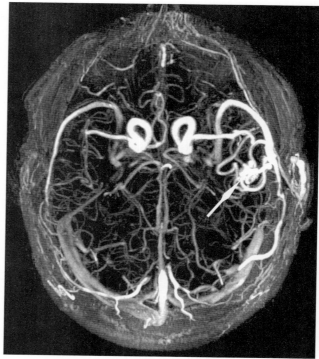

(b)

Fig. 13.25 Arteriovenous malformation. (a) MRI scan (T2-weighted) showing signal void from fast-flowing blood in the vascular malformation(arrows). The high signal area (arrow head) is due to a previous haemorrhage. (b) MR angiogram showing the malformation in the left parietal region (arrow).

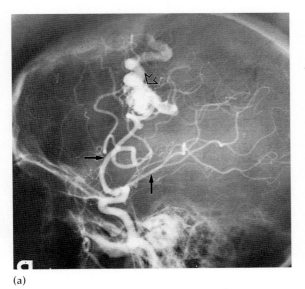

(a)

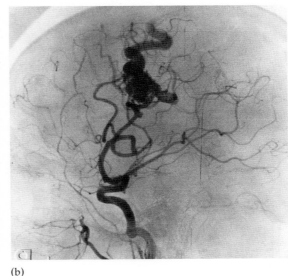

(b)

Fig. 13.26 Arteriovenous malformation. (a) Carotid angiogram showing a collection of large abnormal vessels (large open arrow) supplied by the middle cerebral artery (horizontal arrow.) On this injection the posterior cerebral artery (vertical arrow), but not the anterior cerebral artery, has filled. (b) Subtraction. With this technique the shadowing due to the bones has almost been eliminated so that the contrast-filled vessels stand out more clearly.

puncture is only essential if there is evidence of raised intracranial pressure, focal neurological signs or change in conscious level; the CT scan may show hydrocephalus in such patients.

Encephalitis is caused by infection, usually viral or by an immune reaction to infection. CT and MRI show unilateral or bilateral focal abnormal areas, often in a characteristic distribution appearing as low attenuation on CT and high signal on a T2-weighted MRI scan (Fig. 13.27).

An *abscess* can be caused by pyogenic, tuberculous, fungal or parasitic organisms. Necrosis and pus formation occur in the centre of the abscess, which appears as low density on CT. The wall of the abscess enhances with intravenous contrast and may be surrounded by oedema giving an appearance known as ring enhancement (Fig. 13.28a). Similar changes are seen with MRI.

Patients with AIDS have a high incidence of opportunistic brain infection. Herpes encephalitis may give a near

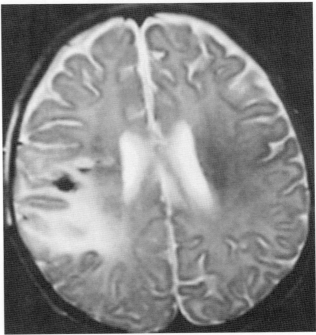

Fig. 13.27 Encephalitis. T2-weighted MRI showing a high signal area in the right parietal area due to herpes simplex.

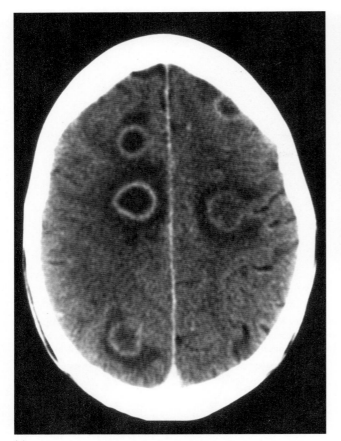

(a)

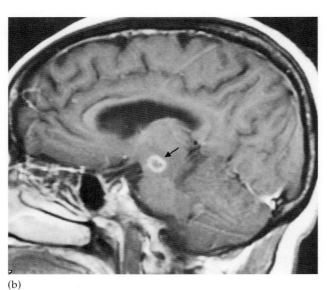

(b)

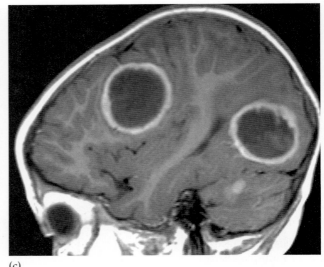

(c)

Fig. 13.28 Cerebral abscess. (a) Post contrast CT scan showing several abscesses which have central low density and marked enhancement at the edge of the abscess. (b) Small cerebral abscess in a patient with AIDS. MRI scan T1-weighted, post contrast shows a ring enhancing lesion in the upper brain stem (arrow). (c) Magnetic resonance imaging scan, T1-weighted post contrast, showing fungal abscesses in a child treated for leukaemia.

diagnostic appearance of enhancing areas at CT, or altered signal intensity on MR scanning, in the temporal lobes. Multiple ring enhancing round lesions on CT or MRI are typical of toxoplasmosis or other cerebral abscesses (Fig. 13.28b and c). Progressive multifocal leucoencephalopathy (PML) is due to the JC virus, which causes regions of demyelination. These are seen as oedematous areas of brain with no surrounding abnormal enhancement. Fungal infections such as cryptococcosis may occur, as may also mycobacterial infections.

Multiple sclerosis

Magnetic resonance imaging is the key imaging modality for multiple sclerosis. It is useful not only in diagnosis, especially if this is uncertain clinically, but also to assess the progress of the disease.

Plaques of demyelination are seen in the white matter, particularly in the periventricular regions as areas of high signal on a T2-weighted scan (Fig. 13.29). Contrast enhancement occurs with acute plaques because of inflammation and breakdown of the blood–brain barrier, but enhancement is not seen with subacute or chronic lesions.

Ageing

Changes are seen on CT and MRI in elderly patients, which often bear little or no correlation with the clinical state of the patient. Atrophy of the brain occurs resulting in dilatation of the ventricles and widening of the cortical sulci. Ischaemia gives rise to low attenuation areas in the deep white matter on CT, particularly well seen in the periventricular regions and small infarcts in the brain substance, particularly in the basal ganglia and capsular regions. Similar changes are seen at MRI.

Dementia

With the increasing number of elderly patients in the population the problem of dementia is going to intensify. Patients with dementia are imaged to exclude a treatable lesion such as hydrocephalus, tumour or subdural haematoma.

In Alzheimer's disease, the commonest form of dementia, both CT and MRI show dilated ventricles, widened cortical sulci and ill-defined white matter abnormalities (Fig. 13.30). Atrophy of the temporal lobes occurs before generalized atrophy. In multi-infarct dementia there are multiple areas of infarction of varying size. These two types of dementia can also be diagnosed with a radionuclide scan using ^{99m}Tc-HMPAO, an agent which crosses the blood–brain barrier.

Head injury

The aim of imaging is to identify those patients with brain injury, and, importantly, those with intracranial haematoma that may require urgent neurosurgical treatment. Such changes may occur with normal skull films, and CT is now the accepted method of investigation. Guidelines have been promulgated for those patients needing CT: a reduced conscious level, suspected fracture, vomiting, seizure or focal neurology.

In the rare event of CT being unavailable and in a skeletal survey for non-accidental injury, a fracture may be demonstrated on a skull x-ray as a translucent line with straight edges. Fractures must be distinguished from lines due to vascular markings or sutures (Fig. 13.31).

In an unconscious patient with a head injury with a high risk of a cervical spine injury, a CT of the cervical spine is carried out with the head CT scan, as adequate x-rays are difficult to achieve in the unconscious patient.

Computed tomography in head injury

Computed tomography is performed without intravenous contrast administration and it is essential to view the scans on both brain and bone window settings. Computed tomography can distinguish between extracerebral and intracerebral lesions and can separate those patients with compressing haematomas who require immediate surgery. CT can also demonstrate fluid levels in the sinuses and mastoid air cells suggesting a facial or skull base fracture, air in the orbits and in severe head injury, air in the cranial cavity. Examination on bone windows can demonstrate fractures of the skull vault, face or skull base.

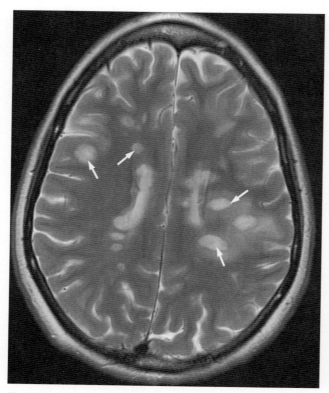

Fig. 13.29 Multiple sclerosis. MRI scan, T2-weighted, showing plaques of demyelination as high signal in the white matter. Arrows point to representative plaques.

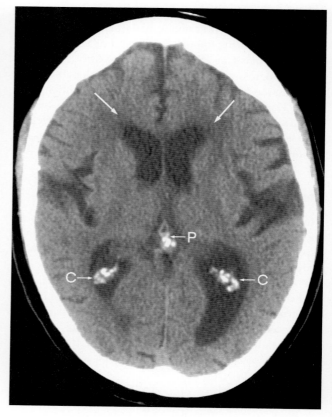

Fig. 13.30 Cerebral atrophy. The ventricles are dilated with rounded anterior horns and the cortical sulci are widened. Ischaemic changes are seen as periventricular white matter lucency (arrows). Normal calcification is seen in the pineal (P) and choroid plexuses (C).

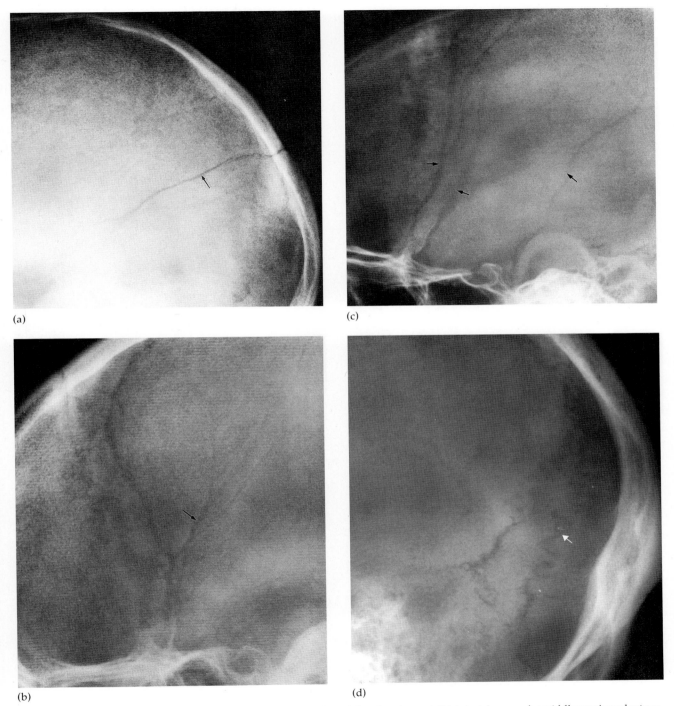

Fig. 13.31 Linear markings in the skull vault. (a) Fracture line with straight edges (arrow). (b) Arterial groove for middle meningeal artery (arrow) – line with straight edges occupying a recognized site. (c) Venous channels: wider, more undulating grooves (arrows) – the more posterior groove ends in a venous star. (d) Suture: shows regular interdigitations (arrow).

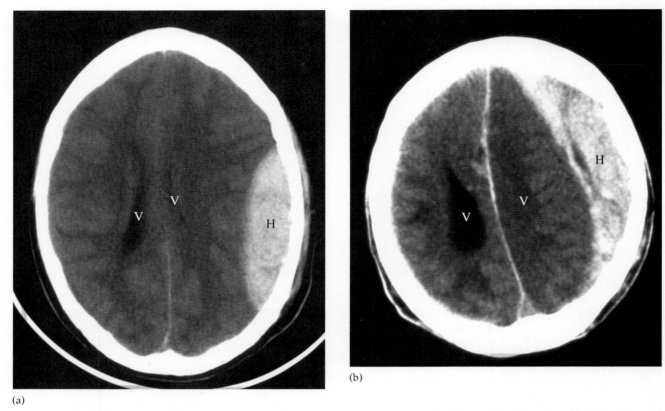

(a)

(b)

Fig. 13.32 Acute extracerebral haematoma. (a) Extradural haematoma. CT scan showing a high-density lentiform area. (b) Subdural haematoma showing a high density area paralleling the surface of the brain. Note the ventricular displacement in both cases. H, haematoma; V, ventricle.

Extracerebral haematomas

Extracerebral haematomas show a high density for about 1–2 weeks following the injury (Fig. 13.32), but after 3–4 weeks the density decreases to become lower than that of the brain (Fig. 13.33). In the intervening period, haematomas pass through a phase of being isodense with the brain and are, therefore, less obvious on CT scans taken without contrast. Nevertheless, they should be suspected if there is midline or ventricular displacement. The displacement may not be obvious if the haematomas are bilateral.

Extradural haematoma is seen as a lens-shaped, smoothly demarcated, high-density area situated over the surface of the hemisphere associated with a skull fracture (Fig. 13.32a).

Subdural haematoma conforms to the shape of the underlying brain and occurs most commonly over the convexity of the brain, but can also arise along the falx and tentorium (Fig. 13.32b). A fracture somewhere in the skull may or may not be present.

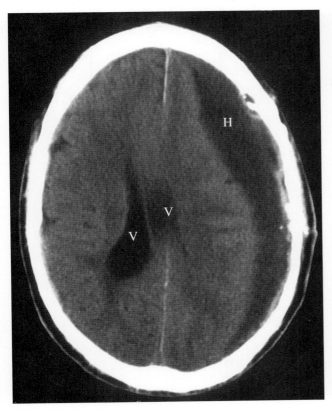

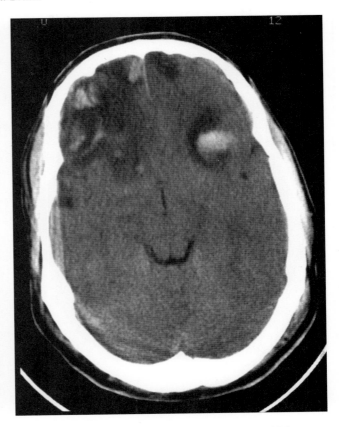

Fig. 13.33 Chronic subdural haematoma. CT scan a month after injury shows the haematoma (H) as a low density area. Note the ventricular displacement. V, ventricle.

Fig. 13.34 Contusion. CT scan showing bilateral frontal lobe contusions. The low density is due to oedema; the high-density areas are focal haemorrhages.

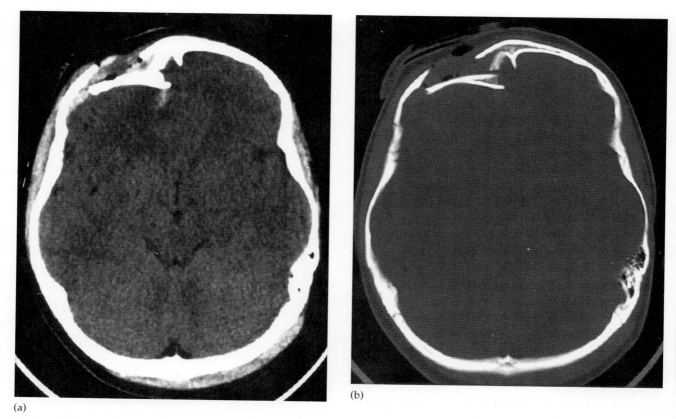

(a)

(b)

Fig. 13.35 Depressed fracture. (a) Brain. (b) Bone window settings. The depressed fracture and bone fragments are more clearly seen on the bone window settings. Such fractures may require surgical elevation.

Intracerebral lesions

Oedema. Post-traumatic oedema may cause the whole brain to swell with homogeneous low density and compression of the ventricles.

Contusions are bruises of the brain which appear as areas of low attenuation and may be associated with high-density areas due to haemorrhage (Fig. 13.34).

Intracerebral haematomas are seen as areas of high density, which may be multifocal. There may be mass effect causing displacement of the ventricles and accompanying brain oedema.

Fractures

Fractures of the skull base or vault should be looked for on bone window settings (Fig. 13.35). Fractures of the skull vault should not be confused with sutures. Assessment should be made of any depression of the fracture, involvement of the paranasal sinuses, sphenoid, petrous and occipital bones as various neurological complications may occur with such fractures.

14

Sinuses, Orbits and Neck

Sinuses

On plain radiographs the normal sinuses are transradiant because they contain air. Plain films have a role in showing mucosal thickening, fluid levels, bone destruction and fractures. However, in sinus disease computed tomography (CT) is often the preferred technique as it gives much better images of the sinuses. Magnetic resonance imaging (MRI) also demonstrates the sinuses well, but is rarely needed as the primary investigation.

Thickened mucosa can be recognized providing there is some air in the sinus (Figs 14.1 and 14.2), by noting the soft tissue density between the air in the sinus and the bony wall. The mucosal thickening may be smooth in outline or it may be polypoid. Polyps may be sufficiently large to extend into the nasopharynx.

Allergy and infection both cause mucosal thickening and it is impossible to say radiologically which condition is responsible. Such changes may also be seen in asymptomatic people.

Acute sinusitis is often diagnosed and treated clinically, but CT is recommended if symptoms persist. Both CT and MRI can elegantly demonstrate mucosal thickening and fluid levels as well as displaying the bony walls of the sinuses. Sinus anatomy is ideally demonstrated with coronal CT sections. This information shows the drainage sites of the frontal, ethmoid and maxillary sinuses into the middle meatus and is a great aid for the surgeon planning endoscopic sinus surgery (Fig. 14.2).

The opaque sinus

The sinus becomes opaque when all the air is replaced.

The causes of an opaque sinus are:
- *Infection or allergy*. The air in the sinus is replaced by fluid, or a grossly thickened mucosa, or a combination of the two.
- *Mucocele*. Mucoceles are obstructed sinuses. Secretions accumulate and the sinus becomes expanded. A frontal sinus mucocele may erode the roof of the orbit and cause exophthalmos. Computed tomography clearly shows the size and extent of a mucocele.
- *Carcinoma of the sinus or nasal cavity*. In all opaque sinuses, particularly the antra, special attention should be paid on CT to the bony margins, because if these are destroyed the diagnosis of carcinoma becomes almost certain

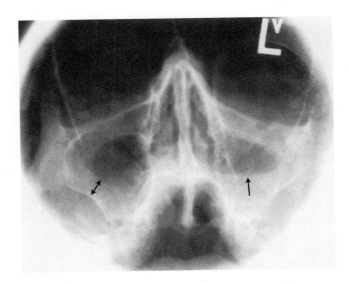

Fig. 14.1 Mucosal thickening and a fluid level. In the right antrum thickening of the mucosa (arrows) results in the sinus no longer having a thin outline. The horizontal line in the left antrum on this erect film (arrow) indicates a fluid level which remains horizontal even when the patient's head is tilted.

Diagnostic Imaging, 6th Edition. By Peter Armstrong, Martin Wastie and Andrea Rockall. Published 2009 by Blackwell Publishing. ISBN: 978-1-4051-7039.

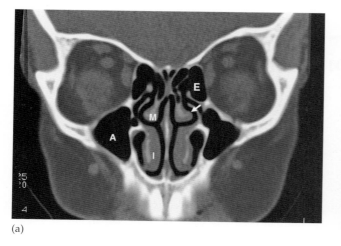

(a)

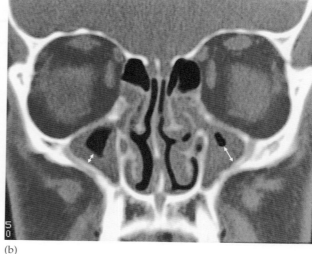

(b)

Fig. 14.2 Coronal CT scan. (a) Normal sinuses. Note the excellent demonstration of the bony margins. The arrow points to the middle meatus into which the maxillary antrum, frontal, anterior and middle ethmoid sinuses drain. The region where all these sinuses drain is known as the osteomeatal complex. A, maxillary antrum; E, ethmoid sinus; I, inferior turbinate; M, middle turbinate. (b) Sinusitis. Mucosal thickening prevents drainage of the sinuses. Both antra are almost opaque. The arrows indicate mucosal thickening in the antra.

(Fig. 14.3). Computed tomography is superb at visualizing bone destruction, but its greatest value is in demonstrating tumour invasion, by showing the extent of any soft tissue mass which may extend beyond the sinus cavity. The same features can also be seen with MRI. Computed tomography and MRI have an important role in treatment planning and in assessing the response to radiotherapy.

Nasopharynx

Computed tomography and especially MRI give excellent visualization of the nasopharynx and can demonstrate the presence of tumour, the most common being a nasopharyngeal carcinoma as a mass disrupting the symmetry of the nasopharynx. Imaging can detect any spread into the skull base and lymphadenopathy in the neck (Fig. 14.4).

Orbits

Computed tomography and MRI clearly demonstrate the anatomy of the orbits. Imaging is indicated in all patients

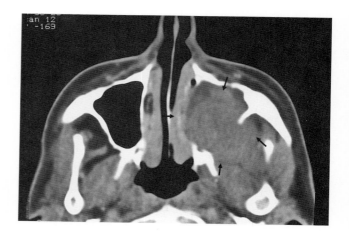

Fig. 14.3 Carcinoma of the antrum. CT scan showing a large mass arising from the left antrum destroying its bony walls and extending into the adjacent soft tissues. The arrows point to the extent of the tumour. The opposite antrum is normal.

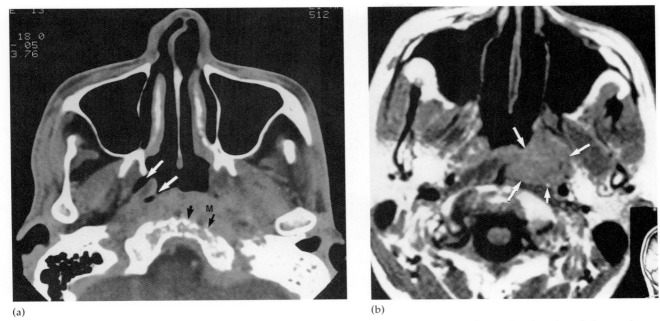

(a)   (b)

Fig. 14.4 Nasopharyngeal carcinoma. (a) CT scan showing a mass (M) in the nasopharynx on the left extending into the soft tissues of the postnasal space and eroding the skull base (black arrows). Note how the tumour obliterates the fossa of Rosenmuller and eustacian recess which are shown on the normal right side (white arrows). (b) MRI scan in another patient clearly showing the extent of the tumour (arrows).

with exophthalmos because it is possible to distinguish between masses arising within the orbit, masses arising outside the orbit and thyroid eye disease. With an intra-orbital mass, its relationship to the optic nerve can be determined.

The main causes of intraorbital masses include various tumours, including tumours of the optic nerve (Fig. 14.5), vascular malformations and granulomas. The most common orbital masses originating outside the orbit, which often present with exophthalmos, are tumours or mucoceles of the frontal or ethmoid sinuses (Fig. 14.6), and a meningioma arising from the sphenoid ridge.

In thyroid eye disease, there is enlargement of the extraocular muscles (Fig. 14.7) which is frequently bilateral and may affect one, several, or all the eye muscles. There is also infiltration of the fat behind the eye which adds to the exophthalmos. When severe, these changes can lead to compression of the optic nerve in the apex of the orbit.

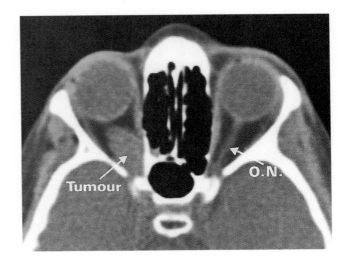

Fig. 14.5 Optic nerve glioma. CT scan showing a soft tissue mass arising from the optic nerve. The opposite orbit demonstrates the normal anatomy. O.N., optic nerve.

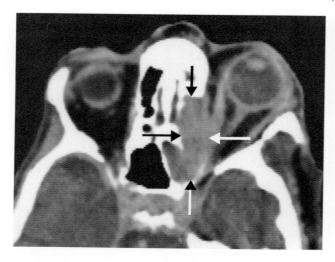

Fig. 14.6 Carcinoma of the ethmoid sinus invading the orbit and causing proptosis. The tumour is arrowed.

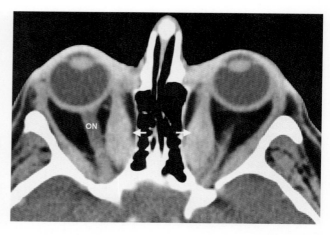

Fig. 14.7 Thyroid eye disease. CT scan through the orbits showing enlargement of the extraoccular muscles, particularly the medial rectus (arrows). ON; optic nerve.

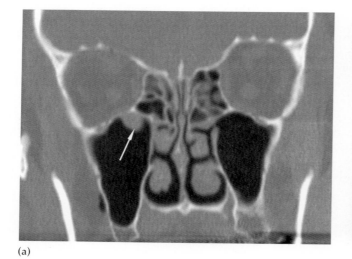

(a)

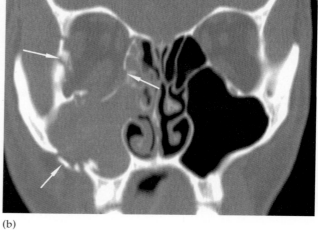

(b)

Fig. 14.8 Blow out fracture of the orbit. CT coronal reconstruction. (a) A patient with a blow to the eye showing a soft tissue opacity in the roof of the antrum (arrow). It is difficult to appreciate the fracture of the orbital floor. (b) A patient with trauma to the side of the face showing disruption of the floor of the orbit and fractures of the lateral and medial walls of the orbit, as well as the lateral wall of the antrum (arrows). There is herniation of orbital contents into the antrum which is opaque.

Blow out fracture

A direct blow to the eye raises the intraorbital pressure and can result in a fracture of the orbital floor, which is the weakest part of the orbit. The break in the orbital floor allows herniation of orbital contents into the antrum, which may result in diplopia. Imaging is best performed as CT coronal reconstruction of the sinuses which shows a crescentic soft tissue mass in the roof of the antrum, which should not be confused with mucosal thickening (Fig. 14.8a). A fracture of the orbital floor may also be visible.

Orbital floor fractures also occur with trauma to the side of the face when there may be fractures of the medial wall of the orbit, the lateral wall of the antrum and the zygomatic arch. Bleeding into the antrum may result in a fluid level or complete opacification of the antrum (Fig. 14.8b).

Salivary glands

Magnetic resonance imaging is the preferred method for the investigation of masses thought to be in the salivary glands, because the signal intensity of masses is often very different from the normal salivary tissue. The commonest salivary gland tumour is a benign adenoma. Magnetic resonance imaging is excellent for demonstrating the presence of a mass (Fig. 14.9) and its relationship to the facial nerve, important information if surgery is contemplated, but MRI is often not able to predict the nature of the mass.

Sialography

Calculi, which occur most commonly in the submandibular duct or gland, normally contain calcium and can, therefore, be seen on plain films.

To show the duct system, a sialogram is performed by injecting contrast into the ducts of the salivary glands. Only the submandibular and parotid glands have ducts that can be cannulated (Fig. 14.10). Stones and strictures in the ducts can be identified. Dilatation of small ducts, which is known as *sialectasis*, may occur with obstruction to the main duct (Fig. 14.11) but may also be seen without obvious obstruction. The main salivary gland ducts can also be visualized using MRI.

Neck

Computed tomography, MRI and ultrasound can be carried out to investigate a mass in the neck, to stage a primary tumour arising in the neck and to determine the presence and extent of enlarged cervical lymph nodes. With a neck mass, ultrasound is recommended as the first line investigation. Ultrasound may demonstrate the extent of the mass and Doppler studies will indicate its vascularity, though

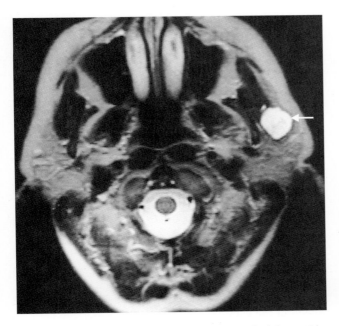

Fig. 14.9 MRI scan showing a high signal mass in the left parotid (arrow), which proved to be an adenoma.

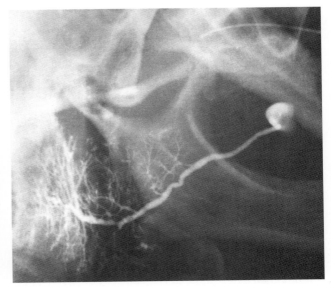

Fig. 14.10 Normal parotid sialogram. Note the long duct of even caliber and the fine branching of the ducts within the gland.

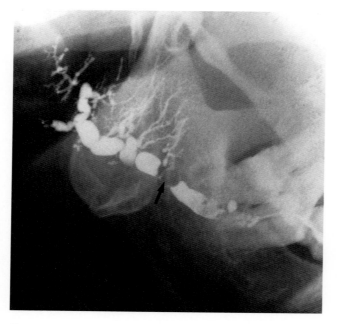

Fig. 14.11 Sialectasis. There is dilatation of the ducts due to a stone (arrow) in the main parotid duct.

ultrasound often cannot predict the cause of a mass. A fine needle aspiration is often combined with the ultrasound examination using the ultrasound as a guide for the most appropriate place for the aspiration.

For CT, intravenous contrast enhancement is necessary as this opacifies the many vessels that might otherwise be mistaken for small lymph nodes. The thyroid gland, which is situated on either side of the trachea, normally enhances quite markedly after intravenous contrast administration.

MRI is the best method of imaging the neck because of the superior contrast between normal soft tissues and tumour. Unless the mass is cystic, e.g. a branchial cleft cyst or cystic hygroma, or contains fat, it may be difficult to determine its nature using CT or MRI, although the size, shape and position may help in this regard.

Computed tomography can demonstrate enlarged lymph nodes in the neck that are too small to palpate or are in sites not amenable to clinical examination. Enlarged nodes may

be due to lymphoma, metastases (Fig. 14.12) or infection, but their appearance on CT, MRI and ultrasound is similar irrespective of the cause.

Larynx

The larynx is best examined with MRI because of the excellent demonstration of soft tissues and the ability to produce images in the coronal plane. Alternatively, CT can be employed (Fig. 14.13). Direct inspection by laryngoscopy reveals a great deal of information about the larynx, particularly in regard to the vocal cords. However, imaging can provide additional information regarding the extent of the tumour, its spread outside the larynx, particularly into the subglottic space, which cannot be inspected directly, and any lymph node involvement.

Thyroid imaging

The thyroid is normally imaged by ultrasound (Fig. 14.14), which has largely superseded nuclear medicine techniques using ^{99m}Tc pertechnetate or ^{123}I. However, nuclear medicine does have an important role in patients with thyroid carcinoma (see below). Computed tomography is not often used to examine the thyroid except in the case of a retrosternal goitre.

The commonest reason for imaging the thyroid is to determine the nature of a thyroid nodule, in particular to try and exclude malignancy. Ultrasound determines whether a nodule is cystic or solid or a mixture of both. Cysts are invariably benign and complex solid/cystic lesions are usually benign (Fig. 14.15). A solid mass could be a carcinoma or an adenoma. Ultrasound may show that the nodule is part of a multinodular goitre by demonstrating an enlarged gland with several nodules of varying size. The risk of malignancy in a multinodular goitre is little higher than in the general population.

Most solitary nodules do not take up radionuclide and are referred to as cold nodules and may be a cyst, adenoma or carcinoma.

The use of fine needle aspiration with cytological examination of the aspirate has increased considerably because of the limitations of imaging. Many centres advocate aspiration as the initial investigation of a thyroid nodule

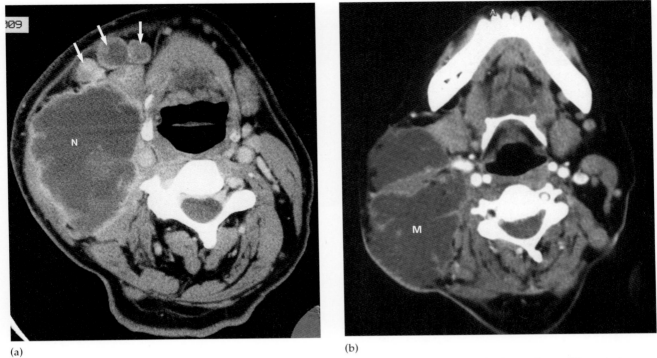

(a)

(b)

Fig. 14.12 Lymphadenopathy. (a) There is a large lymph node (N) and several additional enlarged nodes (arrows) caused by metastases from a carcinoma of the floor of the mouth. (b) The lymph node mass (M) in this patient was due to infection.

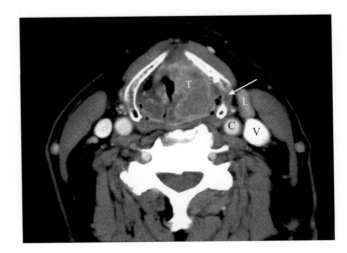

Fig. 14.13 Carcinoma of the larynx. A large tumour (T) in the larynx has destroyed the vocal cords and invaded the thyroid cartilage (arrow). A lymph node metastasis is present (L). C, carotid artery; V, jugular vein.

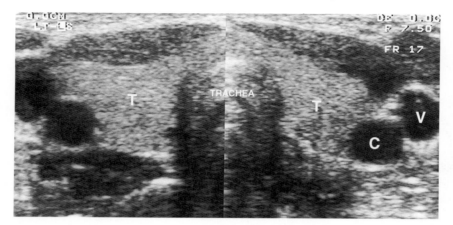

Fig. 14.14 Normal ultrasound of thyroid. The two lobes of the thyroid (T) lie on either side of the trachea. The carotid artery (C) and jugular vein (V) lie lateral to the thyroid gland.

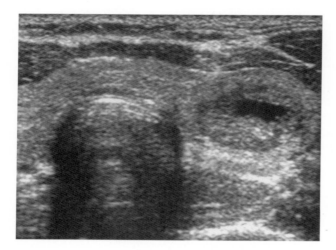

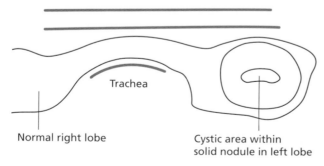

Fig. 14.15 Thyroid nodule. Ultrasound showing a colloid nodule in the left lobe of the thyroid with solid and cystic areas. The right lobe of the thyroid is normal.

because both solid and cystic lesions require confirmation of the diagnosis. Aspiration is sometimes performed under ultrasound guidance (Fig. 14.16).

Thyroid masses may extend retrosternally into the mediastinum, and imaging with CT can be used to determine whether such a mass is due to thyroid tissue, its extent and any tracheal compression (Fig. 14.17).

Iodine-131 has an important role in the management of thyroid cancer. After thyroidectomy an ^{131}I-scan is performed to detect any residual thyroid tissue in the neck. Imaging for metastatic spread at presentation is of no avail as the metastases do not take up sufficient radionuclide. However, after the thyroid tissue has been ablated by surgery or by a therapeutic dose of ^{131}I, thyroid stimulating hormone (TSH) levels rise and stimulate any functioning metastatic or recurrent tumour, which may be identified by radionuclide imaging (Fig. 14.18). Any metastases, recurrent tumour or residual thyroid tissue may subsequently be treated with a therapeutic dose of ^{131}I.

Parathyroid imaging

The usual cause of primary hyperparathyroidism is a parathyroid adenoma, which may be detected on ultrasound as a mass lying behind the thyroid.

A parathyroid adenoma will take up thallium-201 when injected intravenously. The thyroid, which overlies the

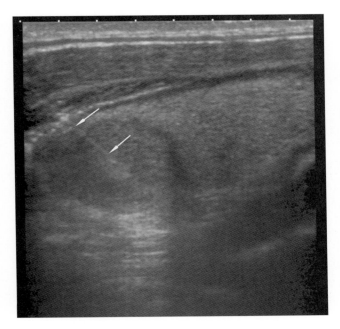

Fig. 14.16 Thyroid carcinoma. Under ultrasound guidance, a biopsy needle (arrows) is introduced into a solid mass in the right lobe of the thyroid which was shown on histology to be a medullary cell carcinoma.

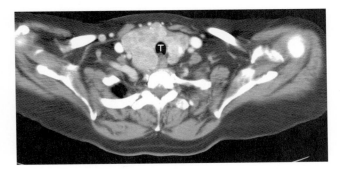

Fig. 14.17 Multinodular goitre. The enlarged thyroid almost surrounds the trachea (T) and enhances avidly after intravenous contrast showing many nodules of varying size.

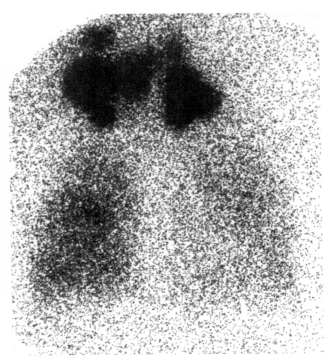

Fig. 14.18 Carcinoma of the thyroid. Iodine-131 scan in a patient who had undergone thyroidectomy for carcinoma of the thyroid and then developed tumour recurrence in the neck and lung metastases. The patient was subsequently cured with a therapeutic dose of ^{131}I.

parathyroids, also accumulates thallium, but, if the thyroid is imaged using ^{99m}Tc, the thallium and technetium images can be subtracted electronically from one another so that the uptake of thallium in the thyroid is removed and the resulting image is that of the parathyroids. The normal parathyroid glands are too small to be visualized, but even a small adenoma can be detected (Plate 7). An alternative technique is to use ^{99m}Tc-sesta-MIBI, which is taken up by the thyroid and parathyroids. A parathyroid adenoma can be visualized as the radionuclide 'washes out' more slowly than the surrounding gland. Localization of a parathyroid adenoma prior to surgery for hyperparathyroidism is important because about 10% of adenomas occur in an ectopic position, often in the mediastinum.

15

Vascular and Interventional Radiology

Vascular radiology encompasses the diagnostic and therapeutic interventions that involve the arterial and venous system. Interventional radiology is a subspeciality of radiology in which minimally invasive procedures are carried out under image guidance.

DIAGNOSTIC ANGIOGRAPHY

Prior to undertaking any intervention, it is important to have an accurate assessment of the extent and distribution of disease whether in the venous or, more commonly, the arterial system. In the past, this could be obtained with a diagnostic angiogram though increasingly non-invasive techniques such as Doppler, computed tomography (CT) and magnetic resonance (MR) angiography are being used.

Arteriography

Arteriograms are performed via a catheter which is introduced into the blood vessel using the 'Seldinger technique' illustrated in Fig. 15.1. Contrast (usually iodinated contrast but occasionally carbon dioxide) is injected through the catheter, which opacifies the target vessel. Accurate images are obtained by digitally subtracting the background image prior to injection, from the image obtained during injection (digital subtraction arteriography or DSA). The result is a road map of the vascular tree without distortion by bones, bowel gas or soft tissues, which would normally appear on a plain x-ray (Fig. 15.2). At the end of the procedure, the

Diagnostic Imaging, 6th Edition. By Peter Armstrong, Martin Wastie and Andrea Rockall. Published 2009 by Blackwell Publishing. ISBN: 978-1-4051-7039.

catheter is pulled out. A few minutes compressing the puncture site with the fingers is enough to stop the bleeding in most patients. The advantages of the Seldinger technique are that it is easy and quick to perform, that the hole in the artery is no bigger than the catheter, and that catheters of any length may be used. There are several indications for arteriography, listed in Box 15.1.

Magnetic resonance angiography

Magnetic resonance angiography is a very useful non-invasive technique, which can demonstrate both arteries and veins. Images of the vascular system can be obtained using special sequences that depend on the signal obtained from flowing blood or via an injection of a contrast agent (gadolinium-DTPA) into a peripheral vein (Fig. 15.3).

MR angiography is particularly useful for showing the aorta and its branches (Fig. 15.4a), aortic dissection, the portal vein (Fig. 15.4b) and for demonstrating carotid artery disease, peripheral vascular disease, renal and mesenteric artery stenosis. Aneurysms and vascular malformations can also be detected in the intracranial circulation.

Box 15.1 Major indications for arteriography

- Diagnosis of vascular diseases: vascular occlusive disease, aneurysm, arteriovenous fistula, arteriovenous malformation.
- Diagnosis or localization of vascular tumours (e.g. insulinoma, parathyroid adenoma).
- Pre-operative definition of vascular anatomy (e.g. organ transplant, local tumour resection, revascularization).
- Diagnosis and treatment of vascular complications of disease, trauma or surgery.
- Performance of vascular interventional procedures (e.g. percutaneous transluminal angioplasty, stenting, embolization or transcatheter infusional therapy).

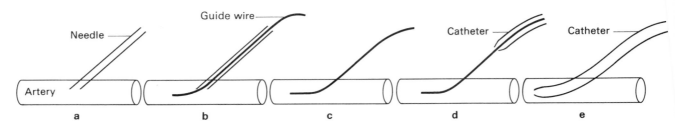

Fig. 15.1 Seldinger technique for catheterizing blood vessels. The femoral artery or vein are the usual vessels used. (a) A needle is inserted through the skin into the blood vessel. (b) A guidewire is passed through the needle into the lumen of the vessel. (c) The needle is withdrawn, leaving the guidewire in the lumen of the vessel. (d) A catheter is threaded over the guidewire and passed into the lumen of the vessel. (e) The guidewire is withdrawn, leaving the catheter in position in the lumen of the vessel.

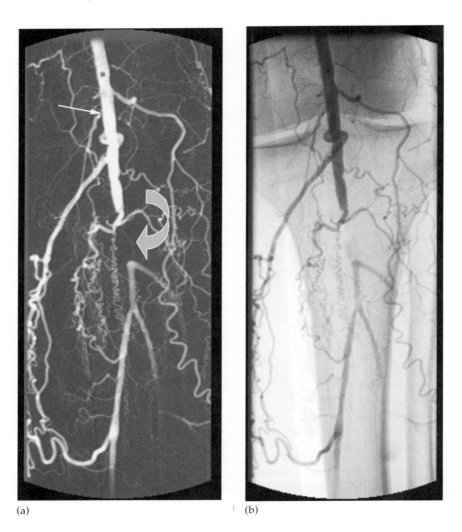

(a)   (b)

Fig. 15.2 Digital subtraction arteriogram (DSA) following an intra-arterial injection of contrast medium. (a) On the subtracted image the bones and soft tissues are barely visible compared to the unsubtracted image (b). The angiogram shows a patent popliteal artery (thin arrow) with a short segment occlusion proximal to the trifurcation (curved arrow).

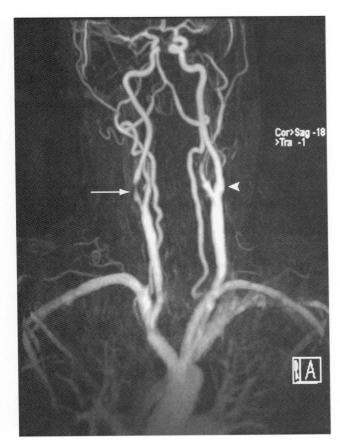

Fig. 15.3 MR angiography of the carotid arteries shows a short stenosis in the right internal carotid artery (long arrow). A normal internal carotid artery is seen on the left (arrowhead).

CT angiography

Spiral CT, particularly multidetector CT, enables large areas of the body to be scanned quickly. After an intravenous injection of contrast, many thin sections can be obtained so reconstruction in the coronal and sagittal planes can be performed to give optimum visualization of the vessels.

CT angiography is particularly useful for visualizing the aorta and its branches for suspected aneurysms (Fig. 15.5) including any rupture or leakage. CT pulmonary angiography demonstrates the pulmonary arteries and can detect pulmonary emboli (see Chapter 2, p. 22, CTPA with thrombus). The peripheral arteries can also be visualized by CT angiography, as can the cerebral vessels.

Ultrasound of the arterial system

Ultrasound has an important role to play in diagnosing arterial disease both in the carotid arteries and peripheral vessels and is commonly the primary imaging modality used in assessment. The common, internal and external carotid arteries can be readily visualized in the neck. The location or size of any atheromatous plaques and the severity of any luminal narrowing can be determined. With colour Doppler imaging, a stenosis in the artery can be visualized and an occlusion will show as an absence of flow (see Plate 2). Because a stenosis disrupts the normal flow pattern, analysis of the flow velocity waveform can give further information regarding the degree of stenosis. Imaging of the iliac vessels may be difficult due to overlying bowel gas, but evaluation of the abdominal aorta is invariably successful and can easily be performed during an outpatient assessment.

Ultrasound venography

Duplex ultrasound has now largely replaced contrast venography for the detection of venous thrombosis. With a venous thrombosis, intraluminal echogenic material is visible and the veins lose their normal compressibility; thrombus-free veins should be compressible by direct pressure using the ultrasound transducer. Colour Doppler scanning shows that there is a lack of spontaneous flow in the affected veins (Plate 9). Ultrasound can readily visualize the external iliac, common femoral and popliteal veins, although it can be sometimes difficult to visualize the calf veins. In practice, this is often not clinically significant as calf vein (i.e. below knee) thrombosis may not be treated.

Contrast venography

Contrast venography is routinely used for the evaluation of the upper limb veins, as it enables imaging of

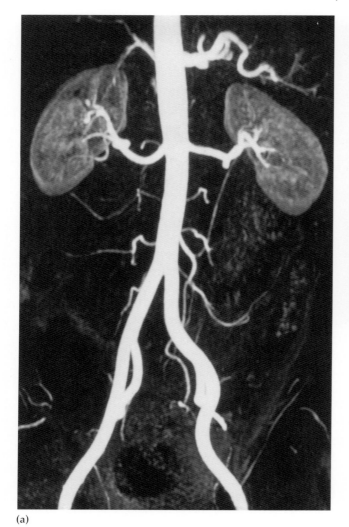

(a)

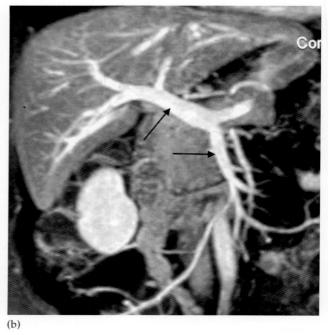

(b)

Fig. 15.4 MR angiography. (a) Contrast angiogram showing a normal abdominal aorta and its branches. (b) Contrast angiogram showing the superior mesenteric (horizontal arrow) and portal veins (upward pointing arrow).

the central veins with the arm in a neutral and abducted position allowing a functional evaluation. A large volume of contrast medium is injected into a vein on the arm or the hand. The contrast is forced into the deep venous system of the upper limb by means of a tourniquet. Thrombi

may be seen as filling defects in the opacified veins, and any stenosis or occlusion in the central veins is well demonstrated.

Venography in the lower limb is seldom used, having been superseded by ultrasound.

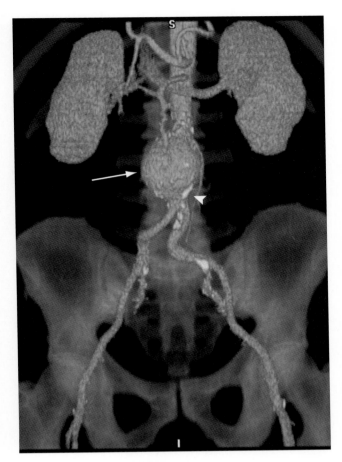

Fig. 15.5 CT angiogram. Reconstruction from many thin axial sections following an intravenous injection of contrast demonstrates an aortic aneurysm (arrow). Calcification is seen in the wall of the arteries (arrowhead).

INTERVENTIONAL RADIOLOGY

Radiologists carry out various percutaneous techniques under imaging control, including dilating stenoses, occluding vessels, draining abscesses and other fluid collections, and obtaining biopsy samples. These procedures greatly assist and may modify surgery, or even replace it altogether. They are carried out with the help of a variety of imaging modalities, notably fluoroscopy, angiography, ultrasound, CT and, more recently, MRI. Interventional radiology is usually performed under local anaesthesia, causing only relatively minor discomfort to the patient, allowing many procedures to be performed as 'day cases'. Only the basic principles of the interventional techniques in widespread use will be described here.

Angioplasty

Arterial stenoses and even occlusions may be traversed with a guidewire. A balloon catheter can be passed through the abnormal site, which has been previously determined by arteriography (Fig. 15.6). The stenosis is then dilated by inflating the balloon (Fig. 15.7). This percutaneous technique, which usually uses the femoral artery as an access route, has been widely employed in peripheral vascular disease and gives results as good as bypass surgery, particularly for iliac and superficial femoral artery disease. Short stenoses are the ideal lesions to treat with angioplasty. Angioplasty is routinely used in renal artery stenosis to treat patients with poor renal function, flash pulmonary oedema or renal vascular hypertension, mesenteric arteries to treat mesenteric ischaemia and is being increasingly used for carotid artery stenoses. Complete occlusions (as opposed to stenoses in a patent vessel) in peripheral vessels of the lower limb can also be treated by a technique known as subintimal angioplasty, the principle being to create a new channel through the diseased segment in the subintimal plane (i.e. within the wall of the vessel) rather than to re-cannalize the original lumen (Fig. 15.8).

Therapeutic embolization

Arteries can be occluded by introducing a variety of materials through a catheter selectively placed in the vessel. Metal coils covered with thrombogenic filaments, gelatin foam, small particles made of polyvinyl alcohol and cyanoacrylate glues that solidify on contact with blood, have all been used for therapeutic embolization. These techniques have been used primarily to control bleeding. Once arteriography has demonstrated the bleeding site, the offending vessel can then be embolized. Arterial embolization is also of use in patients with tumours, e.g. renal cell carcinoma, to reduce tumour vascularity prior to surgery, or inoperable tumours to treat intractable pain and bleeding (Figs 15.9 and 15.10). Vascular occlusion has also been successfully used in treating arteriovenous malformations in various organs, most notably the brain and the lungs (Fig. 15.11). Embolization of

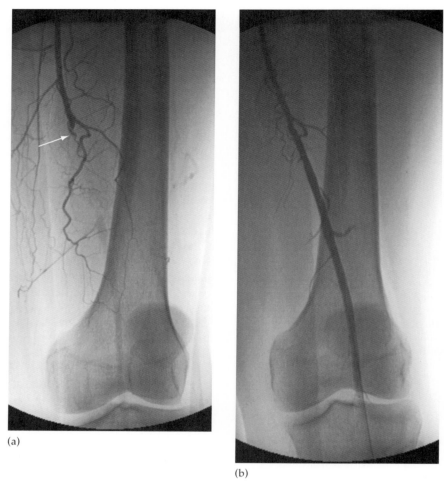

(a)

(b)

Fig. 15.6   Percutaneous transluminal angioplasty. (a) Preliminary arteriogram shows an occlusion in the left superficial femoral artery (arrow). (b) Following the angioplasty, the lumen has been restored.

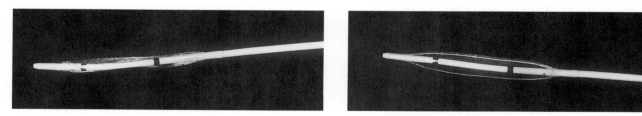

Fig. 15.7   Percutaneous angioplasty balloon catheters. The left image shows the catheter prior to inflating the balloon. The right image shows the catheter with the balloon distended as it would be if it were inside the artery.

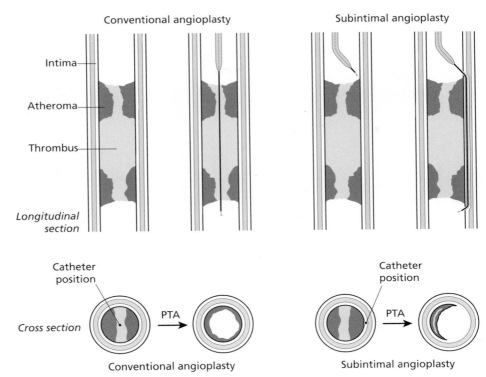

Fig. 15.8 Diagram demonstrating technique of subintimal angioplasty. In subintimal angioplasty, the catheter is passed into the subintimal plane of the vessel, not in the lumen of the vessel. The balloon is then inflated. The principle is to create a new lumen in the subintimal plane rather than re-open the native lumen.

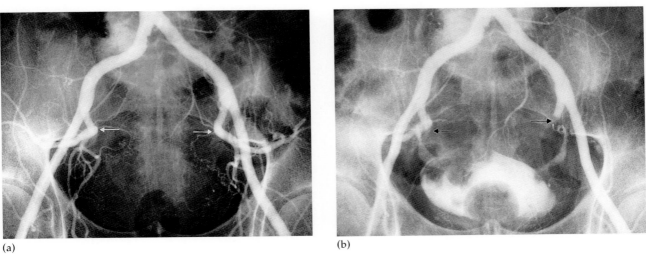

(a) (b)

Fig. 15.9 Therapeutic embolization. (a) Arteriogram prior to embolization showing patent internal iliac arteries (arrows) in a patient with uncontrollable bleeding from a large bladder tumour. (b) Following embolization, both iliac arteries are occluded. The arrows point to the level of occlusion.

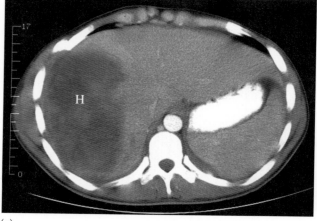

(a)

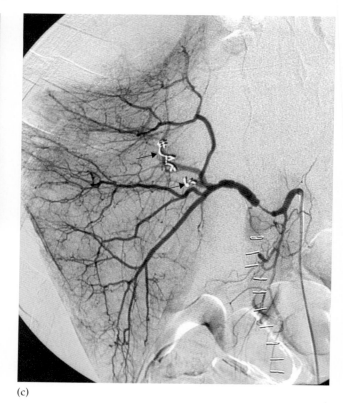

(c)

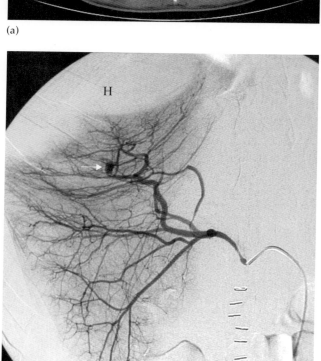

(b)

Fig. 15.10 Therapeutic embolization. (a) CT scan in a patient with a large intrahepatic haematoma (H) following a road traffic accident. (b) Selective hepatic anteriogram shows a false aneurysm (arrow) which was the site of bleeding. Note the haematoma (H) compressing the liver substance. (c) A branch of the hepatic artery supplying the aneurysm has been occluded with coils (arrows) and the aneurysm no longer fills.

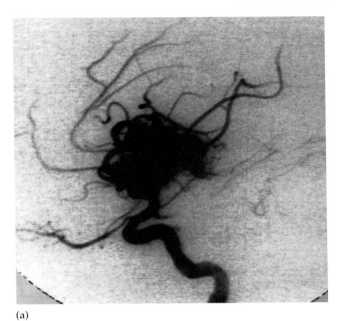
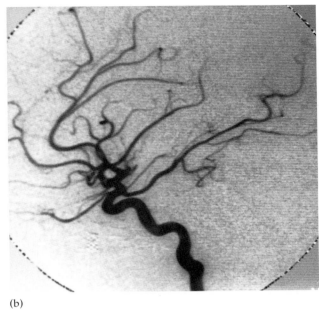

(a)   (b)

Fig. 15.11 Arteriovenous malformation occlusion. (a) Carotid angiogram showing large arteriovenous malformation. (b) After occlusion of the feeding vessels with cyanoacrylate glue the malformation is obliterated.

aneurysms on the intracranial arteries is being increasingly undertaken, thus avoiding craniotomy (Fig. 15.12).

Therapeutic ablation

In some cases, metastatic liver lesions and certain other primary tumours can be ablated percutaneously using a variety of physical techniques such as heating (using radio-frequency, laser or electrocautery), freezing (cryotherapy) or injecting a noxious agent such as ethanol into the tumour. The size and location of the tumour help to determine which method may be appropriate. The treatment is performed under image guidance using ultrasound, CT or MRI. One of the most frequently used of these techniques is thermal ablation of hepatic metastases.

Vascular catheterization for infusion

Arterial catheters can be accurately placed for infusion of cytotoxic or radioactive agents directly into malignant tumours (e.g. hepatocellular carcinoma in the liver), a technique known as transarterial chemoembolization, and for the infusion of fibrinolytic agents to dissolve fresh clots from the vascular system a technique known as thrombolysis.

Vascular stents and filters

Stents are expandable metal cylinders that can be embedded in plastic and collapsed to enable them to be inserted through an artery or vein (Fig. 15.13). Stents are commonly used in the treatment of arterial stenosis and occlusion in coronary, renal and peripheral arterial disease. Covered metal stents can be used to 'exclude' aneurysms, either in small vessels, or, increasingly, in the thoracic or infrarenal aorta, a technique known as endovascular aneurysm repair or EVAR (Fig. 15.14). Due to the size of the deployment system of these large stent grafts, they are normally introduced through a femoral arteriotomy. Stents can also be introduced through the femoral vein and placed across a stricture in the superior vena cava to overcome the distressing symptoms of superior vena caval obstruction,

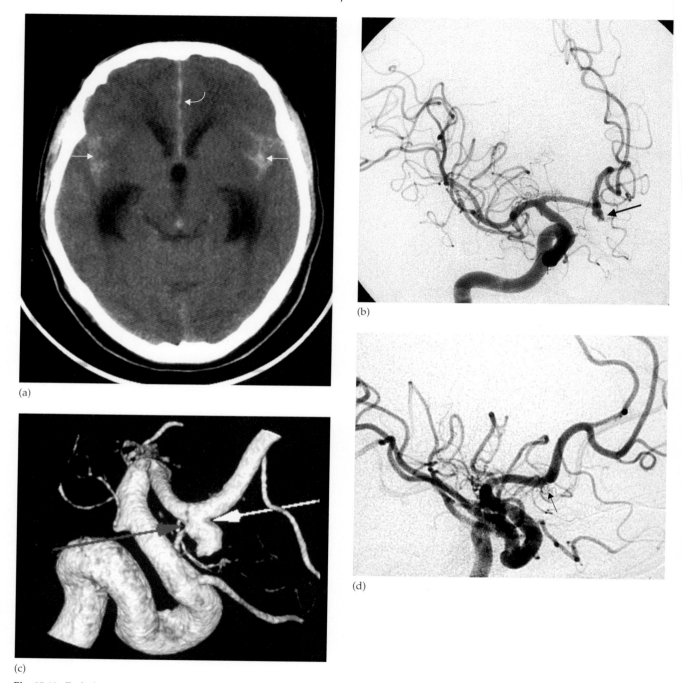

(a)

(b)

(c)

(d)

Fig. 15.12 Embolization. (a) CT scan in a patient with a subarachnoid haemorrhage showing high-density blood in the Sylvian fissures (arrows) and anterior hemispheric fissure (curved arrow). There is also hydrocephalus. (b) Right internal carotid angiogram showing an anterior communicating artery aneurysm (arrow). (c) The arrows on the three-dimensional formatted image point to the neck of the aneurysm. (d) The aneurysm is obliterated after it is occluded with metal coils (arrow).

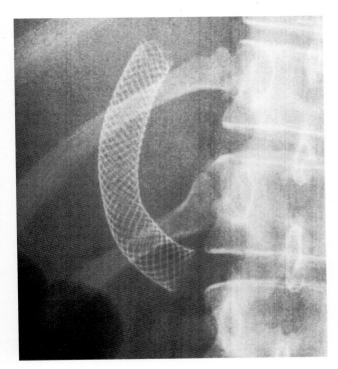

Fig. 15.13 Stent which has been placed in the liver to make a connection between the portal and systemic venous system in the TIPSS procedure.

which is usually caused by a malignant tumour in the mediastinum.

Inferior vena caval filters can be introduced percutaneously through the femoral vein. The filters trap emboli originating from leg or pelvic vein thrombi (Fig. 15.15). They are used in patients who are at risk of pulmonary embolism that cannot be managed satisfactorily with anti-coagulation or where anti-coagulation is contraindicated.

Percutaneous needle biopsy

Needle biopsy techniques are particularly useful for the non-operative confirmation of suspected malignancy.

Under fluoroscopic, ultrasound or computed tomographic guidance (Fig. 15.16), a needle is passed to the desired site and a small amount of tissue is removed. Most intrathoracic or intra-abdominal sites can be sampled. With a fine aspiration needle (20–22 gauge), material can be obtained for cytology. This needle can pass through blood vessels, vascular masses, loops of bowel and solid organs with only minimal risk of infection or bleeding. Apart from a small pneumothorax with intrathoracic biopsy, complications are extremely rare. To obtain material for histological study a larger needle (14–18 gauge for soft tissues, 10–13 gauge for bone) is used. The larger needles require specific approaches to avoid damage to intervening structures and require stricter indications than fine needle aspiration.

Percutaneous drainage of abscesses and other fluid collections

Specially designed drainage catheters can be introduced percutaneously into abscesses or other fluid collections. The catheters vary in diameter from 6–14 French depending on the nature of the fluid to be drained. The larger catheters may have a double lumen to assist with irrigation of an abscess cavity. They are introduced under the control of whichever imaging modality is most convenient; the essential feature is that the operator must know exactly the location of the abscess and must know that the route chosen for introduction of the catheter will be safe (Fig. 15.17). Ultrasound, CT and fluoroscopy are the usual methods.

Once the catheter has been placed in an abscess, it is usually necessary to allow the pus to drain for several days. Irrigation of the tube and the abscess cavity is often essential for continued effective drainage. Thus, the placement of the tube may be only the first step in successful percutaneous abscess drainage.

The technique is suitable for most abdominal abscesses, though the success with some forms of abscess is considerably greater than with others. For example, percutaneous drainage is usually successful for liver and intraperitoneal abscesses, but much less satisfactory for pancreatic abscesses (Fig. 15.18) particularly if they follow pancreatitis and if abscesses are multiple or multiloculated. A similar technique can be employed to insert a chest tube to drain a pleural effusion or empyema.

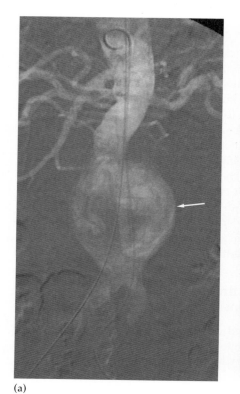

(a)

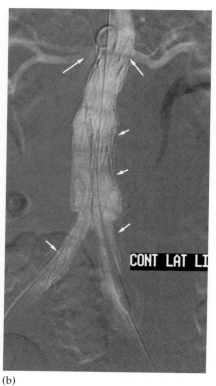

(b)

Fig. 15.14 (a) Digital subtraction arteriogram of abdominal aorta showing large aneurysm (arrow). (b) Digital subtraction arteriogram post stent graft. The covered stent (short arrows), acting as an endoskeleton, has excluded the aneurysm from the circulation by creating a seal proximally below the renal arteries (long arrows) and distally in the iliacs. This depressurizes the aneurysmal sac and reduces the risk of rupture.

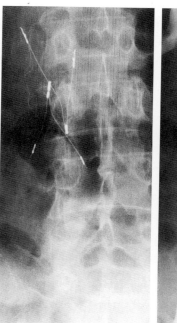

(a)

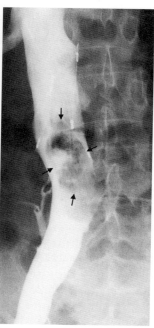

(b)

Fig. 15.15 Inferior vena cava filter. (a) Plain film showing the bird's nest filter in place. (b) An inferior vena cavogram shows a large thrombus (arrows) trapped by the filter.

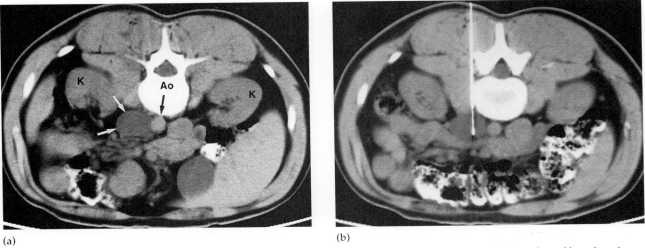

(a)   (b)

Fig. 15.16 Needle biopsy of an enlarged para-aortic lymph node under CT control with the patient prone. (a) An enlarged lymph node (arrow) is seen to the left of the abdominal aorta (Ao) at the level of the kidneys (K). (b) The tip of an 18-gauge cutting needle has been placed in the enlarged lymph node. The tissue obtained confirmed that the lesion was a metastasis from a germ cell tumour of the testis.

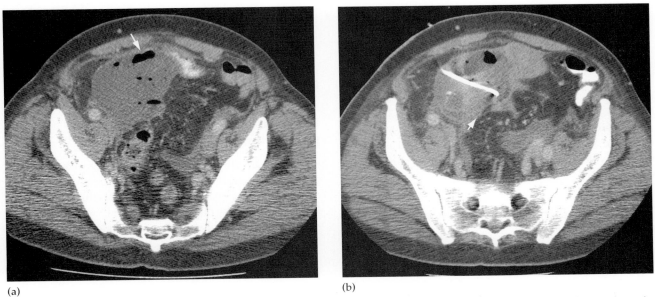

(a)   (b)

Fig. 15.17 (a) An abdominal abscess in the right iliac fossa secondary to appendicitis. Small pockets of air are seen in the collection (arrow). (b) A percutaneous drainage catheter (partially seen) has been inserted into the collection (arrowhead) which is decreasing in size.

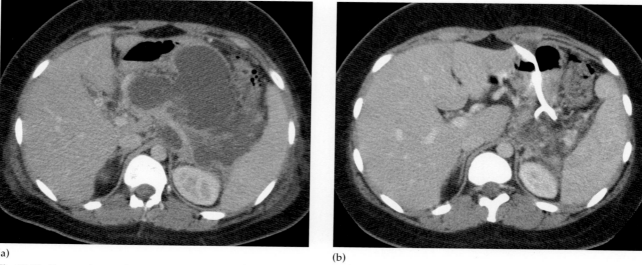

(a)   (b)

Fig. 15.18 Pancreatic pseudocyst drainage. (a) CT scan showing a collection involving the body of the pancreas which developed following acute pancreatitis. (b) A drainage catheter has deliberately been inserted through the stomach into the collection (to encourage development of an internal rather than a cutaneous fistula), which has decreased significantly in size.

Transjugular liver biopsy

In patients with diffuse liver disease, particularly cirrhosis, there may be problems with blood coagulation with a risk of uncontrolled bleeding after a percutaneous biopsy. To overcome this problem, a biopsy is performed via the hepatic veins so if bleeding occurs it enters the vascular system. The jugular vein is punctured in the neck and, under fluoroscopy, a special biopsy catheter is passed through the superior and inferior vena cavae and advanced into a hepatic vein where a biopsy of the liver parenchyma is taken.

Transjugular intrahepatic portosystemic shunt (TIPSS)

Patients who have portal hypertension with bleeding gastro-oesophageal varices or intractable ascites may benefit from the creation of a communication between the portal and systemic venous system to lower the portal pressure when other attempts to treat the varices such as sclerotherapy or banding have failed. This communication may be conveniently performed percutaneously under ultrasound guid-

ance. The internal jugular vein is punctured and a catheter passed through the heart into a hepatic vein. Using a special needle introduced through the lumen of the catheter, the catheter can be passed from a hepatic vein into a portal vein. Once this portosystemic connection has been established, it is kept open with a permanent stent (Figs 15.13 and 15.19).

Interventional radiology of the gastrointestinal tract

Oesophageal, duodenal or colonic stent placement and percutaneous gastrostomy may be performed endoscopically, radiologically or as a combined procedure (Fig. 15.20). Expanding metal stents are usually placed across malignant strictures but newer removable covered stents are increasingly used in the treatment of benign strictures.

Radiologically inserted gastrostomy (RIG as opposed to PEG, percutaneous endoscopic gastrostomy) is carried out to avoid long-term nasogastric or parenteral feeding. The stomach is distended by gas delivered through a nasogastric tube to make it an easier target. Under fluoroscopy, the anterior abdominal wall is punctured and a special gastrostomy tube introduced which is then anchored in the stomach.

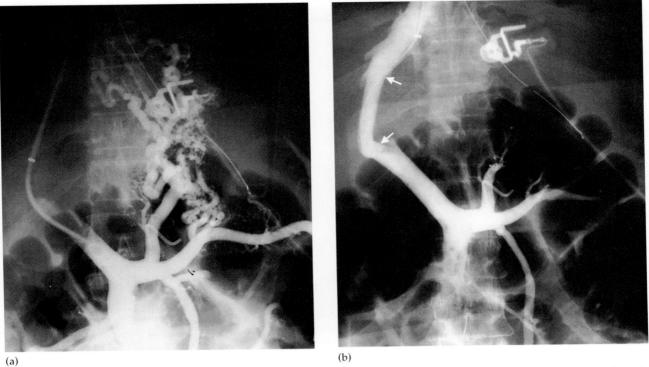

(a)   (b)

Fig. 15.19 Transjugular intrahepatic portosystemic shunt (TIPSS). (a) A catheter has been passed from the jugular vein in the neck through the heart into a hepatic vein and then pushed through the liver parenchyma into a portal vein. A retrograde injection is made outlining the portal vein and its tributaries. Note the gastro-oesophageal varices. (b) A connection between the portal vein and a large hepatic vein has been established and a stent inserted. Its position is shown by the arrows. Note the varices no longer fill (in part due to deliberate occlusion).

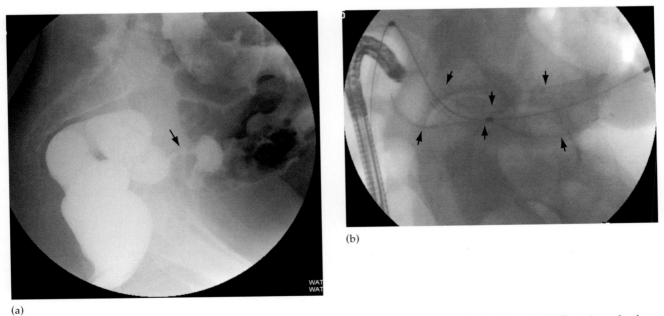

(a)

(b)

Fig. 15.20 (a) A single contrast, water-soluble enema, demonstrates a stricture in the distal sigmoid colon (arrow). (b) The stricture has been crossed using endoscopic and fluoroscopic guidance, and stented (arrowheads). This will allow decompression of the bowel, allowing the patient to undergo elective rather than emergency surgery.

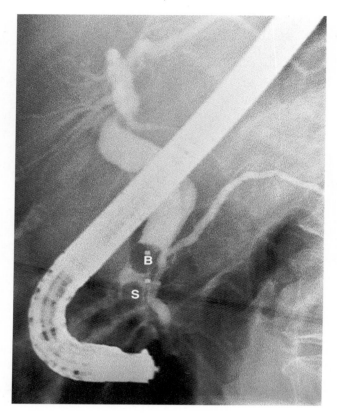

Fig. 15.21 Endoscopic removal of stones in the common bile duct (CBD). A balloon catheter has been passed into the CBD after endoscopic intubation of the papilla of Vater. The stones were then pulled out of the CBD. B, balloon; S, stone.

Interventional radiology of the urinary tract

Internal drainage of an obstructed urinary system is undertaken by the insertion of double-J stents with the proximal end placed into the pelvicalyceal system and the distal end in the bladder, thus bypassing the obstruction. These stents are usually placed via a cystoscope, the catheters being passed into the ureteric orifice under direct vision. Alternatively, the double-J stents for long-term internal drainage may be introduced percutaneously via the loin under ultrasound and fluoroscopic control. Short-term drainage (24–48 hours) can be achieved by simply puncturing an obstructed kidney under ultrasound or fluoroscopic control, passing a guidewire through the needle, and exchanging the needle for a small catheter in order to establish temporary external drainage. This procedure, known as percutaneous nephrostomy, is used almost exclusively to establish drainage in such emergency situations as acute obstruction following extracorporeal shock-wave lithotripsy or to drain an acute pyonephrosis.

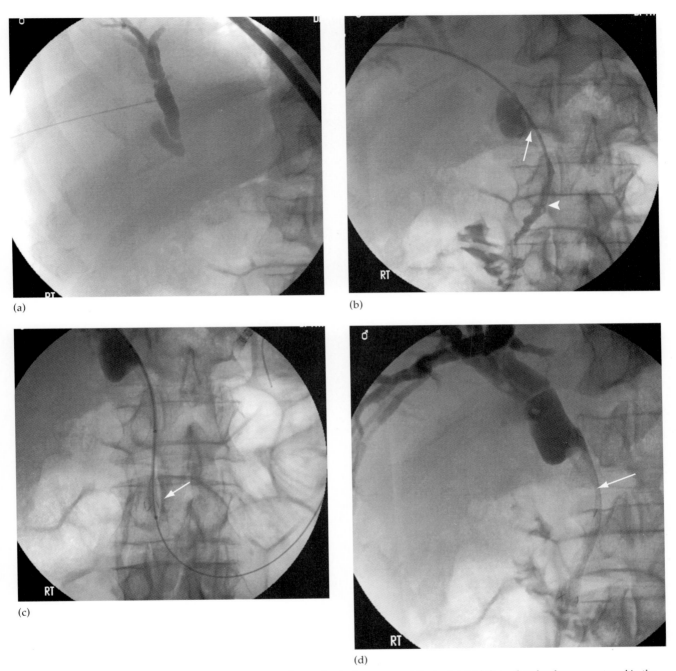

Fig. 15.22 Percutaneous insertion of a stent to bypass an obstruction in the common bile duct. (a) A biliary duct has been punctured in the liver and contrast injected to delineate the biliary tree. (b) A guidewire is inserted through the needle over which a catheter is passed to cross the stricture (arrow) and thence through the ampulla into the bowel. Note the decompressed common bile duct distal to the stricture (arrowhead). (c) A self-expanding metal stent is then inserted over the guidewire (arrow) and deployed across the stricture. Note the radio-opaque marker delineating the distal end of the stent. (d) Completion cholangiogram demonstrates free flow of bile through the stent (arrow) into the duodenum.

Interventional radiology of the biliary tract

The last decade has seen an explosion of techniques designed to drain an obstructed biliary system. The methods used can be broadly divided into those in which the drainage tube is introduced endoscopically, which is the common approach, and those in which it is introduced percutaneously, usually when the endoscopic route has failed.

The two most common causes of bile duct obstruction are tumours, notably carcinoma of the pancreas or cholangiocarcinoma, and stones in the common bile duct. If the obstruction is due to stones, then endoscopic removal of the stones and sphincterotomy of the papilla of Vater is a frequently chosen procedure (Fig. 15.21).

Many patients who present with malignant bile duct obstruction cannot be offered a surgical cure. Non-operative stenting and drainage procedures for patients in whom curative surgery is impossible have, therefore, become far more frequent in recent years. Patients may live for a considerable time with biliary stents in place, particularly if the responsible tumour is slow-growing, as is the case with many cholangiocarcinomas. Usually the stent is introduced at ERCP by cannulation of the papilla of Vater and passing the stent retrogradely up the common bile duct through the tumour so that bile from the obstructed biliary tree drains into the duodenum. If this approach is not successful, the stent can be placed over a guidewire that has been introduced percutaneously through the liver into a dilated bile duct. The guidewire can be manipulated through the tumour into the duodenum via the common bile duct and the stent can then be passed over the guidewire (Fig. 15.22).

Appendix

CT Anatomy of Abdomen

The normal appearances of the abdomen and pelvis of an adult female are shown in this appendix. The levels of the sections chosen are illustrated in the two diagrams. Each section is 5 mm thick. Gastrografin was given orally twice: 15 minutes and 1.5 hours beforehand. Intravenous contrast was injected during the examination.

Ao   Aorta
C   Colon
D   Diaphragm
Duo   Duodenum
Duo III Third part of duodenum
GB   Gall bladder
IVC   Inferior vena cava
K   Kidney
Ps   Psoas muscle
SB   Small bowel
SMA   Superior mesenteric artery
SMV   Superior mesenteric vein
S   Spleen

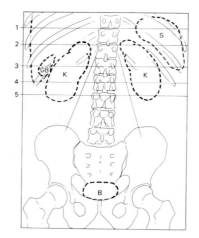

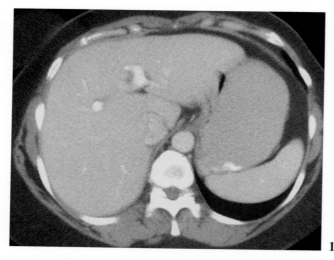

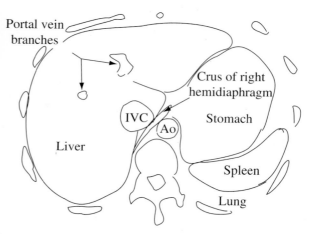

Portal vein branches

Crus of right hemidiaphragm

IVC

Ao

Stomach

Liver

Spleen

Lung

1

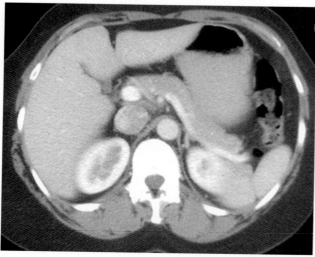

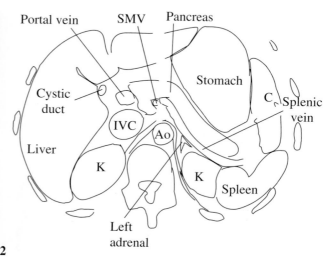

Portal vein   SMV   Pancreas

Cystic duct

IVC

Ao

Stomach

C   Splenic vein

Liver

K

K

Spleen

Left adrenal

2

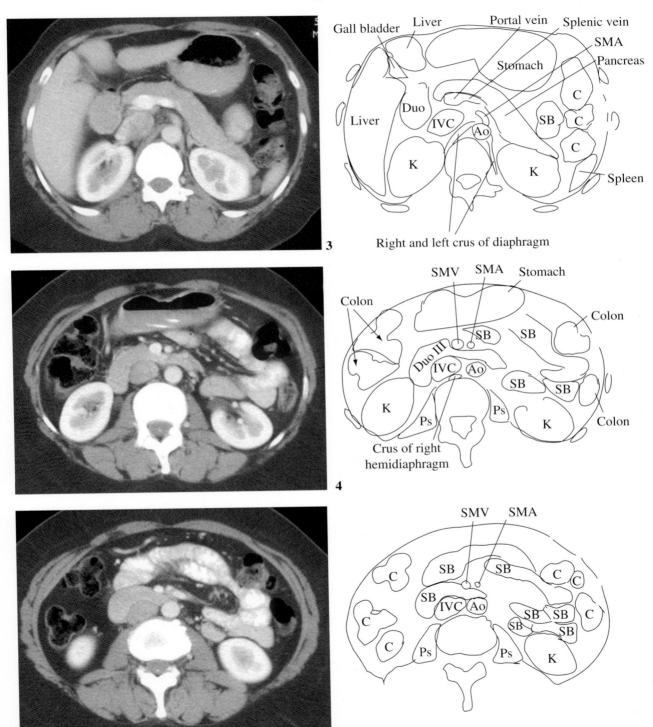

3

Gall bladder — Liver — Portal vein — Splenic vein — SMA — Pancreas

Stomach

Liver — Duo — IVC — Ao — C — SB — C — C — K — K — Spleen

Right and left crus of diaphragm

4

SMV — SMA — Stomach

Colon — Colon

Duo III — SB — SB — Colon

K — IVC — Ao — SB — SB

Ps — Ps — K — Colon

Crus of right hemidiaphragm

5

SMV — SMA

C — SB — SB — C — C

SB — IVC — Ao — SB — SB — C

C — SB — SB

C — Ps — Ps — K

Ao	Aorta
B	Bladder
C	Colon
K	Kidney
IVC	Inferior vena cava
Ps	Psoas muscle
SB	Small bowel
SMA	Superior mesenteric artery
SMV	Superior mesenteric vein

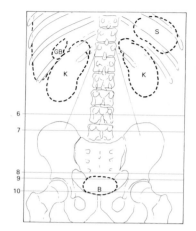

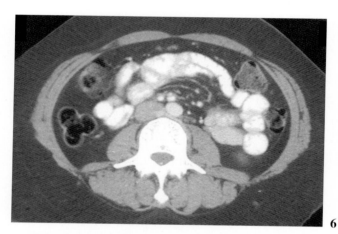

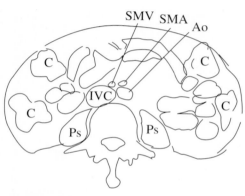

6

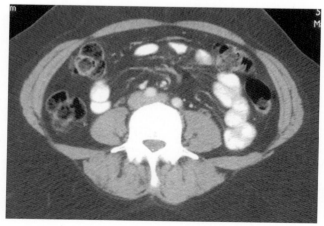

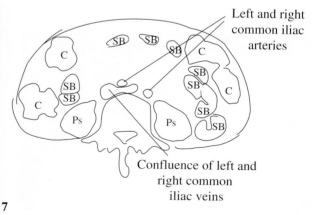

7

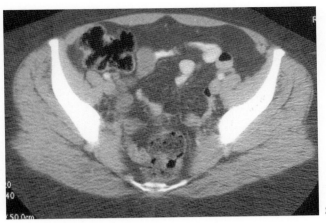

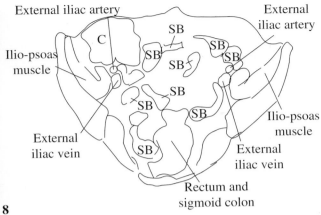

External iliac artery

External iliac artery

Ilio-psoas muscle

C

SB

SB

SB

SB

SB

SB

SB

SB

SB

SB

SB

Ilio-psoas muscle

External iliac vein

External iliac vein

Rectum and sigmoid colon

8

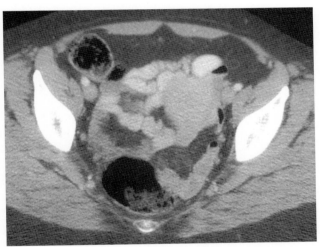

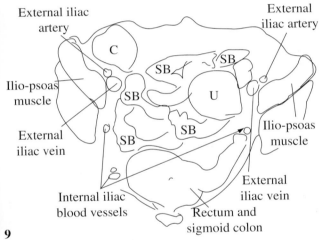

External iliac artery

External iliac artery

Ilio-psoas muscle

C

SB

SB

SB

SB

U

SB

Ilio-psoas muscle

External iliac vein

External iliac vein

Internal iliac blood vessels

Rectum and sigmoid colon

9

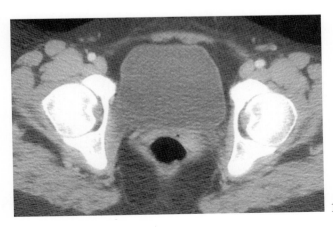

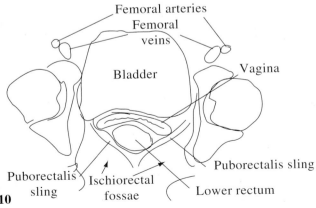

Femoral arteries

Femoral veins

Bladder

Vagina

Puborectalis sling

Ischiorectal fossae

Puborectalis sling

Lower rectum

10

Index